MOVING TOWARD
BALANCE

MOVING TOWARD
BALANCE
8 WEEKS OF YOGA WITH RODNEY YEE

RODNEY YEE WITH NINA ZOLOTOW

PHOTOGRAPHS BY MICHAL VENERA

RODALE

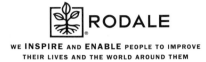

RODALE

WE **INSPIRE** AND **ENABLE** PEOPLE TO IMPROVE
THEIR LIVES AND THE WORLD AROUND THEM

Printed in the United States of America
Rodale Inc. makes every effort to use acid-free ∞,
recycled paper ♻.

Book design by Patricia Field

FOR MORE OF OUR PRODUCTS

WWW.RODALESTORE.COM
(800) 848-4735

We're always happy to hear from you. For
questions or comments concerning the editorial content of this book, please write to:
Rodale Book Readers' Service
33 East Minor Street
Emmaus, PA 18098
Look for other Rodale books wherever books
are sold. Or call us at (800) 848-4735.

For more information about Rodale
magazines and books, visit us at
www.rodale.com

**Library of Congress Cataloging-in-Publication
Data**

Yee, Rodney.
    Moving toward balance : 8 weeks of yoga
with Rodney Yee / Rodney Yee with
Nina Zolotow ; photographs by Michal Venera.
        p.   cm.
    Includes index.
    ISBN 0–87596–921–6 paperback
    1. Yoga.   I. Zolotow, Nina.   II. Title.
RA781.7 .Y438   2004
613.7'046—dc22   2003026817

Distributed in the book trade by St. Martin's Press

2 4 6 8 10 9 7 5 3 1 paperback

Contents

An Offering

I remember the feeling that I had after my first yoga class—my entire being felt balanced and at ease. Walking down the street afterward, I felt for the first time like I was truly connected to the world. Today, I still feel that my yoga practice cleanses me on every level; when I am finished, my mind, body, and heart are like the air after a wonderful rainstorm. This clarity, aliveness, and exhilaration are all qualities that allow me to be more present in everything I do.

I was a ballet dancer in those days, and leading the life of a performer created both physical and emotional strain. In ballet, your state of mind depends mostly on how well you do something: You are either very happy because you mastered a new trick or defeated because things didn't go well. What surprised me about practicing yoga was that I could have a class where my body felt capable and alive or where my body felt restricted and lousy, but it didn't matter. I would always leave feeling better—more balanced, more clear, more free.

Soon this weekly treat of a yoga class began to creep into my dance world. I began to do yoga on a daily basis, taking class about three times a week and practicing at home on my own the other days. In 1985, I began to teach yoga in tandem with performing because several friends were becoming interested in what I was doing. My wife, Donna, and I would clear out our apartment each Tuesday and teach a handful of friends what we were learning. That year, our class grew in number from 5 to 18, and I began to realize that I had found my calling: teaching something I loved to people I loved. I felt almost like a missionary out to save the world with this amazing, transformational practice. Looking back, it seems natural that I was drawn to teaching, as many members of my family are teachers as well.

Over the years I've come to know—both through my own practice and through my students—many of the obstacles that can prevent a person from taking on a yoga practice. We have designed this book as mindfully as possible to help you work past those obstacles and lead you to include yoga as a natural part of your daily life. We also present modifications to the poses to encourage you to take the postures with ease and steadiness. Whatever physical capabilities, mental attentiveness, or emotional awareness you possess, this book can lead you through your own doorway to the practice of yoga. As Nina and I were writing together, I realized that I was distilling the knowledge I have accumulated and honed over more than 20 years into what I consider to be the most potent and accessible practices that will help transform and balance your life. This book is an offering not only of my service but also of my desire to share the practice that has made and continues to make such a difference in my life.

—Rodney Yee

On Taking a Chance

Between fall 2003 and spring 2004, with the help of two wonderful yoga teachers, Jason Crandell and Baxter Bell, I took three different groups of yoga practitioners through the eight-week program presented in this book. We presented the program as "The Home Practice Course" at Piedmont Yoga Studio and offered it to yoga students of any level who were interested in starting or re-igniting a home practice. My initial goal in offering these series courses was simply to test the program on a wide range of students, male and female, young and old, absolute beginners and advanced practitioners. I wanted to be sure that both the overall program itself and the specific sequences of poses were realistic and accessible for all types of students. However, after just a few weeks of observing students and listening to their weekly reports, it became obvious that I was witnessing something exciting. Week after week, students came into class and reported not just feelings of physical and emotional well-being, but various insights that they had experienced during their week of home practice, insights about the nature of yoga. Some began to realize for the first time that, Hey, this yoga thing is something much, much bigger than an exercise system. Others began to comprehend just how much a daily yoga practice could enrich their lives. "There's some magic in the program," I began to say (and I hardly ever use words like that).

Now after saying good-bye to our third group of students, I can see that this "magic" has two causes. First, the program is very well designed. It allows you to delve deeply each week into different aspects of yoga postures, breath awareness, and meditation. Taking the time to focus this way on backbends for one week and restorative poses for another leads you to understand the physical, emotional, and psychological effects of a specific aspect of yoga in a way that just can't happen during a single class. Second, practicing at home five days a week for eight weeks for the first time inevitably brings a visceral understanding of both yoga practice and yoga philosophy that no number of years of taking classes can provide. As someone who considers her own yoga practice a vital part of her life, witnessing this awakening in so many students was sweet.

I realize, of course, that embarking on the eight-week program in this book on your own is somewhat more daunting without having me and Jason or Baxter there to hold your hand through it. However, I honestly believe that if you do take on this program—either by yourself or with a group of friends—it will work the same magic on you that it did on our students. Rod and I have worked hard to include in this book everything we know—and everything we've learned from our friends and students—that might help inspire you to start practicing yoga and encourage you to make yoga a permanent part of your life.

(Oh, and, yes, I did get the feedback that I wanted and we did end up streamlining the program in various ways due to student comments. Thanks, everyone!)

—Nina Zolotow

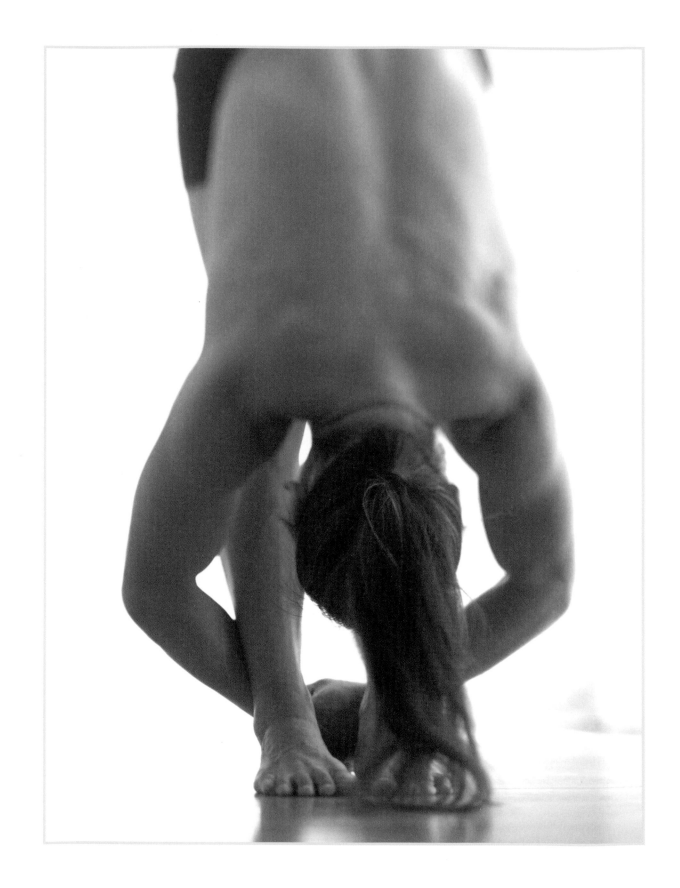

About Yoga and Balance

Yoga is an ancient discipline in which physical postures, breath practices, meditation, and philosophical study are tools for achieving liberation. In my interpretation, achieving liberation in yoga means learning how to be present with everything that arises, whether it is pain or pleasure, sadness or joy, failure or success. And to be present with whatever arises, I believe we must not only be aware of what is arising but we must also be able to see all things that arise as equal, with detachment.

The way we achieve this state of detachment is by honing our attention. In *The Yoga Sutras by Patanjali* (one of the most important ancient yoga texts), translated by T. K. V. Desikachar, the first sutra defines yoga as follows:

YOGA IS THE ABILITY TO DIRECT THE MIND EXCLUSIVELY TOWARD AN OBJECT
AND SUSTAIN THAT DIRECTION WITHOUT ANY DISTRACTIONS.

Focusing on any given object, such as any part of your body, your breath, or the flame of candle, brings your mind into the present moment where you let go of any thoughts of the past or the future. Learning to focus your mind on your body as well as your breath as you practice your postures and to feel, observe, and be present with all your sensations is what distinguishes the practice of yoga from an exercise system.

So in hatha yoga, whether you are practicing Downward-Facing Dog, Triangle Pose, or Headstand, your body and your breath are the objects toward which you direct your mind. And learning how to sustain your focus on your body and your breath is a key to this practice.

YOGA IS NOT AN EXTERNAL EXPERIENCE.
IN YOGA WE TRY IN EVERY ACTION
TO BE ATTENTIVE AS POSSIBLE
TO EVERYTHING WE DO. . . . AS WE
PERFORM THE VARIOUS ASANAS WE
OBSERVE WHAT WE ARE DOING
AND HOW WE ARE DOING IT. . . .
IF WE DO NOT PAY ATTENTION TO
OURSELVES IN OUR PRACTICE,
THEN WE CANNOT CALL IT YOGA.

—T. K. V. DESIKACHAR, *THE HEART OF YOGA*

By focusing on your body and your breath in your yoga practice, you learn to be fully present. And when you are totally involved in listening and responding to the present moment, nothing else exists. There's no room for the past. There's no room for the future. You're engaged in the present moment.

In this book you will learn physical postures that will help balance and purify your body, breath practices that even out your subtle body, and meditation practices that train and discipline your mind. All these studies— physical postures, breath practices, and meditation— are the practices that move you toward the *balance* that is yoga.

Of course for most of us, moments of being completely present are very rare. Obsessions and anxieties distract us from the present. Am I doing it right? What if I hurt myself? Why am I so bad at this? Will I ever be able to do this pose? What should I cook tonight for dinner? But when we practice yoga, we *aim* for complete awareness. And that process alone teaches us many things about who we are and what it is that will move us toward balance.

So this is a very practical book in which I am asking you to learn about yoga by practicing it at home, either alone or with a partner, for eight weeks. This is because I believe that to truly understand yoga you have to do it on your own. Taking yoga classes provides many benefits, of course, but I have observed time and time again that it is when people start to practice at home that the real insights occur. In class, you follow the teacher's instructions and move at the pace your teacher sets for you. At home you learn to listen to your body and breath, to move at your own pace, and to begin to develop your intuition about how to balance your body as well as many different aspects of your life.

When I teach, I can tell just by watching who is practicing at home and who is not. People who are not practicing at home simply try to fit their bodies into my instructions as if they were following orders and are mainly concerned about whether or not they are doing it "right." But people who are practicing at home are inquisitive about instructions and test them out in their own bodies, asking themselves, "How does this feel?" and "What effects is this having?" Their home practice has trained them to focus their minds on their bodies in a way that no amount of time in the classroom could.

So as a yoga teacher, I love it when people begin to practice at home. However, it is often difficult for many people to make the transition from taking yoga classes to practicing at home. With no guidance, they roll out their yoga mats and ask themselves, "Now what?" This book is specifically designed to help you make that transition. It provides a structured program that will guide you into a deeper understanding both of yoga and of your own relationship to it.

However, as you practice your first poses on your own, I want you to try to cultivate an attitude of playfulness and acceptance. Being present during your practice means allowing yourself to be aware of whatever physical sensations, emotions, and thoughts are currently arising. And if you approach your practice with a sense of curiosity, rather than self-judgment or competitiveness, you will not only find it easier to motivate yourself to practice, but you will also be able to be more present during the times when you do practice.

> IF I TELL YOU SOMETHING, YOU WILL STICK TO IT AND LIMIT YOUR OWN CAPACITY TO FIND OUT FOR YOURSELF.
>
> —SHUNRYU SUZUKI, *Not Always So*

Ultimately, your practice will not and should not look like any formula I could give you. I encourage you to be creative and spontaneous, to rekindle your curiosity about who you are and be unafraid of the exploration of your body. The mysteries of the self are as deep and wide as those of the universe, and I hope the practices that I am introducing you to will lead you toward your own innate, ever-changing balance.

ASPECTS OF BALANCE

Each week during the eight-week program, you will explore in depth one of the following eight aspects of balance as you practice related postures, breath awareness, and meditation.

Being Present

Being present in yoga is being aware of your physical sensations, emotional movements, and thought patterns. The act of engaging your mind in a physical sensation that is arising or the way the breath is moving is a great way to train your mind to be present. For all of us, the nature of the mind is one of constant wandering. But as we channel our mental energies into the present moment, we have such a better chance of responding to what is taking place with all of our faculties.

Awakening Connection

Awakening connection in yoga means seeing how a single object is connected to everything and to all movement that is taking place at any given point in time. Balance means not only being in the present moment, but seeing your contextual relationship with your environment. When we study a wild animal, we study it in the context of what it does in its environment, and we see it in how it balances an entire ecosystem. Only in this way can we begin to understand how any individual thing is balanced within itself and within the world at large. So our individual balance is often synonymous with our balance within the context of the whole, whether that is our whole body, our whole life, our whole family, or our whole community.

Opening into Vulnerability

Opening into vulnerability in yoga means emotional acceptance of whatever physical sensations, intellectual thoughts, or emotional movements are taking place. When you open into vulnerability, you observe your tendencies to close down and allow yourself at least the willingness to be responsive to what's taking place. If you are not willing to be vulnerable to what's outside yourself, there is no possibility to be in balance. The truth of the matter is whatever is outside is affecting you and you are also affecting your environment. Being conscious of this enables you to move toward a true balance that acknowledges your connection to the world at large.

Allowing Receptivity

Allowing receptivity in yoga means both having a willingness to be open and a willingness to absorb what you have allowed in. So if opening into vulnerability is unlocking and opening your windows, receptivity is sitting in front of the open window and receiving whatever weather comes in, whether that means feeling a light rain on your skin or allowing the sunlight to hit you directly on the face. As Rumi says, "The dark thought, the shame, the malice, meet them at the door laughing, and invite them in." Allowing receptivity moves you toward balance because you are able to receive with equanimity all that is arising, whether it is beautiful or disgusting, joyful or frightening.

Facing the Unknown

Facing the unknown in yoga means becoming comfortable with not knowing, which is the moment-by-moment scenario of our lives. Living with the illusion that you can control the future eventually moves you away from being present. Instead of observing what is taking place and responding to it, you interpret reality from the view of your expectations and desires for the future. However, if you can move toward becoming comfortable with not knowing, you can be present with whatever is arising, whether or not it is what you expected or hoped for.

Turning Inward

Turning inward in yoga means giving yourself time to feel and listen to what is arising and moving inside your own body, mind, and breath. So much of our lives are based on meeting external expectations. From our earliest years in school, we are asked how we are going to play the game, what are we going to be when we grow up. And people even laugh at us when we say something that comes from deep inside. So using your yoga as a time to really listen to the shifts and changes of your desires, emotions, and ideas may help you balance your inner world and your outer world. For example, in your yoga practice, having a moment of meditation before you practice gives you time to listen inward so that you can design a practice that correlates with your internal moods, feelings, and sensations. I believe that you move toward balance only when your external expressions coordinate with what is arising internally.

Changing Orientation

Changing orientation in yoga means taking a different point of focus. By changing your point of focus, you gain different perspectives on the world and on yourself. Sometimes things look out of balance simply because of the orientation from which we are viewing them. For instance, a natural forest fire may initially look devastating, but in the long-term view of that environment, it may be the perfect event, the event that is in balance. One of the main goals of yoga is to unveil the illusion of separation, which means to

enable you to see yourself in a much larger context. If you see the children of different countries as your own children, what effect does that have on your actions in the world? The practice of changing orientation dislodges our habitual viewpoints and our habitual conclusions about what the world is and who we are. This may allow us to move toward balance by making external changes to restore balance or by simply learning to perceive the natural balance that already exists.

Moving toward Balance

Moving toward balance in yoga means moving toward physical, intellectual, and emotional contentment. You move toward balance in your body by learning how to listen more minutely to the language of your body both in and out of the yoga room. When you learn to understand the language of your body, your body begins to tell you what it needs to be healthier and more at ease. You move toward balance in your mind because in your practice you learn to focus more and more on the present moment. This moves you away from a judging mind and toward a mind that is constantly noticing and adapting to what is taking place, creating a sense of contentment with things as they are. You move toward balance in your heart as you become more familiar with its language and more willing to feel what you feel and not repress it. So balance comes not with the control of your mind, body, or emotions, but with your ability to relax with them. The ability to relax in any given situation enables you to use all of your faculties in response to both the internal and external changes so that you can navigate as mindfully and skillfully as possible.

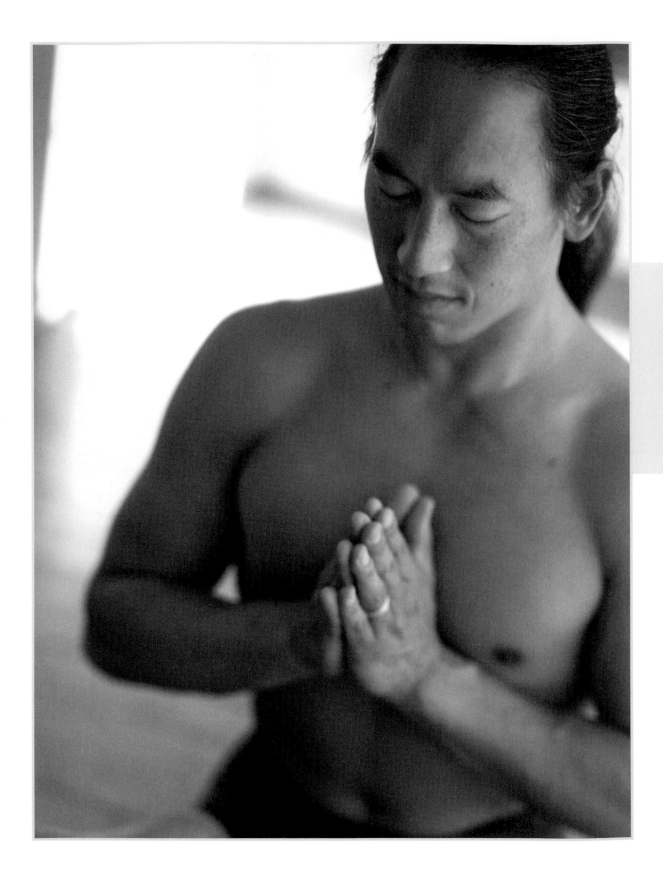

Part 1:

Before You Practice

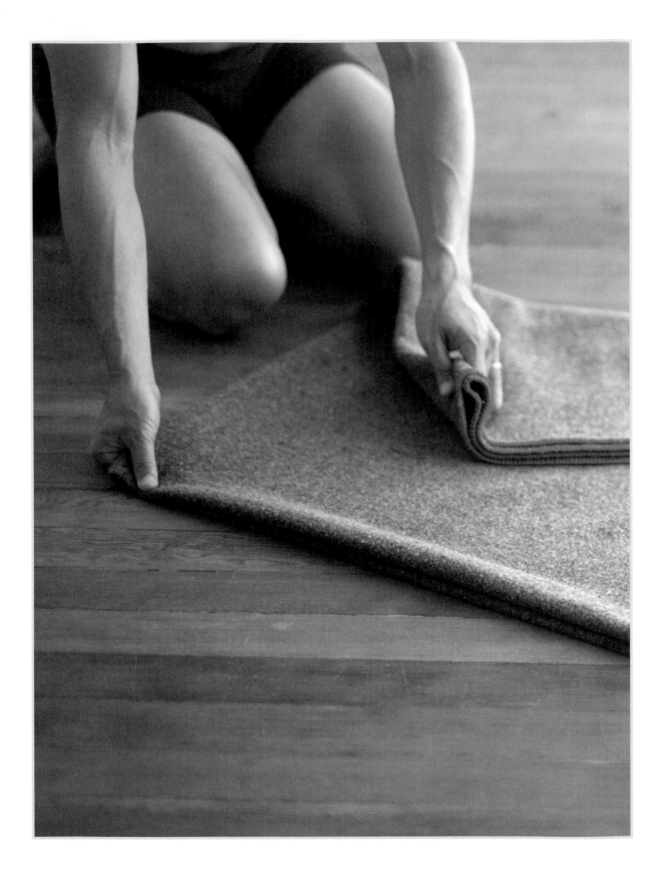

DO NOT KILL THE INSTINCT OF THE BODY FOR THE GLORY OF THE POSE. DO NOT LOOK AT YOUR BODY LIKE A STRANGER, BUT ADOPT A FRIENDLY APPROACH TOWARDS IT. WATCH IT, LISTEN TO IT, OBSERVE ITS NEEDS, ITS REQUESTS, AND EVEN HAVE FUN. PLAY WITH IT AS CHILDREN DO, SOMETIMES IT BECOMES VERY ALIVE AND SWIFT. TO BE SENSITIVE IS TO BE ALIVE.

—VANDA SCARAVELLI

Preparing to Practice

BEFORE YOU START OUR EIGHT-WEEK PROGRAM OF HOME YOGA PRACTICE, THERE ARE A FEW SIMPLE things you'll need to do: Find the time and place to practice yoga, assemble your yoga props, and learn about your body and your breath. This chapter provides information about these topics and concludes with some special advice—for those of you who may need it—on how to motivate yourself to practice.

FINDING THE TIME AND PLACE TO PRACTICE YOGA

For many people, finding the time to practice yoga at home is the main problem they must solve in order to embark on our eight-week program. Therefore, it is a good idea to sit down now, look over your schedule (if you have one), and figure out where you're going to fit in about 1 hour of yoga practice, six days a week. To manage this, you may need to consider waking up earlier than usual, asking your partner to take charge of the children at specified times, or juggling your work and home commitments around a bit. Once you have decided when to practice, you might even consider marking it on your calendar to establish this practice time as a fixed priority in your life for the next eight weeks.

MORNING PRACTICE

Most people prefer to practice yoga early in the morning before going off to work or school. The early morning is a beautiful time to practice because the world is calm and peaceful, and there are very few distractions.

Practicing yoga in the morning can also set the tone for your entire day. So if you generally feel better after doing yoga—more centered, calm, or filled with energy—why not allow yourself to begin your day with that orientation?

Finally, many people find that going straight from bed into practice is the only way to ensure that they actually do practice on a given day because they find that if they put off practicing until they get home from work, things get in the way and they never get around to it.

OTHER PRACTICE TIMES

On the other hand, some people have things they need to do in the morning (getting to work early, nursing a baby, or getting children off to school, for example). And other people simply find that the morning doesn't work for their particular bodies or personalities. It is worth experimenting to find what works for you, rather than simply doing something because of your preconceived notions of the "best" or "right" time to practice. Some practitioners do find that practicing in the late afternoon or even just before bed are the best times for them.

WHERE TO PRACTICE

After identifying the times when you want to practice, you need to find a space in which to practice. Although a few people are lucky enough to have an unused room that they can turn into a designated "yoga room," many people live in small houses or apartments and have to make do with some corner of the living room, bedroom, or even the kitchen. In some cases, using a combination of different spaces or areas in your home can be effective (for example, you may have a wall in one room where you do against-the-wall poses and another space in a different room where you practice your freestanding poses). Many everyday people have been able to develop rich and rewarding home practices within the confines of small, crowded spaces.

Flooring

If you have any options, consider the type of floor on which you will be practicing. Your first choice should be a wood floor, if one is available. If your home is carpeted,

I like starting early in the morning when it's still kind of nighttime and the world is still settled down for its rest. Sometimes while I practice, I'm aware of the sky lightening as the sun comes up. At first the songbirds are chirping, later the neighbors' lights shine through the curtains as they rise for the day. And then there's the roar of traffic from the busy street a block away and the sounds of the rest of the household awakening.

—LOUISA SPIER

The more I've been doing my home practice, the more I'm coming back to a daily practice time that is much more authentic for me, and it's not the morning. I want to sleep in the morning, and when I wake up, if I have a lot of energy, I want to take a walk or go to a café or do something social. And if I'm really tired, I'd rather stay in bed and read. So even though I think the morning is a really beautiful time to practice, it's not what I as a person desire, even though it may be what I as a yoga practitioner—the image of a yoga practitioner, that is—desire.

—JASON CRANDELL

I worked it out where there was this one wall in my bedroom that became the inversion wall. I moved a few things around to clear a space—especially after kicking over a lamp while trying to learn Handstand. And for most other poses, for a long time, I would just use the kitchen floor. It's not a serene room, but I knew that at certain times, I wasn't going to be in anyone's way in there and it was the only place that was big enough to do certain poses, so I would just roll the mat out there.

—DEBBI HERSH

it is best to practice on the most tightly woven carpet, such as industrial carpet, rather than on loose, cushy carpet, which is very difficult to balance on. In addition, if the surface is too soft, you get very slow feedback, so your body responses are also slow, which can be damaging to your joints. The worst surface you can practice on is concrete; however, marble and tile are actually quite good and you may even prefer them to carpeting.

ENHANCING YOUR ENVIRONMENT

If you are lucky enough to be able to dedicate a room or corner of a room to yoga, consider putting some effort into creating an environment that will make you more likely to want to practice and to focus on yoga while you are in it. Some people set up altars, display photographs of teachers or inspiring spiritual figures, or burn candles or incense. For other people, creating an inviting environment may be as simple as doing yoga in front of a window with a good view or in a room that has beautiful natural light.

If you have more than one possibility in your home, try to find your yoga space the way a cat finds a place for a nap. Where do you *want* to practice? Maybe you have a big spare room but that space between your bed and the wall feels like the place where you want to lay down your mat, so why not practice there? And even if you do have a designated yoga room, on some days you may feel like practicing in a different space. Go with your intuition and lay down your mat wherever you wish. Various rooms or spaces in your home may be more appealing during different seasons or at different times of day.

ASSEMBLING YOUR PROPS

The basic set of props that you'll need to do the daily practices in this eight-week program includes:

- One yoga mat (a thin sticky mat, not a padded exercise mat)
- Two blocks (wood, cork, or foam)
- One strap (with a buckle, if possible)
- One sturdy chair (with an opening below the chair back large enough for you to fit through)
- One round yoga bolster
- Two densely woven single blankets

You can find yoga props for sale at many yoga studios as well as on several Web sites. However, if you do not wish to make a major investment in buying "official" yoga props, you can make do in many cases by using things you already have around the house.

YOGA MAT. If you buy only one yoga prop, buy a yoga mat (also known as a sticky mat). A yoga mat provides you with the best surface on which to practice yoga and keeps you from slipping around, especially when you start to sweat. (Note that if you find that your brand-new sticky mat is more slippery than sticky and that practicing on it is worse than practicing on the floor, try washing the mat with soap and water. Some new mats have oil on them, which needs to be removed to restore their stickiness.)

YOGA BLOCKS. You will be using blocks to support different parts of your body, such as your hands or pelvis. For example, you may sit on a block while doing a seated twist or place both hands on blocks in Upward-Facing Dog.

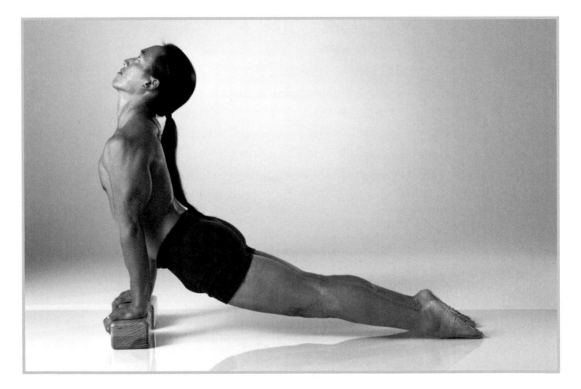

If you have a choice between wood, cork, or foam, go with the wood, as wood provides the best support. If you do not have blocks, you can use books or small boxes. However, be sure to use something that is firm rather than squishy so it can easily support the weight of your body. And make sure that for those poses requiring two blocks, as in the photo above, that the two props you use are the same size.

YOGA STRAP. You will be using the strap primarily to reach parts of your body, such as your toes, that you cannot reach without help. At other times, you will buckle the strap into a loop and use the loop to bind your arms together.

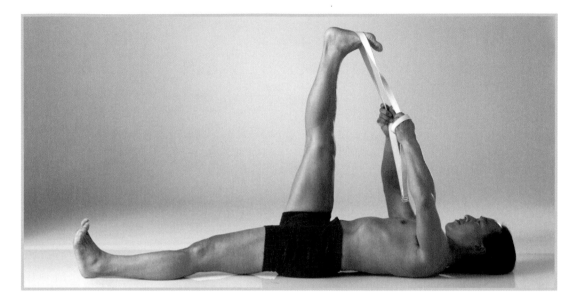

If you do not have a yoga strap, you can use a tie or sash. For those times when you need to make a loop with the strap, you will have to tie your sash.

CHAIR. You will use the chair to rest your head on while you are in seated and standing positions, and in a few cases, to support your body. You can use any chair, except one that has wheels. In addition, the chair should have an opening below its back that is large enough to fit your hips through. A sturdy chair is preferable because you don't want the chair to collapse or fall. An inexpensive folding chair was used for the photographs in this book.

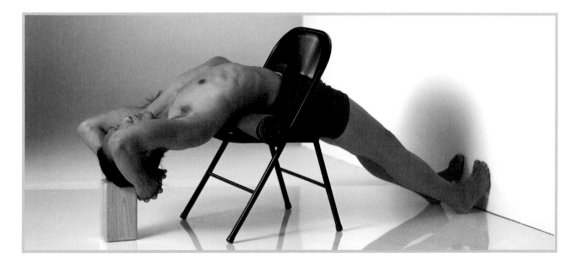

Some taller or heavier practitioners remove the backs from metal chairs like these so they can fit their bodies through the opening more easily.

YOGA BOLSTER. You will be using the bolster to support your body in reclined positions and to rest your head on while you are in seated positions.

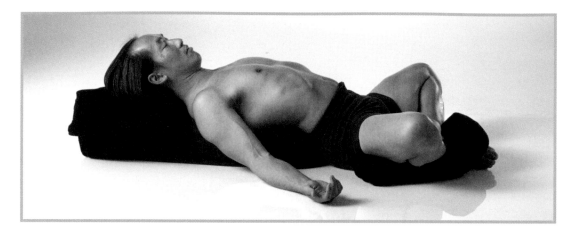

If you do not have a bolster, you can roll a folded blanket to create a bolster substitute or you can use a stack of blankets folded into thin rectangles.

BLANKETS. You will be using blankets to sit on and to support and cushion your body in various ways. If possible, use single-bed-size blankets of densely woven fabric, such as wool or cotton. Squishy or fluffy blankets, such as comforters or polar fleece blankets, do not provide the necessary support that you will need, as your body weight flattens them.

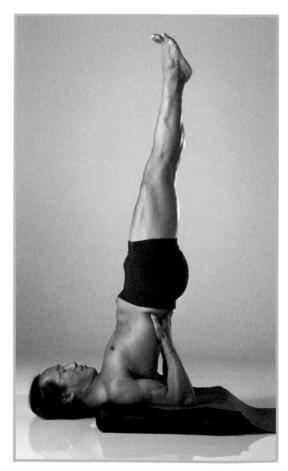

BLANKET FOLDING

For reasons that still seem a bit mysterious, folding blankets properly for yoga practice is a bit difficult for many beginners. It is important, however, for you to have neat, carefully folded blankets because a well-folded blanket provides an even, symmetrical surface to support your body. But a sloppy, unevenly folded blanket can throw your body out of alignment, making it worse than not using a prop at all. Therefore, take a deep breath and work as slowly as necessary.

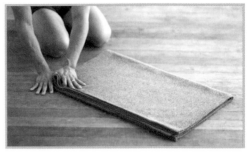

BASIC RECTANGLE. The basic rectangle is a folded blanket that you can sit on, kneel on, or use for Shoulderstand. It is also the starting point for creating a bolster substitute as well as for folding in half when you need a smaller prop to support your head or your pelvis.

To create the basic rectangle:

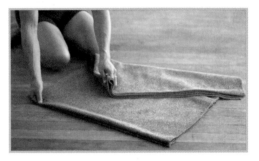

1. From the short edge of the blanket, fold the complete blanket in half so the two short edges come together into a neat rectangle (approximately 62 × 40 inches).

2. From the short edge of this rectangle, fold the blanket in half again so the two short edges come together in a smaller rectangle (approximately 31 × 40 inches).

3. From the short edge of this rectangle, fold the blanket in half again so the two short edges come together into a smaller rectangle (approximately 31 × 20 inches).

MAKING BLANKET ROLLS. Depending on the thickness you want, you can create a blanket roll by using one blanket to make a thinner roll or two blankets to make a thicker one.

To create single-blanket roll:

1. Fold a blanket three times into a neat basic rectangle (described above).

2. From the short edge of the basic rectangle, roll the blanket into a single tight roll.

To create a double-blanket roll:

1. Create a tight single-blanket roll as described above.

2. Take a blanket that you have folded into a single basic rectangle, and place the single-blanket roll on top of it, at the short end. Now, roll the basic rectangle around the single-blanket roll.

Making a Rectangular Stack. To create a stack of thin rectangular blankets as shown below, you need two blankets that have been folded three times into basic rectangles (described on page 9).

To make a rectangular stack:

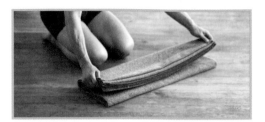

1. From the long edge of the basic rectangle, fold the first blanket so that the long sides come together into a long, narrow rectangle.

2. Repeat for the second blanket.

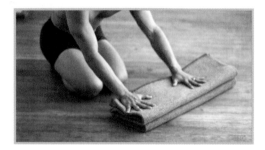

3. Now you have two long, narrow rectangles. Stack the second long, narrow rectangle on top of the first long narrow rectangle so that their thick folded edges are directly opposite each other.

LEARNING ABOUT YOUR BODY AND YOUR BREATH

Throughout the eight-week program, this book refers to various parts of your anatomy with which you may or may not be familiar. Each week during the program, the book will focus on three particular areas of your body. But for now, you may wish to get a general overall view of the body and learn some of the anatomical terminology that will be used throughout the book. Look over these photographs now—and come back to them whenever you wish throughout the eight-week program—to locate various parts of your body and clarify the relationships between them.

During the eight-week program, there will be information about bones, muscles, and joints. In all cases, it is good to touch these areas and even to massage them so you can become viscerally acquainted with them. During the practices, you will both observe these areas and manipulate them to understand their relationships with the rest of your body. By making a particular part of your body a point of focus, you will notice how it feels, how it functions in your body, and how it interconnects with the rest of your body. Focusing on a particular part of your body during your practice also helps train your mind, providing a seed of meditation. Although this book presents some of the key body parts to focus on during the eight-week program, realize that you yourself can select any part of the body to study while practicing your poses.

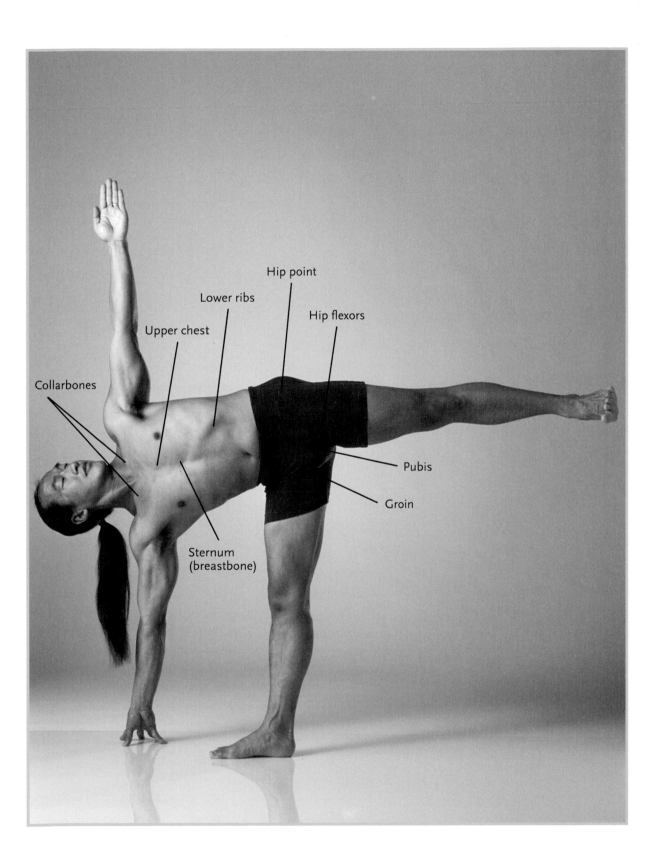

Collarbones

Upper chest

Lower ribs

Hip point

Hip flexors

Sternum
(breastbone)

Pubis

Groin

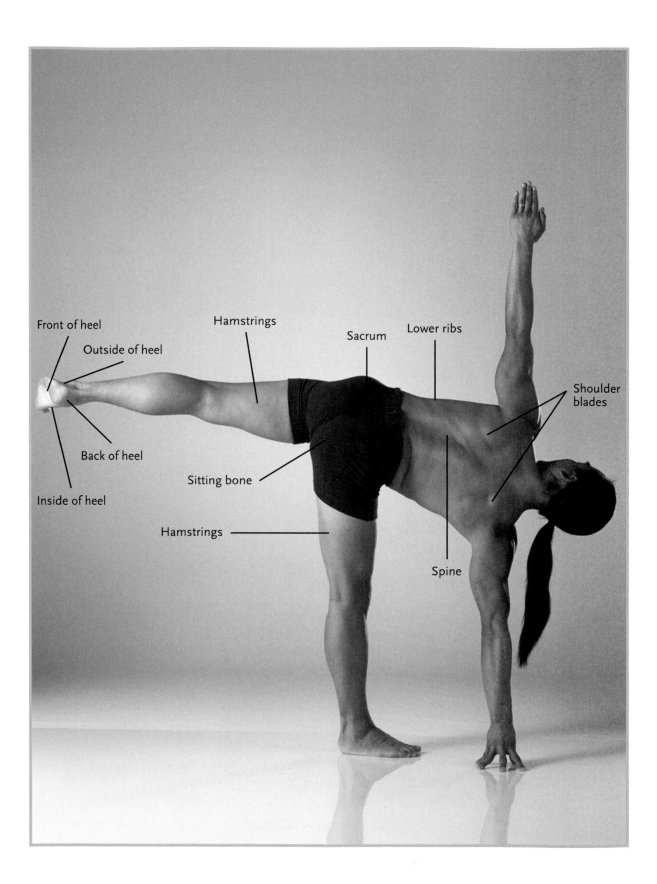

Front of heel

Outside of heel

Hamstrings

Sacrum

Lower ribs

Shoulder blades

Back of heel

Sitting bone

Inside of heel

Hamstrings

Spine

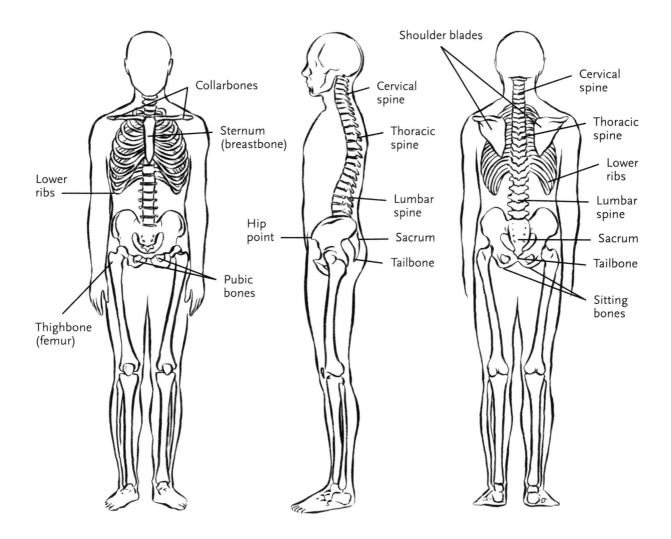

Collarbones

Sternum
(breastbone)

Lower
ribs

Pubic
bones

Thighbone
(femur)

Shoulder blades

Cervical
spine

Thoracic
spine

Lumbar
spine

Hip
point

Sacrum

Tailbone

Cervical
spine

Thoracic
spine

Lower
ribs

Lumbar
spine

Sacrum

Tailbone

Sitting
bones

BREATHING IN YOGA POSES

Students often ask how they should breathe while doing yoga poses. The answer is to simply allow yourself to breathe freely. Do not force or hold your breath. The rate of your breath will vary depending on the type of pose you are doing. For example, your breath may be slow in Relaxation Pose while it is quite rapid in a backbend. This is natural, so don't try to force your breath into a given pace (though reminding yourself not to hold your breath is always a good idea).

Timing Your Breath

In the sequences in this book, the timing for a given pose is specified either as a time span (seconds or minutes) or as a number of breaths. For those poses whose timings are specified in breaths, simply count your breaths to the specified number. For those poses whose timings are specified as a time span, you should first time your breath to determine how many breaths you typically take per minute. When you practice the pose, you can then count your breaths up to the number that you typically take for the given time span. For example, if you take 15 breaths per minute in an active pose and the sequence specifies 30 seconds in Triangle Pose, you would count 8 breaths as equal to 30 seconds.

Before you start the program, it is a good idea to take the opportunity to time your breath in two different poses, once for a quiet, seated pose, such as Seated Crossed-Legs Pose, and a second time for a very active pose, such as Warrior 1. Simply set a timer for 1 minute and

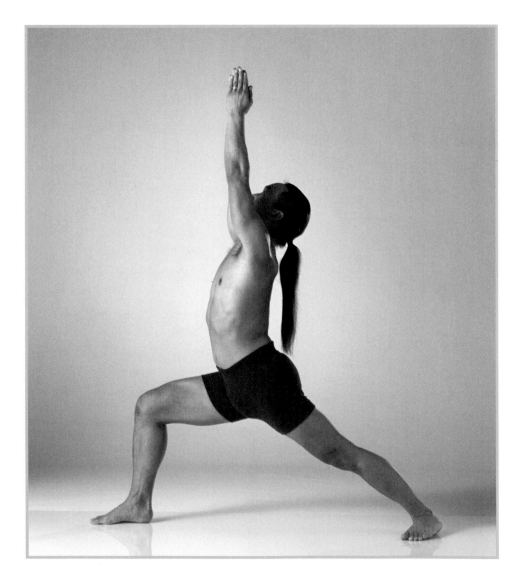

then, as you practice the pose, count how many breaths you complete within 1 minute. You can then use those two counts to estimate for any given pose how many breaths you should take while you are practicing the pose. (Don't worry about being too exact with this. The timings are just general guidelines.)

USING A TIMER. Note that for long holds, such as those more than 1 minute, it may be easier to use a timer or a watch with a countdown function, rather than counting your breaths. This is especially useful for restorative poses, which you can hold for periods of up to 5 or 10 minutes.

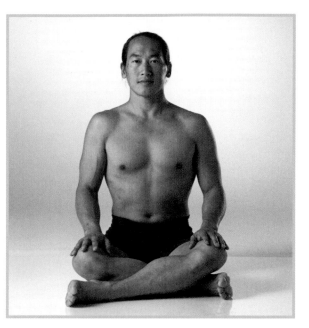

MOTIVATING YOURSELF TO PRACTICE

Often people have a hard time getting themselves to start a new activity, no matter how satisfying or rewarding they know it will be. Our habits of doing certain things on a daily basis and of never doing other things can be very difficult to break. Perhaps you have a daily routine of getting up at a certain time in the morning, going off to work for eight hours, fixing dinner at around the same time every night, and watching TV the last two hours before bed. How are you going to switch over to a new habit of getting up an hour earlier to do yoga or giving up those two hours of TV to practice instead? Sometimes trying to break your old habit of *not practicing yoga* in order to establish a new habit of *practicing yoga* can feel insurmountable. This section presents various ways to motivate yourself to practice and describes a few of the tricks that real practitioners have used to overcome their inertia. Often, tricking yourself into starting a home practice can be the very thing that allows you to make it an integral part of daily life. Maybe some of these suggestions we've included in this section seem like cheating to you, such as playing music or bribing yourself, but in the end, anything that gets you to your mat on a regular basis will help you start the practice of yoga.

Note that the suggestions here are simply gleaned from personal experience and those of fellow practitioners. Follow any or all that appeal to you or develop your own (and maybe even write to Rodney and Nina about your discoveries—rodandnina@wanderingmind.com).

MUSIC. Many people find playing music makes it easier for them to get themselves to the mat. You may wish to play music that puts you into a certain mood, or you may simply wish to play something that is fun to listen to. Fellow practitioners have confessed to playing everything from Japanese pop to Icelandic rock, from classical music to Indian ragas, and from New Age music to punk. It is a recommended, however, that you turn off the music for the end of your practice so that you practice Relaxation Pose, breath awareness, and meditation in silence.

COFFEE AND TEA. It is generally recommended that you do yoga on an empty stomach; however, some people find they just can't start without their morning caffeine. So, yes, if you can't get going in the morning without that cup of coffee or black tea, by all means, go ahead and have it. See page 27 for information about eating before yoga practice.

OTHER PEOPLE. It is a common misconception that practicing yoga is something you must do completely by yourself. Although practicing alone is extremely rewarding, there are many people for whom this may not be possible (for example, people with families or several roommates). Practitioners with families often find their partners and children will wander in and out of the yoga room, maybe because they want help with their homework, assistance in resolving a fight, or simply some company. If this is something you can comfortably tolerate or that you even enjoy (Nina, for example, really enjoys having her son, Quinn, chat amiably with her about his day while she's in a headstand), you may find that allowing other people to be around you while you practice will make it more likely that you actually can fit a practice into your day.

There are also many people who find that practicing yoga with someone else, whether a family member or a friend, is the very thing that allows them to maintain a regular home practice. If this is something that appeals to you, it is definitely worth experimenting with. See "Practicing with a Friend" on page 376 for detailed information about the many ways in which you can practice with others.

While working through the eight-week program in this book, you may find it helpful to join forces with a friend or even a group of friends explicitly for the purpose of completing the course together. You can do some or all of the practices in the book together or simply meet once a week to discuss your thoughts and feelings about the program, and provide each other with support and encouragement. When the eight-week program in this book was taught as a series class at Piedmont Yoga Studio in Oakland, California, some of our students said that the single-most important factor in keeping up their daily practice was knowing that they would be talking each week with their fellow students about the previous week of practice.

I've heard you're supposed to find a place away from family pets but I can't bear to shut out my puppy so I let him sit with me while I practice. Sometimes he licks my face or bites my shorts but mostly he's pretty patient.

—HILLARY FOX

PETS. People who own pets often find that although they may be distracting at times, having the company of their pets while they practice can create a casual, comfortable, and playful atmosphere that deepens their enjoyment of their practice.

BRIBING YOURSELF. When asked what motivated them to start practicing, some students confessed that they had made deals with themselves—essentially bribing themselves—to get themselves to start their yoga practice. Rewarding yourself can motivate you to maintain your practice until the habit of doing yoga becomes an integral part of your life. Maybe you'll bribe yourself with purple flowery yoga pants, a night at the movies, 70 percent chocolate, a crossword puzzle book, or a day at the beach. One student said she bribed herself with "Queen and ice cream." But here's the prize-winning cheater, at right.

CULTIVATING ACCEPTANCE. One of the main things that can kill your motivation to practice is worrying about whether or not you are doing the poses or the practice "correctly." Instead, can you observe and respond without judgment? Yoga is meditation in movement, not a competitive sport or an elitist art form. And being present during your practice means allowing yourself to be aware of whatever physical sensations, emotions, thoughts, are currently arising. If you cultivate an attitude of curiosity rather than ambition and competitiveness, you will not only find it easier to motivate yourself to practice, but you will be able to be more observant during the times when you do practice.

Face it, though, no matter how conscientiously you take on an attitude of curiosity and self-acceptance, you're not always going to enjoy yourself when you practice. Some days you may be bored, sad, lonely, angry, or depressed. Many different emotions may arise during a practice, either because you are currently going through some difficulty outside the yoga room or merely because opening up your body in new ways releases pent-up feelings. In either case, simply allow yourself to feel your feelings. If you feel like crying, cry. If you have to get up and punch or throw something, do that (one student did) and return to Downward-Facing Dog. You may eventually find that your practice becomes a kind of refuge, a time when you can safely experience emotions that cannot be expressed so easily at other times during your day.

Every day for a long, long time, I would get out of the warehouse and get home and watch The Simpsons, *the 6:00 and 6:30 episodes. So I bartered with myself that for the 6:00 to 7:00 period, I would, no matter what, five days a week, lay my yoga mat out in front of the TV and do as much yoga as I could. It seemed like a perfect trade, and it didn't seem like it was at cross purposes—it didn't seem like it was ironic or even that funny—it just seemed like it was a reasonable thing to do. And it worked beautifully. And then basically what happened was that I started to become more interested in what my body was doing in that period and* The Simpsons *actually became more of a distraction. It was a natural evolution that I turned it off after a few months.*

—JASON CRANDELL

During my divorce, the mat became the only place I could cry. As soon as I stepped on the mat in Mountain Pose, I wept. It didn't stop me from practicing, and I didn't look forward to practice as that specific release. I would be feeling fine. Then boom. As soon as I focused on my body and breath, the gates were opened for grief. My yoga practice offered me help every day. I didn't have to ask. Just as the perfect mate would know exactly what you want without you having to ask! He could read your mind, your emotions, and your hormones! Unfortunately, my mat can't hold my hand at the movies.

—SUSAN OREM

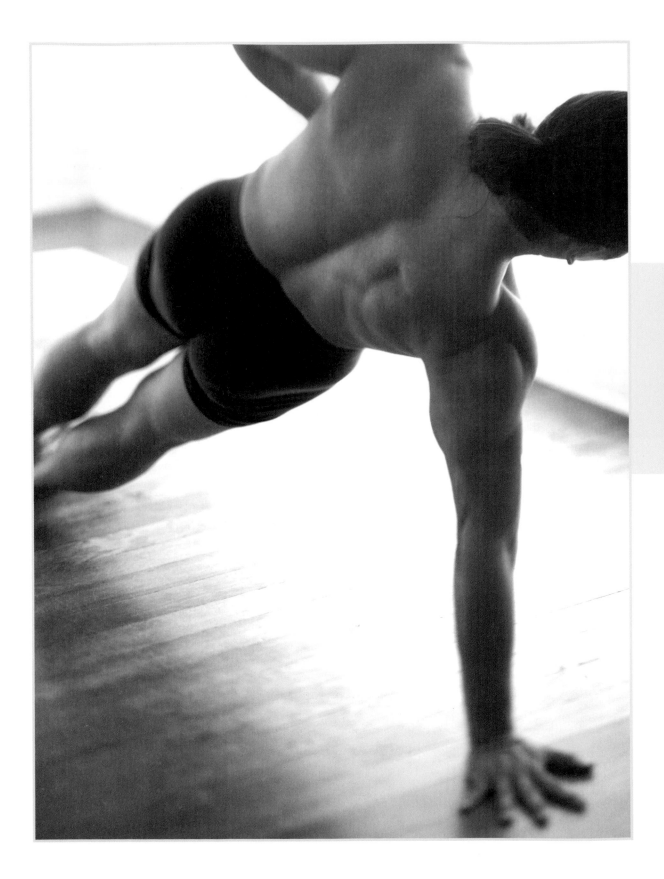

PART 2

8 Weeks of Yoga

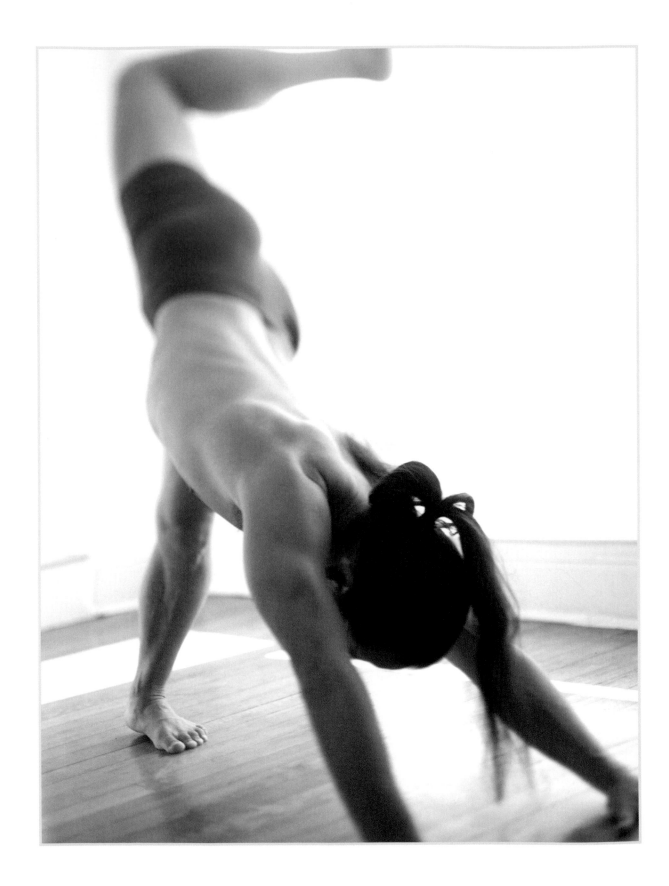

JUST BEING LOW DOWN IN A ROOM TENDS TO CLEAR THE MIND. MAYBE IT'S BECAUSE BEING ON THE FLOOR IS SO FOREIGN TO US THAT IT BREAKS UP OUR HABITUAL NEUROLOGICAL PATTERNING AND INVITES US TO ENTER INTO THIS MOMENT THROUGH A SUDDEN OPENING IN WHAT WE MIGHT CALL THE BODY DOOR.
—JON KABAT-ZINN, *WHEREVER YOU GO, THERE YOU ARE*

About the 8-Week Program

THIS CHAPTER PROVIDES GENERAL INFORMATION ABOUT THE EIGHT-WEEK YOGA HOME PRACTICE program, describing how to use the book to guide yourself through the eight weeks of practice. It also provides background information about meditation and breath awareness, both of which you will be asked to practice during the program. The chapter concludes with a set of questions that our students typically have about the program, along with our answers to them.

ABOUT THE PROGRAM

The yoga program in this book provides you with six different days of yoga practice for each of the eight weeks in the program. If it is possible for you to practice six days a week, it is recommended that you do so because immersing yourself in yoga for eight weeks will have a profound effect on you in the long run and will help you acquire the habit of doing yoga on a daily basis. You can take any day off during the week that you wish, though it is best, if possible, to take the same day off each week to establish a routine.

If it is not possible for you to practice six days a week, you can take longer to do the program. In this case, work through all the practices specified for a given week before moving on to the next week's practices (rather than skipping practices in order to complete the program in eight weeks). For example, it is better to take two weeks to practice the lessons in Week 1 than to skip over any of the lessons for that week and move on to Week 2.

This program was designed to be used by a wide range of yoga practitioners, from absolute beginners to experienced, long-term practitioners. For those of you who are new to yoga, we provide modified versions of each of the poses so you can practice the easiest form of each pose, if needed. However, if you find particular poses or lessons within the program overly challenging, take it easy on yourself. Feel free to skip over anything that you do not feel ready for—you can always return to it sometime in the future. For example, you may not feel ready at this time to take on Handstand or Headstand, but when you do feel ready, you can return to those poses and the practices designed to teach them to you. Don't be hard on yourself if there is something you cannot do or are not yet ready for. Try not to use your yoga practice as another way to judge yourself or to find yourself wanting, whether you find a pose too difficult or skip an entire day of practice.

Each weekly lesson consists of the following:

- Introduction
- Day 1
- Days 2 through 5
- Day 6
- Poses of the Week

It is recommended that at the beginning of each week, you look briefly through the entire week's program to familiarize yourself with the overall focus of that week. Then, before starting Day 1, take time to go over the anatomy lesson. This will prepare you to work with more understanding in the poses being highlighted during the coming week.

INTRODUCTION

The introduction to each week contains philosophical background on a particular aspect of yoga and explains how the specific poses you will be exploring in the coming week relate to that aspect of yoga. The introduction also contains an anatomy lesson that asks you to investigate the three particular areas of the body you will be focusing on during that week's practices. It is recommended that each week you take the time not only to read through this section but also to follow the instructions for exploring the various parts of your anatomy. Be playful as you move your body in order to learn both about the location of a part of your body as well as its relationship to the rest of your body.

DAY 1

Day 1 contains a practice that teaches you the new poses for the coming week. Look over the photos in the practice, from start to finish, before beginning to follow the instructions.

LEARNING THE VARIATIONS. Day 1 presents three versions of every new pose. It is recommended that you—regardless of your level of experience—try all three versions as instructed. Then after trying all three versions, you can choose the version you want to work with primarily in the coming week. When you evaluate the three different versions of a pose, try to find the version that fully engages your mind yet does not inhibit your breath.

At this time, highlight or bookmark any particular poses or versions of poses that you like especially or that you find intriguing. These notations will become useful when you are ready to create your own sequences as described under "Creating the Sequence That You Love" on page 354.

Day 1 also includes very detailed anatomical instructions for each of the three versions of the new poses. For some beginning practitioners, this may feel like too much to take in at once. If so, simply choose a single instruction to focus on. You can always return to this alignment information at any time in the future when you are interested in finding new aspects of the pose to focus on. In fact, the information in these sections should be a valuable resource for years to come.

LISTENING AND RESPONDING. In this book, you are ultimately learning to listen to your body. So no matter how detailed the instructions are for a given pose, find some time for experimenting. Try dropping all the instructions for a few moments and simply feel the totality of the pose.

DAYS 2 THROUGH 5

Days 2 through 5 for each week provide you with unique sequences, designed specifically to deepen your understanding of a particular pose or two. Before starting to practice, look quickly over the photos of each pose in the sequence to get an overall feeling for the day's lesson.

As you move through the practice, you will be instructed either to do a particular version of a pose (for example, "Practice version 1 of Downward-Facing Dog") or any version of a pose (for example, "Practice Downward-Facing Dog"). If a particular version of a pose is specified, you should practice that version, if it is accessible to you. In this case, the photograph next to the pose name will indicate which version you should practice. If no version is specified, you can practice any of the three versions that you wish even if it is different than that shown in the photograph.

At this time, highlight or bookmark any sequences that you like especially or that you find intriguing. These notations will become useful when you have completed the program and are looking for sequences to repeat. See "Creating a Personal Practice" on page 349 for further information on this.

DAY 6

Day 6 of each week is set aside for focusing on breath awareness and meditation. Many of you will be tempted to skip these days, thinking that if you are not doing poses, you are not "doing yoga." However, if you can open your mind to exploring these branches of yoga, you will find the lessons very rewarding. A number of our students have said how glad they were that this program introduced them to the daily practice of breath awareness and meditation.

Breath Awareness

PRANAYAMA. One of eight branches of yoga practice is *pranayama,* the natural absorption of the life force, or *prana,* into the body and mind. There are many *pranayama* practices, all of which, in my opinion, are quite advanced work. The tradition in which I have been trained highly recommends that you have some mastery of the *asana* practice (the postures) before you start a *pranayama* practice. The reason for this is that working with the breath is one of the essential aspects to both our mental and physical balance. When working with these subtle and powerful practices, it is easy to get off course without proper supervision and instruction, which can lead to both physical and psychological imbalances. However, the breath awareness practices that I have selected for the program in this book are all benign practices, which you can use to begin your experiment with your breath and which can lead you toward a *pranayama* practice.

PRACTICING DAILY. I recommend that you do your breath awareness exercises daily, at the end of each practice. This will enable you to gain the sensitivity required to listen to the breath. For many of you, focusing on the breath may initially seem too subtle. Most of you will notice your mind wandering and some of you may even find yourself falling asleep. With persistence and care, your mind will begin to steady itself on the subtle language of the breath. As this begins to happen, this conversation between the breath, the body, and the mind can become one of your most intimate and cherished relationships.

RELAXATION AND ABSORPTION OF BREATH. One of the most important things I want to teach you about in this book is the relationship between relaxation and your ability to absorb the breath. Almost all the breath awareness exercises are done in a restorative pose (though a few are done in seated poses). This is because the main prelude to any of the breath awareness exercises is *deep relaxation.* Keep in mind that in your breath awareness practices, you are not trying to do anything special with the breath, but instead are trying to let the breath return to its natural state, without the overlay of your breathing *habits.* On most days, meditation follows the breath awareness exercise because it is breath awareness that begins to steady and focus your mind. On the days you start with sitting meditation before the breath awareness exercise, you will be using the meditation to cultivate deep relaxation and understanding of posture. This will allow your observation of your breath to be more keen and have the possibility of coming from a place of deep quietness.

Meditating on your breath is a practice you can do in your everyday life, whether at home in the presence of your family, at work with your co-workers, or alone out in nature.

At any time, returning your mind to the sound and feeling of your breath can help center you and bring you back to the present moment.

Meditation

Many of us have the idea that when someone meditates, the mind is quiet, the body is at ease, and everything is "peaceful." Therefore, many people can't even imagine themselves meditating. But anyone who has meditated can tell you that everyone has to deal with the wandering mind, aching body, bleeding heart, and anxious breath. And by spending some quiet time observing the impermanence of all of your sensations and thoughts, you can digest and release past experiences. You notice that the quiet spaces in between the mental noise expand and open up.

TIME TO DIGEST. Initially, the meditation practices in the eight-week program may be the most challenging part of the program for you. Furthermore, many of you may find it difficult to justify taking the time to sit and do "nothing." But consider that after you eat a large meal, you usually don't even think about eating more, even if your favorite food is sitting next to you. Most of you are already full of experiences, thoughts, emotions, and physical sensations. But you may have become habitual about immediately running on to the next activity, being somewhat afraid of and unacquainted with solitude, relaxation, and quietness. The benefits of meditation are surprising and fulfilling. Even when you are sitting with agitation and frustration, the net result of having that time to observe but not react to difficulties is profound. Learning to sit with difficulty is so beneficial because it gives you a chance to respond appropriately instead of reacting habitually.

MONKEY MIND. Even within 10 minutes, your body may run through numerous complaints, and focusing on your breath may seem futile due to what is called the "monkey mind," a mind that is continually jumping from one thing to the next. But with consistency of practice, you will develop your ability to concentrate on your breath and in doing so will learn how to channel one of your greatest assets: your mind.

POSES OF THE WEEK

At the end of each week are full-page photographs of the new poses for the week, labeled with alignment pointers. For every pose, there is also a "point of play," which is a movement that you can practice to teach yourself about finding balance in the particular pose. These pose pages are designed for reference, providing you with both visual and written cues that you can return to at any time when you want to learn more about a particular pose or find new aspects of a pose to explore.

TYPICAL STUDENT QUESTIONS

Do I really have to try all three versions of every pose?

Yes, as long as the version is possible for you. Each version has something different to teach you about the posture itself. And it is beneficial for flexible beginners and even advanced practitioners to back up on occasion and feel the more supported versions of the pose.

Do I really need to use yoga props?

Yoga props are so useful for enabling you to find steadiness, ease, and correct alignment in your poses that it is strongly recommended that you give them a try. Many times students compromise their alignment by trying to go too deep in the pose; for example, many beginners try to put their hands on the floor in Triangle Pose and end up jamming their hips and spine, whereas using a block under the bottom hand allows them to keep their spines more fully extended.

In addition, using yoga props will enable some less flexible people to practice poses that might otherwise be inaccessible. For example, many people cannot get into Reclined Hero Pose without using either a chair or a bolster. In a case like this, using a prop will enable you to receive the physical and emotional benefits of a pose that you might otherwise not be able to practice. In addition, the restorative versions of certain poses, such as the restorative version of Reclined Cobbler's Pose, require props. In restorative poses, props enable you to relax more deeply in the poses as well as to stay in the poses for long periods of time (for example, up to 10 minutes in Reclined Cobbler's Pose). Props are also useful because some of the physiological benefits from the poses come after a certain period of time. For example, in restorative poses, sometimes it takes you 2 to 3 minutes just to settle into the pose, with the real, deep relaxation coming only after that settling period.

Props can also teach you the proper architecture of the pose, educating your body to align itself correctly in many different other poses. For example, in Supported Relaxation Pose, the bolster will teach you to lift and open your chest. You can then transfer the visceral understanding you gained from lying over the bolster to any pose where you lift and open your chest.

People who are not used to dealing with props in their yoga practice may at first find them somewhat awkward and even annoying; however, with time you will become more comfortable using them and will learn to appreciate the many benefits that they provide. Of course, if you are in a situation where you want to practice yoga and props are not available, such as out in nature, feel free to go ahead and practice without them.

Can I eat before doing yoga?

Traditionally it is recommended that you do yoga on an empty stomach (four hours after a full meal or two hours after a light meal). However, if you find that your blood sugar plummets when you practice and that you cannot make it through a practice on an empty stomach, you may wish to try eating a piece of fruit or some yogurt before practicing. Feel free to experiment to find out what is best for you.

Also, you may have medical needs to consider. One fellow practitioner is a Type 1 diabetic, and she must accommodate this in her yoga practice as well as in her daily life. So she never follows the "rules" about minimal eating and always has a substantial breakfast prior to her morning practice.

What if I don't have enough time to do the complete practice?

If you don't have enough time to do a complete practice, it is better to do all the poses in the sequence for shorter periods of time than to skip over poses in the sequence. However, if, for some reason, you must stop halfway through a practice, always try to practice the restorative poses at the end of the sequence before going on to your next activity. See "Shortening a Practice" on page 350 for further information on this.

Many people will be tempted to shorten a practice by eliminating the Relaxation Pose from the end of the practice. It is strongly recommended, however, that you do not do this. Relaxation is the time when your body assimilates all the information from your practice and gives you time to make a smooth transition from your practice to your next activity. Learning how to relax is one of the most important yoga lessons.

Does it matter what I wear?

You can wear whatever you wish, as long as the clothing does not restrict your movements. However, you should always practice with bare feet (and that means no socks or stockings!). Bare feet keep you from sliding all over your mat and allow your feet to be more sensitive. Also, if it's warm enough, it is better to practice wearing as little as possible, so you can see your skin. Noticing whether or not your skin is receptive and even is one of the best ways to balance your work.

What if I feel pain while doing a pose?

Whenever you feel pain in a pose, back up in the pose until there is only a minor sensation of the pain. And then ask yourself: Which muscles can I relax? Which muscles can I contract to relieve the pain? The pain in your body can be a great resource to teach you how to improve the alignment and action of a pose.

There are some types of pain that are more dangerous than others. For instance, joint pain is more dangerous than muscle pain. Whenever you have joint pain, you definitely need to back out of the pose until you can figure out how to move without causing the pain. Ideally, in every pose, you should adjust the pose until there is a feeling of evenness of breath, mind, and sensation running throughout your entire body.

See "When You Are Injured" on page 362 for information on working with injuries.

Can I still keep taking yoga classes?

It is a good idea to continue taking class about once or twice a week to maintain your connection with your current yoga teacher while at the same time leaving time in your schedule to practice yoga on your own.

If what your teacher tells you about a pose contradicts what this book says, follow your teacher's instructions while in class. At home, you have the option of following the instructions exactly as they are in our book or modifying them according to your teacher's style. Try experimenting with both versions of a pose—your teacher's and our book's—to see which you prefer and which works best for you. In the end, it is your body and your yoga practice.

How should this practice relate to my other exercise programs?

You do not need to give up your other exercise programs to practice yoga. In fact, in many cases, your yoga practice will complement other physical activities, such as running, walking, cycling, weight lifting, or swimming, because it allows you to move, open up, and bring awareness to parts of your body that you may normally ignore. Another thing you may wish to consider is that yoga is primarily a spiritual practice, rather than an exercise program. So in many ways, it does not make sense to pit your yoga practice against other physical activities that you enjoy. Consider your priorities instead, as well as your schedule, to determine which activities you can manage to combine within a given day, as well as within a given week.

What if I hurt myself?

Depending on the type of injury you have, you may or may not be able to continue with the entire program. See "When You Are Injured" on page 362 for information on how to deal with injuries in your yoga practice.

What if I get sick?

If you get sick during the eight-week program, whether or not you can continue with the program depends on how sick you are and how you feel. Listen to your body. If you feel up to it, continue with the program as is. However, if your body tells you to take a rest, stop the program for as long as you need to and resume it when you are ready. If you feel well enough to want to practice a bit but are not up to the rigors of the full program, see "When You are Sick" on page 361 for alternatives.

What should I do when I am menstruating?

If you are menstruating during Weeks 1 through 4 of the program, you can practice the sequences during those weeks exactly as specified. However, Weeks 5 through 8 include inverted poses, which you should generally avoid during your period. So if you are menstruating during the time in which you would be doing any part of Weeks 5 through 8, either practice A Moon Practice (see page 360) or take off one or more days to rest. See "Your Monthly Cycle" on page 359 for further information on how to practice during your period.

What if I am pregnant?

If you are pregnant, do not start the eight-week program in this book. Instead, if you wish to start a home yoga practice at this time, it is best that you take a prenatal yoga class from a qualified teacher in your area (or if there is none, practice from a prenatal yoga video or book).

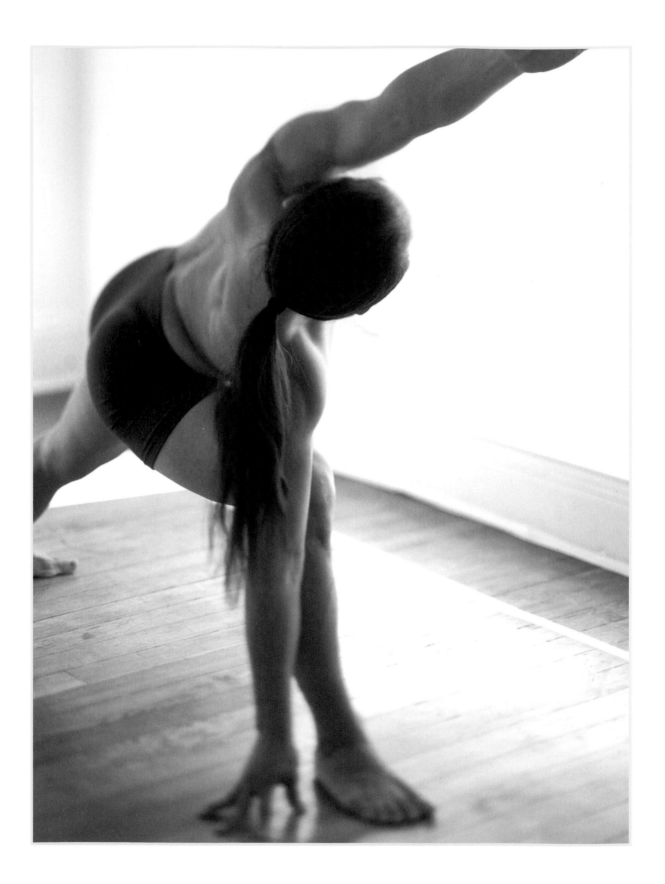

WEEK 1:

Being Present

BEING PRESENT MEANS OBSERVING AND RESPONDING APPROPRIATELY TO WHATEVER ARISES. WHEN YOU LIVE in the present, you have a true connection to what is real, as it arises and falls, fluctuates and changes. In my mind, this allows you to be completely alive. People frequently talk about the value of living in the present. I would like to take this further by asking: How are you *responding* in the present moment? As you balance yourself in the center of your body and the quiet of your mind, you can move easily in any direction, without a preset tendency, and therefore choose how to respond. If your body is always leaning forward, it is not easy to step backward. But the more your body is balanced toward center, the easier it is to move in any direction. Likewise, a mind that is clearer is able to receive and respond to whatever arises, in all its uniqueness.

This week you will focus on the standing poses, vigorous postures that awaken your entire body. In the standing poses, your legs bear the weight of your body, your arms reach with vigor, and your spine is fully extended. Feeling the vibrancy of these postures—the coursing of your blood, the pumping of your heart, the quickening of your breath, the strong work of your legs, back, and arms—calls your mind into the present moment. The act of witnessing your aliveness invests your whole being—your mind, body, breath, and spirit—in the present.

The trick is to allow your mind to be present without being overly determined. Imagine you are a tightrope artist balancing on a narrow wire. To remain focused on all the shifts in your physical balance, including the rise and fall of your breath, you would keep your mind fully engaged in all the fluctuations occurring in the present moment. Your direct connection to the present lies as much in the alertness of your mind as it does in the natural receptivity and relaxation of your body.

The standing poses also awaken your physical connection to the earth. As you engage your leg muscles—some of the largest muscles of your body—your mind is harnessed. And as the soles of your feet—some of the most sensitive parts of your body—come in firm contact with the ground, you renew your connection to the earth, a connection that is essential in creating presence of mind.

About the Standing Poses

Most of us live extremely sedentary lives. But for our bodies to be healthy and happy, we need to move in our full range of motion. Practicing the standing poses is a way to begin this journey. Standing poses awaken your legs back to their natural function, increasing their agility, strength, and alignment. As your legs move and work, your digestive system functions more effectively and your circulatory system is stimulated. Practicing the standing poses is like taking a walk in the brisk winter air after being cooped up all day. The poses invigorate your entire body, which brings ease to your mind.

EMOTIONS. The standing poses stabilize and ground you, getting you out of your head and into your legs and feet. Energizing and moving your legs dramatically changes your internal chemistry, creating a strong feeling of vitality and vibrancy. The standing poses also allow you to rediscover your connection to the earth, which nourishes and soothes you.

FOCUS OF YOUR MIND. In standing poses, focus your eyes on your top hand or, in the upright poses, your front hand. Gaze with receptivity. Instead of concentrating with effort, relax your eyes and softly receive the hand within the context of the other visual stimuli. Focus also on the continual alignment of your body over your feet. In the standing poses your body moves in and out of center.

BALANCING. Few of us feel uncomfortable in the basic standing poses, yet these poses can be the most complicated. This is due to the variety of movements you need to make to align your body in the pose (like singing harmony instead of singing solo). You will find in the standing poses that your body moves in and out of center. Your response to this movement is the act of balancing.

BREATH. In the standing poses, draw your inhalation into the grounding of your legs. Let the tension of your brain and sense organs follow your breath down into your torso, pelvis, and legs. Practice the poses so you can elicit the fullness and ease of your breath. Allow your breath to mimic how you breathe as you walk. Exhale as if your entire being is fading into emptiness, without effort or fear.

ARMS. In the standing poses, your arms find full extension over your head, out to the side, and behind your back. From these simple shapes, you will discover how your arms support your chest and express your heart.

FEET AND LEGS. Learning the standing poses trains your body from the foundation up. Your feet return to their natural strength and responsiveness, and your legs regain their natural strength, alignment, and circulation. Having awareness of your feet and your legs is essential to understanding all the yoga poses.

PELVIS. Your pelvis transfers the information and strength of your legs into your spine. Because we sit in chairs, our hip joints have become stiff and unresponsive. The standing poses help you regain your fluidity and teach you about the relationship of your pelvis to your spine.

SPINE. As you reeducate your lower body, your spine reaps the benefits. In most standing poses, your spine is in fairly simple positions in which you can maintain the natural curves, alignment, and integrity of your spine. The work of both your legs and arms feeds into your spine to create support and fluidity.

SHOULDERS. In the standing poses, your shoulder blades move down your back and firm against your rib cage. Your upper arm bones draw into the sockets. Your collarbones lift and widen from the work of your upper arm bones and your legs. In all standing poses, aim to return to this neutral shoulder state.

ANATOMY LESSON

1. Fronts, backs, outsides, and insides of your heels

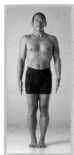

To learn about your heels, sit down and palpate different parts of your feet, maybe even have someone give you a heel massage. After sensitizing yourself in this way, stand up in Mountain Pose and shift your weight to different parts of your heels.

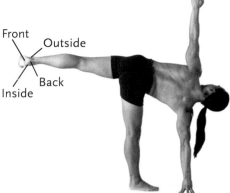

Front
Outside
Back
Inside

2. Sitting bones, tailbone, and pubis

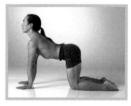

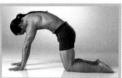

To learn about your sitting bones, tailbone, and pubis, stand in Mountain Pose and touch these areas. Then move back and forth from versions 2 and 3 of Cat Pose to observe the articulations and movements of these three areas.

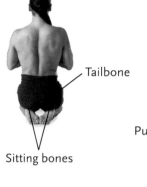

Tailbone

Sitting bones

Pubis

3. Natural curves of your spine

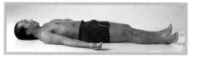

To learn about the natural curves of your spine, lie in Relaxation Pose and observe which parts of your spine touch the floor and which parts of your spine curve up away from the floor. Many of you will be able to insert a flat hand under your lower back and under your neck.

You might also want to stand with your back against the wall and let your buttocks, your shoulder blades, and the back of your skull touch the wall.

To learn more, stand in Mountain Pose as shown above and touch your spine, up and down, as much as possible.

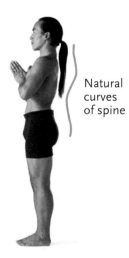

Natural
curves
of spine

DAY 1: LEARNING THE VARIATIONS

When trying all the variations of a standing pose, you will be tempted to go as deeply into the pose as possible. Instead, ask yourself, which variation is more integrated? In which variation do you have a sense of your entire being, with no single element becoming so prominent that it becomes your only focus? The standing poses should be challenging, yet while you do them, you should be able to breathe easily and work all your muscles evenly.

Keep in mind that the poses are intended to teach you more about your posture, your body, your mind, and your breath, and although you will become more skilled over time with the postures, the investigation and inquiry remain important.

MOVING IN AND OUT OF STANDING POSES

This week you will be moving in and out of the standing poses from Mountain Pose. Each time you move from Mountain Pose to another standing pose, notice the position of your feet and the distance between them. This foundation will set up the rest of the pose.

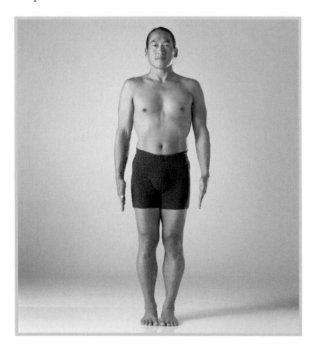

TRANSITION POSE. To move into the wide-stance standing poses, such as Triangle Pose and Warrior 1, begin in Mountain Pose, with your feet and legs together, or, if you prefer, with your feet hips-distance apart. Then, from

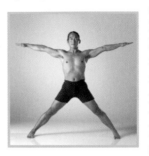

Mountain Pose, bend your legs and jump or walk your feet three and a half to four feet apart and parallel, with your arms extended out to the sides. From this wide-legged position, you will move into the wide-stance standing poses; you'll also return to this transition position when you change sides and when you come back to Mountain Pose.

ADJUSTING YOUR STANCE. At this point, you are ready to adjust your stance. Depending on the particular pose you will be moving into, there are two different foot positions and lengths of the stride between your feet.

SIDE-FACING POSES. For the wide-stance poses where your hips are not facing the front foot (such as Triangle Pose, Warrior 2, and Extended Side Angle), turn your back foot in 15 degrees and your front foot out 90 degrees. Because your hips will not be turned toward your front foot in the final pose, let your stride remain wide. You can calculate the correct distance to take between your feet by bending your front leg so that the angle between your thighbone and your shinbone measures 90 degrees. When your front leg is at 90 degrees, your stride is wide enough

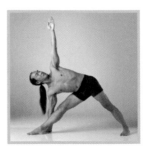

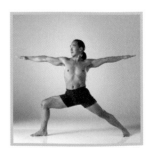

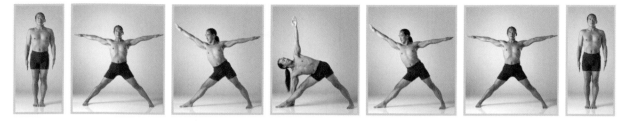

This series of photographs illustrates moving in and out of a side-facing pose, Triangle Pose.

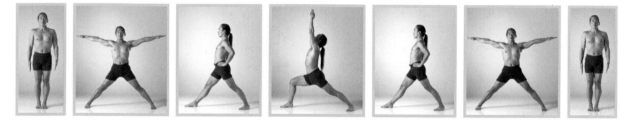

This series of photographs illustrates moving in and out of a front-facing pose, Warrior 1.

if your front shinbone is perpendicular to the floor and your thighbone is parallel to the floor, while your back leg remains straight.

FRONT-FACING POSES.
For the wide-stance standing poses where your hips are facing the front foot (such as Warrior 1 and Pyramid Pose), turn your back foot in 45 to 60 degrees and your front foot out 90 degrees. Because your hips will be turned toward

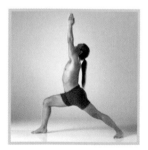 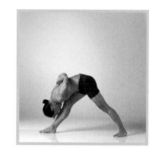

your front foot in the final pose, adjust your stance so your stride is slightly shorter than it is for the side-facing poses.

For any of the standing poses, if you are tired, have a difficult time balancing, or your joints don't feel like opening that much, take a shorter, more comfortable stride. It is important to feel grounded even as you challenge yourself in the standing poses.

To move out of a standing pose, return to the transition pose and then to Mountain Pose.

Note that the sequence in which the poses are introduced in today's practice is important because doing the poses in this order will awaken your body energetically and anatomically, in a gradual and graceful manner. As you move through the practice, try to feel and comprehend the sequencing. Pay special attention to how your pelvis is positioned from one pose to the next.

1. Try all three versions of **MOUNTAIN POSE** *(Tadasana)* for 30 seconds in each version.

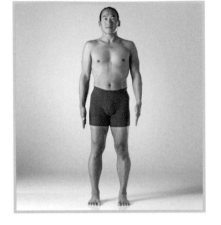

VERSION 1: Feet hips-distance apart

This version with your feet hips-distance apart provides stability; use it to channel the strength of your legs into the length of your torso and the support of your chest. The challenge is to find the full, even extension of the backs of your legs, arising from your evenly grounded heels.

VERSION 2: Feet together, big toes touching, heels slightly apart, thumbs in your armpits, lifting your chest and head

This version allows you to feel the insides of your legs more prominently. From your inner heels grounding, feel the re-bounding energy rising up through your inner legs into the base of your pelvis. As you join your legs together, your stability is de-creased; however, the amount of upward thrust into the length of your spine is increased. With your thumbs in your armpits, press your shoulder blades firmly into place down your back and against your rib cage, and circularly move the front of your armpit skin into the lift and broadness of your collarbones. Bring your aware-ness to your sitting bones and observe the relationship between the placement of your sitting bones and the strength of your legs.

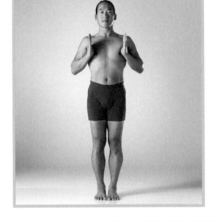

VERSION 3: Full pose, feet together

This version allows you to search for complete evenness in your standing posture. The challenge is to find both the stability from version 1 and the direction of movement from version 2. Search for the subtle balance between the right and left sides of your body with a complete ease of breath. Visualize the curves of your spine and feel how they respond to your breath and to the strength of your legs.

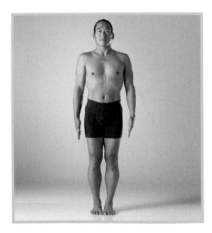

2. Try all three versions of **DOWNWARD-FACING DOG POSE** *(Adho Mukha Svanasana)* for 30 seconds in each version.

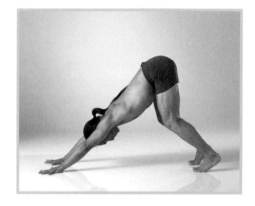

VERSION 1: Knees slightly bent

This version allows you to extend your spine fully, even with tight hamstrings. With bent legs, most of you can lift your sitting bones, bringing a natural curve to your lower back and length to your waist. Search for the full extension of your torso through your shoulders and your arms. Extend your heels downward as you lift your arches upward.

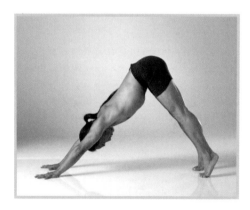

VERSION 2: Rising up onto your toes

Coming up on your toes allows you to feel a strong lift of your sitting bones and pelvis. It also activates your legs while still allowing you to extend your spine and shoulders. Try to feel the full extension of your knees and elbows, with a sharpness of your legs and arms. As you feel the tip of your tailbone curling forward, deepen your groins by allowing your groins to drop toward your sacrum and sitting bones.

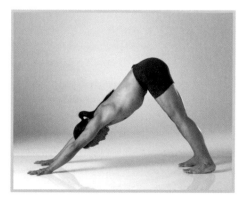

VERSION 3: Full pose, with knees straight and heels touching (or reaching toward) the ground

This version fully opens the backs of your legs. Work your legs strongly down through your heels and thighbones into your hamstrings. Similarly, find the full extension of the insides of your arms into the reach of your index fingers and thumbs. The challenge is to maintain a movement toward a natural sway back without taking the arch into your middle back.

3. Try all three versions of **STANDING FORWARD BEND** (*Uttanasana*) for 30 seconds in each version.

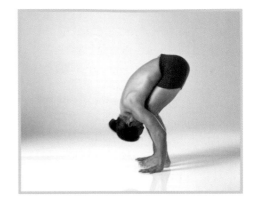

VERSION 1: Knees bent and spine rounded

This version subtracts the pull of your hamstrings, allowing your pelvis to spill forward over your thighs. From here you can allow your spine to release gradually as it is pulled by the weight of your neck and head. Focus on finding the movement of your pelvis over your thighs with space between your belly and the tops of your thighs. Press your right and left heels evenly.

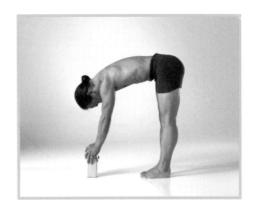

VERSION 2: Knees straight, hands on a block in front of you

This version allows you to open the backs of your legs and to feel the support of your leg bones aligned over your heels. The challenge is to get your pelvis to spill over deeply despite the restriction of the hamstrings. Placing your hands on a block allows you to take some weight off your torso and your lower back so you can release completely, without straining your lower back. Move the depth of your groins into the lift of your sitting bones as the tip of your tailbone curls between your sitting bones.

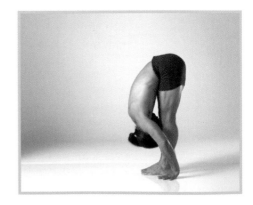

VERSION 3: Full pose, with hands touching the floor alongside your feet

This version is for those of you who can touch your hands on the ground easily when your legs are straight. You can find the full opening of your back body—from the soles of your feet to the back of your skull—by intentionally drawing your body toward your legs and down toward the floor. The challenge is to draw yourself deeply into the pose without feeling congested in your abdomen or throat. Round your spine evenly as you search for full extension.

4. Try all three versions of **TRIANGLE POSE** *(Trikonasana)*, on both right and left sides, for 15 seconds in each version. Stand in Mountain Pose for 10 seconds between versions.

VERSION 1: Bottom hand on the top of your shin, top hand on your hip, and head facing forward

This version helps you learn how to bring your body directly over your front leg while at the same time keeping both sides of your waist long. Use your top hand on your sacrum to help rotate and open your chest. Find the strength of your legs and the foundation they create moving into the length of your spine and openness of your chest. Press the inner and outer heels of your front foot evenly as you move through the outer back heel of your back foot.

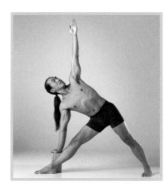

VERSION 2: Bottom hand on a block (at its appropriate height), top arm reaching up, and head turning to look toward your hand

This version allows you to press down with your bottom arm to support the lift of your chest. You learn how to reach your top arm directly above your bottom arm and your chest as you look up, turning your head toward your top hand. The challenge is to allow both your legs and your arms to open your chest fully. As you rotate your chest, deepen both groins.

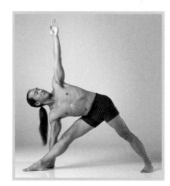

VERSION 3: Full pose, with no props

This version fully opens the hamstring of your front leg, challenging you to maintain the extension of your spine, the lift and broadness of your chest, and the grounding of your back leg. Your arms and legs should feed evenly into supporting and extending your spine. The challenge here is to keep both sides of your waist equal in length as you reestablish the natural curves of your spine.

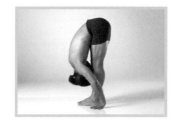

5. Practice **STANDING FORWARD BEND** for 20 seconds. Go only as far as you can feel your breath moving easily throughout the pose.

6. Try all three versions of **WARRIOR 2 POSE** *(Virabhadrasana 2),* on both right and left sides, for 15 seconds in each version. Stand in Mountain Pose for 10 seconds between versions.

VERSION 1: Hands on your hips and front knee bent less than 90 degrees

This version allows you to focus on your foundation, especially on the continual grounding of your back leg. Having your hands on your hips allows you to feel how your legs move into your lifted chest. Play with bending your front leg toward 90 degrees as you keep the strong grounding of your back leg. Ground the four corners of each foot and lift your arches from that grounding as evenly as you can.

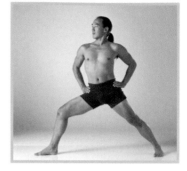

VERSION 2: Front leg bent to 90 degrees and thumbs in your armpits, lifting your chest and head

Your thumbs in your armpits helps you keep the lift of your front chest as well as the length of your waist above your back leg. Move your shoulder blades firmly into your back and broaden them away from your spine. Lengthen your spine from the release of your groins and the tuck of the tip of your tailbone.

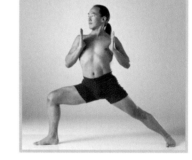

VERSION 3: Full pose, with front leg bent to 90 degrees and arms outstretched

This version supports your chest with fully outstretched arms. Keep a strong awareness in your back arm and back leg. As you anchor your torso from your back arm and back leg, open your hips and chest from that anchoring into your outstretched front arm and the bending of your front leg. From that foundation, lengthen the sides of your waist and let your breath create natural, balanced curves in your spine.

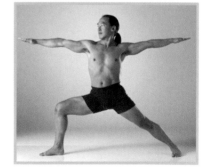

7. Practice **STANDING FORWARD BEND** for 20 seconds. Play with straightening and bending your legs to maximize the breath inside your hips.

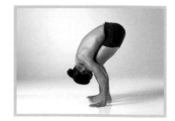

8. Try all three versions of **EXTENDED SIDE ANGLE POSE** *(Utthita Parsvakonasna)*, on both right and left sides, for 10 seconds in each version. Stand in Mountain Pose for 15 seconds between versions.

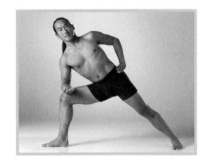

VERSION 1: Elbow of your bottom arm on your knee, upper hand on your sacrum, looking forward

This version allows you to guide your body over your front leg while at the same time keeping both sides of your waist long. It also helps you maintain the grounding of your back leg as you move your body toward your front leg. Place your front shin directly over your front heel and lift both the inner and outer arches of your feet.

VERSION 2: Bottom hand on block (at its appropriate height), top arm over your head, head turning to look toward your upper arm

This version allows you to push into the ground fully to lift your chest. However, coming farther down will make it more difficult to open the hip of your front leg as you keep a connection with your back leg. The reach of your top arm can help you extend both sides of your waist. The challenge is to keep your top arm, pelvis, and back leg lined up in a single plane. Move the sitting bone above your front leg deeper under the plane of your torso.

VERSION 3: Full pose, with bottom hand on the floor

This version challenges you to find the length of your bottom waist while you maintain full contact with your back foot. The tendency is to collapse onto your front arm and leg, so focus on shifting the thrust of your pelvis into your back leg as you move toward the natural curves of your spine. As you rotate your chest toward the ceiling, continue to search for the center of the pose and the release in your hips that will allow your spine to rise.

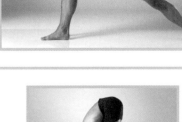

9. Practice **STANDING FORWARD BEND** for 20 seconds. Shift your pelvis forward and backward to maximize the grounding of the fronts of your heels.

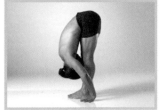

10. Try all three versions of **TREE POSE** *(Vrksasana)*, on both right and left sides, for 15 seconds in each version. Stand in Mountain Pose for 10 seconds between versions.

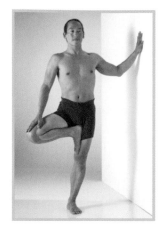

VERSION 1: Standing near a wall, with one hand on the wall and the other hand on your bent knee

This version allows you to discover the foundation of Tree Pose without worrying about balance. Draw your bent-leg foot as high as it will go toward the floor of your pelvis. Press your bent-leg foot into your straight-leg thigh, as you press your straight-leg thigh into your bent-leg foot. To square off your pelvis, press your bent-leg thigh and bent-leg knee toward the ground. Sometimes your bent-leg foot slips. If it does, simply keep it as high as possible (with practice it will get easier to keep it in place). Observe the shape of your feet, grounding both heels and articulating your arches.

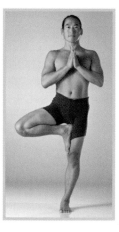

VERSION 2: Your hands in *namaste* (prayer position) in front of your chest

This version allows you to learn how to balance on one foot. The press of your hands together and the press of your bent-leg foot against your straight-leg thigh will give you a strong sense of center. The challenge is to balance fluidly as you soften your breath and your eyes. Equalize the distance between both sitting bones and the floor.

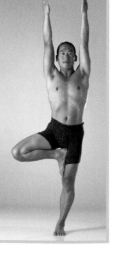

VERSION 3: Full pose, with arms above your head

This version allows you to learn how to maintain the alignment of your pelvis and chest as your arms extend fully overhead. The challenge is to keep your neck soft and your elbows straight while slowly bringing your hands closer together. As you reach your arms over your head, you will tend to increase the backbend in your lower back. To keep this from happening, focus on lengthening the back and sides of your waist.

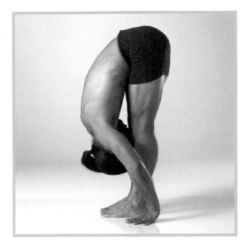

11. Practice **STANDING FORWARD BEND** for 20 seconds. Breathe into your pelvis and your lower back to release tension slowly and elongate your waist.

12. Try all three versions of **WARRIOR 1 POSE** *(Virabhadrasana 1)*, on both right and left sides, for 15 seconds in each version. Stand in Mountain Pose for 10 seconds between versions.

VERSION 1: Hands on your hips, back heel lifted off the ground

This version allows you to move your pelvis without the restriction of the grounding of your back heel, letting you extend your lower back completely from a very strong back leg. The balance will be more difficult without the grounding of your back heel, but there will be more freedom in your lower back. You can learn how to balance from the articulation of your front foot. Press evenly through the inner and outer heel of your front foot.

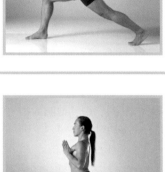

VERSION 2: Back heel grounded and thumbs in your armpits, lifting your chest, keeping your head forward

This version teaches you to lift your chest while you bring down your back heel. To elongate your back even more, lift and turn your chest in one direction and ground and rotate your back leg in the opposite direction. Use your thumbs in your armpits to engage your shoulder blades and extend the sides of your chest. Maintain the depth of your groins as you tuck your tailbone to help lift your front spine.

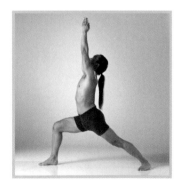

VERSION 3: Full pose, with arms reaching and head looking up

The reach of your arms over your head furthers the extension of your spine and can help lift your chest as well, but also demands much more effort within the pose. The challenge is to create some ease within the pose. Lift your chest fully but soften your neck and eyes. The backbending of your spine will be exaggerated, so keep as much length as possible in the back of your spine.

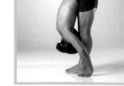

13. Practice **STANDING FORWARD BEND** for 20 seconds. Move your rib cage around to facilitate the ease of your spine.

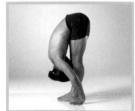

14. Try all three versions of **HALF MOON POSE** *(Arda Chandrasana)*, on both right and left sides, for 15 seconds in each version. Stand in Mountain Pose for 10 seconds between versions.

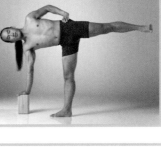

VERSION 1: Back of your body against a wall, looking forward

This version removes the difficulty of balance from the pose so you can focus on alignment. Position your supporting foot at 90 degrees and rotate your supporting leg so that your knee is pointing in the same direction as your foot. Reach through both heels.

VERSION 2: In the middle of the room, bottom hand on a block, looking forward

This version allows you to test your balance in the middle of the room while maintaining the alignment you found in version 1. The challenge is to orient yourself in the center of the room by being acutely aware of your body's internal, physical feedback. You will tend to let your sitting bones and tailbone move into a backbend (sticking your butt out). So, with the rotation of your bottom leg, bring your sitting bones and tailbone back in line with the plane of your torso.

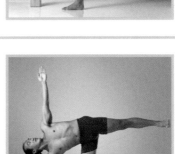

VERSION 3: Full pose, with bottom hand on the floor, looking upward

Balance is more difficult when you look upward. By placing your bottom hand on the floor you challenge your ability to keep your spine extended and your chest spiraling upward. Rely on the contact of your supporting-leg foot and your hand to adjust your balance. The natural curves of your spine will be challenged by your fear of falling and the possible lack of flexibility in your supporting-leg hamstring. Try to find the razor's edge of balance that brings your body into one plane.

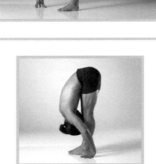

15. Practice **STANDING FORWARD BEND** for 20 seconds. Move your shoulders around and feel your shoulder blades move toward your pelvis, eventually releasing your neck.

16. Try all three versions of **PYRAMID POSE** *(Parsvottanasana)* on each side for 15 seconds in each version.

VERSION 1: Hands on blocks

This version allows you to keep the extension of your spine while you square off your hips and establish a good foundation in your legs. The challenge is to keep your back heel down while you turn your hips toward your front foot and keep your front foot evenly on the ground. Hold your torso as high as needed to alleviate the pull of your front leg's hamstring.

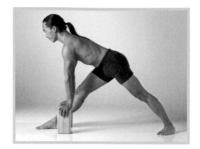

VERSION 2: Hands (or fingertips) on the floor

This version allows you to learn to release into a forward bend while maintaining the anchoring of both legs. The challenge is to keep the extension of your front body even though your spine is rounding. Move slowly into the pose, respecting your limitations. Deepen both groins equally.

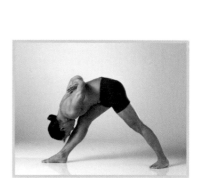

VERSION 3: Full pose, hands in *namaste* behind your back

This version allows you to open your front leg fully while you continue to maintain the full grounding of your back leg, with the added opening of your shoulders. The position of your arms complicates the pose due to the fear created when you do not have your hands available to catch or adjust you. The challenge is one of balance, as many forces are trying to pull you out of center. Continue to make small adjustments by shifting your weight more toward center. In this pose, your spine has a very gentle roundness that extends from your tailbone to the crown of your head.

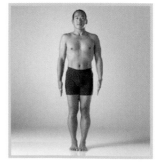

17. Practice **MOUNTAIN POSE** for 15 seconds. Feel the alignment of your back body and how it supports your front body.

18. Try all three versions of **Legs Up the Wall Pose** *(Viparita Karani)* for 1 to 2 minutes in each version.

VERSION 1: Back flat on the ground, buttocks against the wall, legs in crossed-legs position

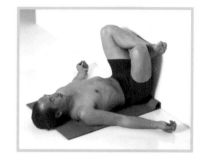

This version allows you to move closer to the wall (or against the wall), without the restrictions of your hamstrings. The challenge is to get as comfortable on the floor as possible, with as much of your back in contact with the ground, spreading from your spine. Keep your feet slightly active, allowing your legs to fold deeply with the pull of gravity.

VERSION 2: Back flat on the ground and legs straight up the wall

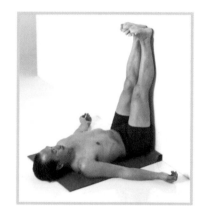

Because your back is fully supported, this version allows you to receive the full effect of an inverted pose and the deep rest of a relaxation pose. The challenge here is to find the right distance from the wall so your sacrum is flat on the ground while your legs are straight. Experiment with different distances until your lower back feels no pull or strain. Release and deepen both your groins.

VERSION 3: A bolster or folded blanket (rectangle) supporting from your upper pelvis to the bottom tips of your shoulder blades (shoulders themselves touching the floor while chest is on the prop)

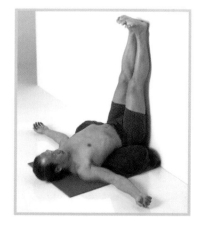

This version opens your heart and lungs and quiets the nervous system due to the position of your neck. An ease comes from deep relaxation in this posture because your upper chest is completely open while your belly is completely soft. The difficulty here is in positioning the bolster so that your chest is open but your sacrum and legs are grounded. Play with the distance of your pelvis from the wall and the position of the bolster. Feeling the support of the bolster, relax the curves of your spine.

19. Try all three versions of **RELAXATION POSE** *(Savasana)* for 2 minutes in each version.

VERSION 1: Support under your head

If your head spills backward when you lie flat on the ground, you cannot find complete relaxation. So until your upper back and neck become more supple, place a thin pillow or folded blanket under your head to keep the back and front of your neck equally extended. Having your head slightly lifted lets your body turn inward, which allows your neck to feel less vulnerable and more at ease. Finding the right amount of lift is crucial to the ease of your entire body. Relax your sense organs, the backs of your eyes, the bridge of your nose, your inner ears, the root of your tongue, and the receptivity of your skin. Soften the soles of your feet.

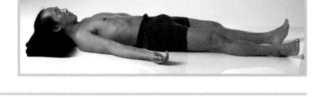

VERSION 2: A blanket roll under midthighs

Often your lower back has some tightness or a varying degree of discomfort. When you use a support under your thighs—which allows your back to be supported and touch the ground—your back muscles feel like they can relinquish their constant job of supporting your lower spine. In this position it is important to keep letting the weight of your legs fall onto the bolster. Soften the muscles around your groins.

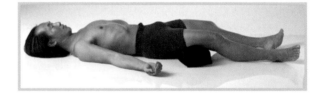

VERSION 3: Full pose, without props

There is nothing like having your body rest in its natural configuration in full contact with the ground. Allow your spine to take its natural curves and continue to let go of the muscles of your entire back body by scanning up and down your back body, noticing where you have any tendency to grip. Keep the direction of your body dropping into the lap of the earth as you keep your mind awake but broad.

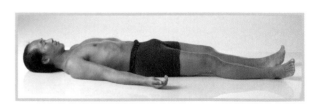

20. For 5 to 10 minutes, practice version 3 of **RELAXATION POSE** and focus on breathing with relaxation in your face.

21. Try all three versions of **HERO POSE** *(Virasana)* for 15 seconds in each version.

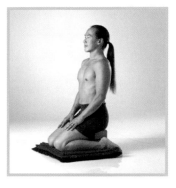

VERSION 1: On a block on top of a folded blanket, with feet hanging off the back of the folded blanket

Using the prop in this way should remove all resistance from your legs and feet, allowing you to sit with the natural curves of your spine. It is important to learn to do this pose with complete ease so that you will take it frequently. Play with the balance of your spine sitting erect with ease and with its natural curves. Soften the fronts of your feet as you draw up through your arches.

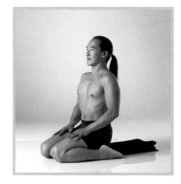

VERSION 2: On the edge of a blanket that has been folded into a long, thin rectangle

This version encourages the fronts of your shins and feet to open completely while giving some compensation for tightness in your hips and quadriceps. The height of your pelvis should be sufficient to allow the natural curves of the spine and ease in your knees, although there is more stretching in the fronts of your shins and the tops of your feet. Feel the activity of your feet creating energetic movement through your legs and into your spine. Sit upright on your sitting bones as directly as possible.

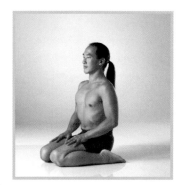

VERSION 3: Full pose, without props

The complete folding of your legs challenges you to soften the muscles of your calves, quadriceps, and the backs of your knees while you maintain the natural curve of your lower back. Practice this version with care and initially for short periods of time. Feel the grounding of your thighs as you keep your pelvis vertical. On your inhalation allow your legs to fold as completely as possible. On your exhalation, elongate and suspend your spine.

22. For 5 minutes, sit in **HERO POSE,** on a prop high enough to keep you comfortable. Meditate on the lift of your chest and the relaxation of your neck and face.

DAY 2: LEARNING MOUNTAIN POSE AND TRIANGLE POSE

This practice teaches you the relationship between Mountain Pose, Triangle Pose, and the other standing poses.

Energetically, Mountain Pose is the axis for all other yoga poses. And all the other poses inform you how to align yourself in Mountain Pose. Looking deeply at your posture and its relationship to your breath and mind is subtle yet profound in Mountain Pose. Your breath and mind illuminate every part of the pose equally. Triangle Pose is one of the most complex yoga poses because you must orchestrate the movement of different parts of your body in several different directions, yet it is also one of the most comfortable and accessible poses.

FOCUS FOR THIS PRACTICE:

- In Mountain Pose, feel the natural curves and elongation of your spine rising from your rooting heels. In the other standing poses, search for similar curves and freedom in your spine as you press your heels down firmly and evenly.

- In Downward-Facing Dog, observe your sitting bones, tailbone, and pubis. Lift your sitting bones as your pubis and tailbone move toward each other.

- In Standing Forward Bend, observe your heels grounding evenly.

   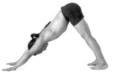

1. Practice version 1 of **Downward-Facing Dog** for 1 minute.

2. Practice any version of **Standing Forward Bend** for 1 minute.

3. Practice version 2 of **Downward-Facing Dog** for 15 seconds.

4. Practice any version of **Standing Forward Bend** for 1 minute.

5. Practice version 3 of **Downward-Facing Dog** for 1 minute.

 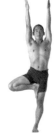

6. Practice any version of **Standing Forward Bend** for 1 minute.

7. Practice **Mountain Pose** for 30 seconds.

8. Practice **Triangle Pose** for 30 seconds on each side.

9. Practice **Mountain Pose** for 15 seconds.

10. Practice **Tree Pose** for 30 seconds on each side.

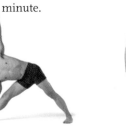 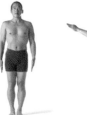 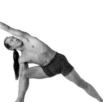 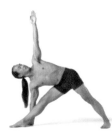 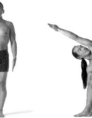 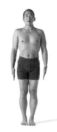

11. Practice **Triangle Pose** for 30 seconds on each side.

12. Practice **Mountain Pose** for 15 seconds.

13. Practice **Extended Side Angle Pose** for 15 seconds on each side.

14. Practice **Triangle Pose** for 30 seconds on each side.

15. Practice **Mountain Pose** for 5 breaths.

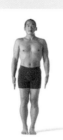
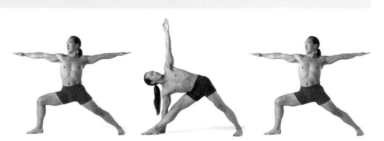

16. Practice **Standing Forward Bend** for 30 seconds.

17. Practice **Mountain Pose** for 5 breaths.

18. Practice the following series of standing poses on the right side and then repeat on the left side: **Warrior 2** for 10 seconds, **Triangle** for 10 seconds, **Warrior 2** for 5 seconds.

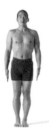
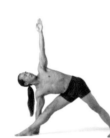
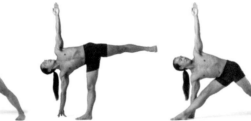
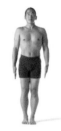

19. Practice **Mountain Pose** for 5 breaths.

20. Practice the following series of standing poses on the right: **Triangle Pose** for 5 seconds, **Half Moon Pose** for 5 seconds, **Triangle Pose** for 5 seconds.

21. Practice **Mountain Pose** for 5 breaths.

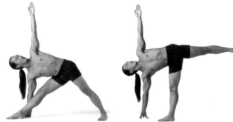
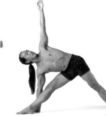
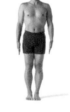
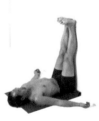

22. Repeat the **Triangle** to **Half Moon Pose** series on the left: **Triangle Pose** for 5 seconds, **Half Moon Pose** for 5 seconds, **Triangle Pose** for 5 seconds.

23. Practice **Mountain Pose** for 1 minute.

24. Practice version 2 of **Legs Up the Wall Pose** for 2 minutes.

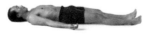

25. Relaxation and Breath Awareness. For 3 minutes, practice **Relaxation Pose** and observe your breath, relaxing the backs of your eyes during your inhalations.

26. Meditation. For 5 minutes, sit in **Hero Pose** and meditate on the relaxation of your thighs toward the ground.

DAY 3: LEARNING WARRIOR 2 POSE AND EXTENDED SIDE ANGLE POSE

Although Warrior 2 and Extended Side Angle Pose differ greatly in the position of the pelvis, the foundations of the legs are the same: back leg fully extended and front leg at 90 degrees. Both postures gather the strength of your legs into your spine and then into the reach of your arms. Many of you will find Warrior 2 one of the most accessible standing poses because your torso is vertical with your legs directly underneath. Extended Side Angle Pose is like mixing Mountain Pose with Warrior 2. This is a wonderful pose for learning how your back leg extends into your spine while opening the hip of your front leg. It is easy to feel how both your arms and your legs affect the length and support of your spine. Whenever I need to center myself and energize myself, I include these two poses in my yoga practice.

This sequence helps you warm up and understand the direction of movement and opening for Warrior 2 and Extended Side Angle Pose. Because your front leg bends to 90 degrees, these poses build considerable strength in your legs and encourage flexibility in the hip joint.

FOCUS FOR THIS PRACTICE:

- In the standing poses, press the outer heel of your back leg into the ground.

- In Mountain Pose, feel your pubis moving toward your tailbone as your inner heels make good contact with the floor.

- In Standing Forward Bend, lift your sitting bones as you tuck your tailbone toward your pubis.

- In Warrior 2, find the natural curves of your spine.

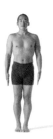
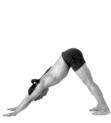
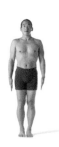
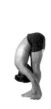

1. Practice **Mountain Pose** for 30 seconds.

2. Practice **Downward-Facing Dog** for 30 seconds.

3. Practice **Mountain Pose** for 10 seconds.

4. Practice **Standing Forward Bend** for 30 seconds.

5. Practice version 3 of **Tree Pose** for 10 seconds on each side.

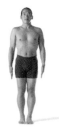
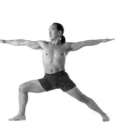
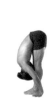
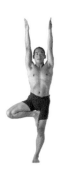

6. Practice **Mountain Pose** for 10 seconds.

7. Practice **Warrior 2** for 30 seconds on each side.

8. Practice **Standing Forward Bend** for 30 seconds.

9. Practice **Tree Pose** for 10 seconds on each side.

10. Practice **Standing Forward Bend** for 30 seconds.

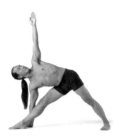

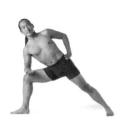

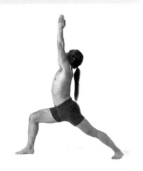

11. Practice **Triangle Pose** for 15 to 30 seconds on each side.

12. Practice version 1 of **Extended Side Angle Pose** for 15 to 30 seconds on each side.

13. Practice **Standing Forward Bend** for 30 seconds.

14. Practice **Warrior 1 Pose** for 15 to 30 seconds on each side.

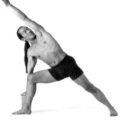

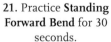

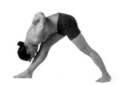

15. Practice **Standing Forward Bend** for 30 seconds.

16. Practice version 2 of **Extended Side Angle Pose** for 15 to 30 seconds on each side.

17. Practice **Standing Forward Bend** for 30 seconds.

18. Practice version 3 of **Warrior 2** for 15 to 30 seconds on each side.

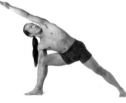

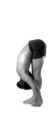

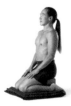

19. Practice **Standing Forward Bend** for 30 seconds.

20. Practice version 3 of **Extended Side Angle Pose** for 15 seconds on each side.

21. Practice **Standing Forward Bend** for 30 seconds.

22. Practice **Pyramid Pose** for 30 to 45 seconds on each side.

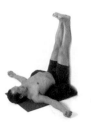

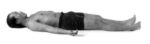

23. Practice **Legs Up the Wall** for 3 minutes.

24. Relaxation and Breath Awareness. For 3 minutes, practice **Relaxation Pose.** Observe the natural pause at the end of your exhalation.

25. Meditation. For 5 minutes, sit in **Hero Pose,** meditating on the release of the front of your shins and the top of your feet.

DAY 4: LEARNING WARRIOR 1 POSE AND TREE POSE

Because of your arm position in these poses, both Warrior 1 and Tree Pose require a lot of effort but they are also exhilarating. It is crucial to learn how to open your upper chest and your arms with increasing relaxation in your neck and sense organs. Both these poses are also difficult balance poses in which you must be relaxed about the fear of falling. Since Warrior 1 has a strong element of backbend, it is important to transpose the length of your spine rising from your legs, which you find in Tree Pose and other standing poses, into it.

The repetition of Tree Pose and Warrior 1 in the following sequence lets your body make its own subtle adjustments to bring understanding and ease in the poses. Standing in Tree Pose many times will help you balance on one leg more successfully each time. Learning how to be in these poses with ease teaches you to be strong in the world through relaxation.

FOCUS FOR THIS PRACTICE:

■ In Tree Pose, find the fronts of both heels, and try to balance on the front of the heel of your standing leg.

■ In Warrior 1, firm your back leg from your back heel, and tuck your tailbone toward your pubis.

■ In Warrior 1, search for the natural curves of your spine that you found in Mountain Pose and Tree Pose.

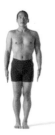

1. Practice **Mountain Pose** for 15 seconds.

2. Practice **Standing Forward Bend** for 30 seconds.

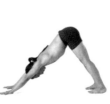

3. Practice **Downward-Facing Dog** for 1 minute.

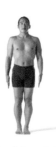

4. Practice **Mountain Pose** for 15 seconds.

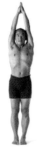

5. Practice **Volcano Pose** (see page 81) for 30 seconds.

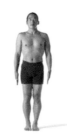

6. Practice **Mountain Pose** for 1 breath.

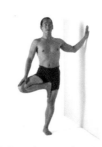

7. Practice version 1 of **Tree Pose** for 30 seconds on each side.

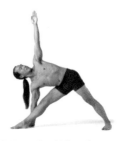

8. Practice **Triangle Pose** for 30 seconds on each side.

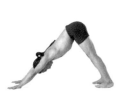

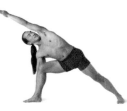

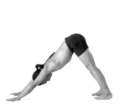

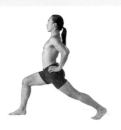

9. Practice **Downward-Facing Dog** for 30 seconds.

10. Practice **Extended Side Angle Pose** for 15 seconds on each side.

11. Practice **Downward-Facing Dog** for 30 seconds.

12. Practice version 1 of **Warrior 1 Pose** for 15 seconds on each side.

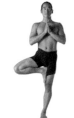

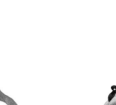

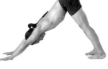

13. Practice **Standing Forward Bend** for 15 seconds.

14. Practice version 2 of **Tree Pose** for 30 seconds on each side.

15. Practice version 2 of **Warrior 1 Pose** for 30 seconds on each side.

16. Practice **Downward-Facing Dog** for 15 seconds.

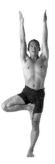

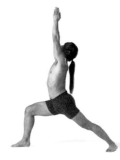

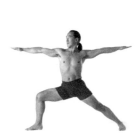

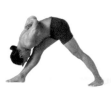

17. Practice version 3 of **Tree Pose** for 30 seconds on each side.

18. Practice version 3 of **Warrior 1 Pose** for 30 seconds on each side.

19. Practice **Warrior 2 Pose** for 30 seconds on each side.

20. Practice **Pyramid Pose** for 30 seconds to 1 minute on each side.

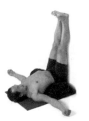

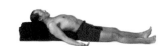

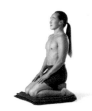

21. Practice **Legs Up the Wall Pose** for 3 minutes.

22. Relaxation and Breath Awareness. For 3 minutes, practice version 3 of **Supported Relaxation Pose** (see page 268) with

your hands on your lower rib cage. Allow your breath to move easily into your side lower ribs.

23. Meditation. For 5 minutes, sit in **Hero Pose** and meditate on the natural curve of your lower back and the length of your waist.

DAY 5: LEARNING HALF MOON POSE AND PYRAMID POSE

Both Half Moon Pose and Pyramid Pose are challenging balance poses, but when you find your ease, they become very quiet, like a half moon in the night. Half Moon Pose is the standing pose that is most like flying. When you align yourself on the skeleton of your bottom leg, there is almost no muscular work and you feel like you are floating. Pyramid Pose—when you get past the tightness in your hamstring and navigate the balance of the pose—is also very internal and nocturnal, feeling like a good night's rest under a down comforter. Both poses require some flexibility in the back of your front leg.

Today's sequence begins with Downward-Facing Dog, Standing Forward Bend, and Triangle Pose before Half Moon Pose and Pyramid Pose to open up the backs of your legs. The transition from Triangle Pose to Half Moon Pose takes some practice. This sequence provides many opportunities to play with the transition as well as the poses themselves. The entire practice works on your foundation—your feet and legs—to bring you a sense of your connection to the earth. Your connection to the earth will allow you to articulate your balance.

FOCUS FOR THIS PRACTICE:

- In Half Moon Pose, build your pose from the placement, orientation, and grounding of your supporting foot.

- In Pyramid Pose, guide your balance with your front foot as you ground and orient yourself from your back foot.

- Even as the natural curves of your spine change from one standing pose to the next, continue to search for an open channel between your tailbone and the crown of your head.

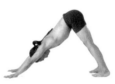 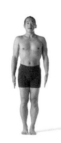 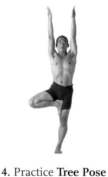 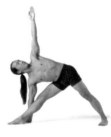

1. Practice **Downward-Facing Dog** for 1 minute.

2. Practice **Standing Forward Bend** for 1 minute.

3. Practice **Mountain Pose** for 30 seconds.

4. Practice **Tree Pose** for 30 seconds on each side.

5. Practice **Triangle Pose** for 30 seconds on each side.

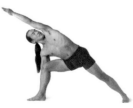 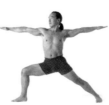 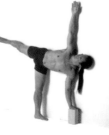 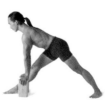

6. Practice **Extended Side Angle Pose** for 30 seconds on each side.

7. Practice **Standing Forward Bend** for 30 seconds.

8. Practice **Warrior 2 Pose** for 30 seconds on each side.

9. Practice version 1 of **Half Moon Pose** for 30 seconds on each side.

10. Practice version 1 of **Pyramid Pose** for 30 seconds on each side.

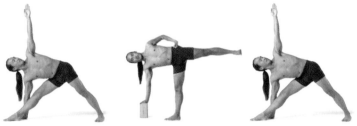 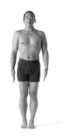

11. Practice **Standing Forward Bend** for 30 seconds.

12. Practice moving from **Triangle** to version 2 of **Half Moon Pose** in the center of the room as follows: **Triangle Pose** for 15 seconds, **Half Moon Pose** for 15 seconds, **Triangle Pose** for 15 seconds.

13. Practice **Mountain Pose** for 30 seconds.

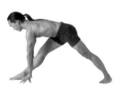 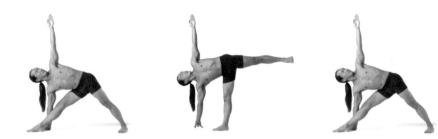

14. Practice version 2 of **Pyramid Pose** for 30 seconds on each side.

15. Repeat the **Triangle** to **Half Moon Pose** series, this time practicing version 3 of Half Moon Pose: Triangle Pose for 15 seconds, Half Moon Pose for 15 seconds, Triangle Pose for 15 seconds.

 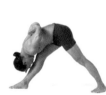 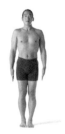 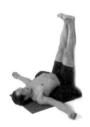

16. Practice **Standing Forward Bend** for 30 seconds.

17. Practice version 3 of **Pyramid Pose** for 30 seconds on each side.

18. Practice **Mountain Pose** for 1 minute.

19. Practice **Legs Up the Wall Pose** for 3 minutes.

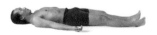

20. Relaxation and Breath Awareness. For 3 minutes, practice **Relaxation Pose**, with normal breathing, focusing on the relaxation of your legs.

21. Meditation. For 5 minutes, sit in **Hero Pose** against the wall, meditating on the fold of your legs and their release toward the ground, with a slight activity in your feet.

DAY 6: BREATH AWARENESS AND MEDITATION

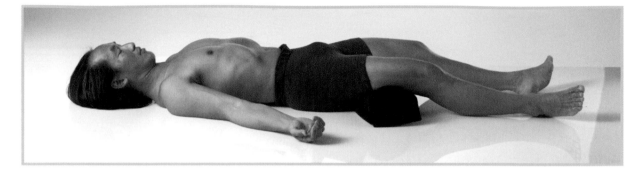

Breath Awareness

Practice version 2 of Relaxation Pose with your hands on your belly for 10 minutes. Feel your natural breath.

RELAXATION POSE. Resting your lower thighs on a rolled-up blanket slightly flattens your lower back, giving your entire spine more support from the ground. Hopefully you can relax deeply in this position. If you cannot relax in this pose—if it makes you feel anxious—practice version 3 of Supported Relaxation Pose as shown on page 268. Always do all breath awareness exercises in the version of Relaxation Pose that is most comfortable for you.

FOCUSING ON YOUR BELLY. As you lie in Relaxation Pose, scan your body to find a deeper sense of relaxation and observe how that feeling of relaxation relates to the shift in your breath. Placing your hands on your belly helps you focus more on the simple rise and fall of your belly as it synchronizes with the rise and fall of your breath. It is also easier to feel your exhalation fading into emptiness when your belly recedes back into your spine. And your inhalation may become smoother because you are watching how your torso easily fills with breath. The more you are able to relax your entire body, the more you will feel the simple rise and fall of your breath throughout your body, as supple as the motions of your relaxed belly.

If you find it difficult to lie in Relaxation Pose and feel your natural breath, persist unless you get anxious. If you get anxious, roll over onto your right side and rest in any comfortable position. It is also common to try to manipulate your breath as you watch it. If this happens, note that you are doing so and reduce the manipulation as best you can.

YOUR NATURAL BREATH. When you first begin to observe your breath, you will observe your habitual breath. As you feel the inhibitions or restrictions that define your habitual breath, ask yourself, How can I free myself from these restrictions?

Giving your mind to your natural breath is like lying on the earth and watching the clouds move through the sky. At first you might think, Oh, this is not really interesting or necessary. But consider how you feel during and after such a time, how refreshed, balanced, and content, after only 5 to 10 minutes of gazing upward at the sky. After more than 20 years of practicing breath awareness and *pranayama,* I come back often to this simple exercise of lying on my back and watching my breath. And I feel that after all this time I am still learning how to take a natural breath. You might wonder, well, why start this at all, if after 20 years someone who has been dedicated to the practice still doesn't feel like he can take a natural breath? My reply is that every time I do this practice, I feel a great sense of relief as I sense my body move into its natural balance and natural state of contentment.

Meditation

For 5 to 10 minutes, sit in Hero Pose. Sit on a prop high enough to keep you comfortable and at ease for 5 minutes, and place a blanket under your shins if desired. Note the gradual deepening of the folding of your legs as you feel the length of your waist and the lift of your chest.

STAYING STILL. Realize that sitting for 5 minutes in any posture with the intention of staying still is going to be difficult, and that any little tweak or sensation in your body is going to seem exaggerated. In general we are used to keeping ourselves busy, and this creates a certain amount of distraction. When you end this distraction as you sit down to meditate, especially in Hero Pose (a position most of you haven't sat in since you were a child), you will probably experience both mental and physical discomfort. You might think that this doesn't sound like it is going to be any fun at all. And you might ask yourself: Why should I put up with this? But I can assure you that after your first 5-minute meditation—whether you have been completely agitated, blissful, or something in between—a magical space will start to open up.

FOCUSING ON POSTURE. In this meditation, I'm asking you to observe the gradual deepening of the folding of your legs while you feel the length of your waist and the lift of your chest. In this practice, you are using a simple but profound meditation technique in which you take a specific aspect of your body

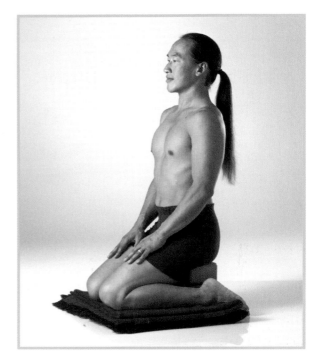

posture and keep bringing your mind back to it. The moment your mind wanders, your body begins to collapse or drop into its habitual unconscious posture. By bringing your mind back to the length of your waist and the lift of your chest from the grounding of your legs, you learn how to focus on your posture in the present moment. This will carry over throughout your day. Your mind will tend to gather back into your body and continue to notice the way you're holding your chest and the way you lengthen your waist from the strength of your legs.

MOUNTAIN POSE

Mountain Pose allows you to feel the subtle balance
and evenness of your entire body.

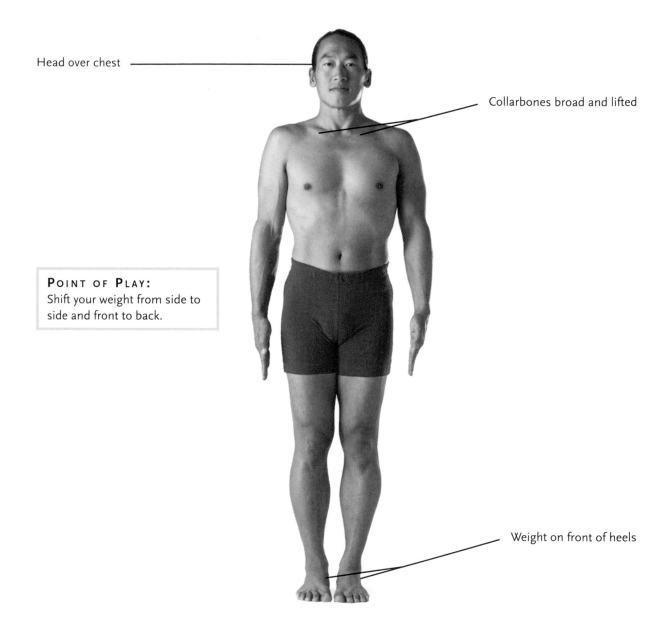

Head over chest

Collarbones broad and lifted

POINT OF PLAY:
Shift your weight from side to
side and front to back.

Weight on front of heels

DOWNWARD-FACING DOG POSE

Downward-Facing Dog Pose elongates your spine
from the dynamic work and opening of your legs and arms.

POINT OF PLAY:
Bend and straighten your legs.
Lift your heels up and lower
them down. Drop your lower
ribs, and center them.

Waist long

Lower ribs centralized

Shoulder blades moving
toward pelvis

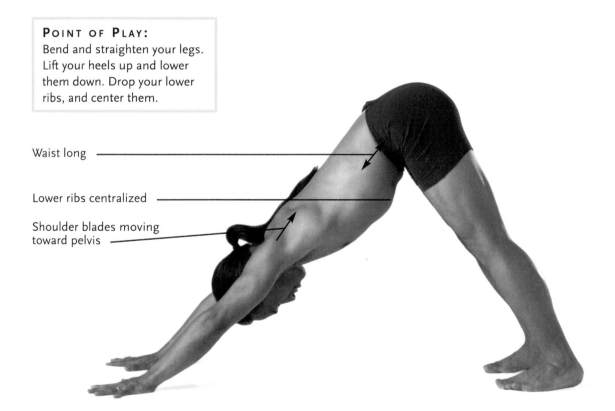

STANDING FORWARD BEND

Standing Forward Bend restores your body in an easy inverted position
while releasing the tension from your back body.

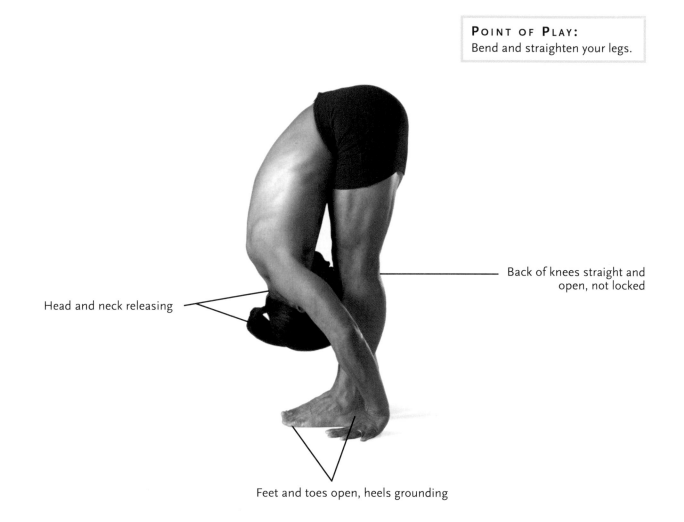

Back of knees straight and
open, not locked

Head and neck releasing

Feet and toes open, heels grounding

TRIANGLE POSE

Triangle Pose is one of the archetypal standing poses in which you will encounter balance, strength, openness, and ease.

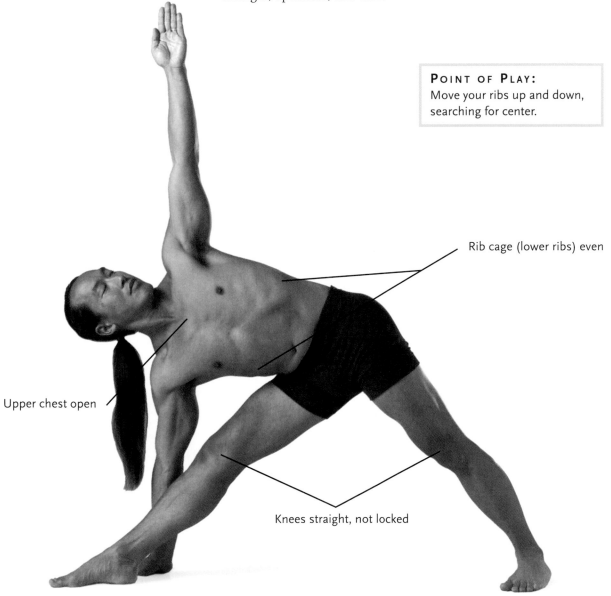

Rib cage (lower ribs) even

Upper chest open

Knees straight, not locked

WARRIOR 2 POSE

Warrior 2 Pose allows you to sense—emotionally and physically—the vibrancy and strength emanating from the posture.

POINT OF PLAY:
Move your upper torso from side to side, searching for center.

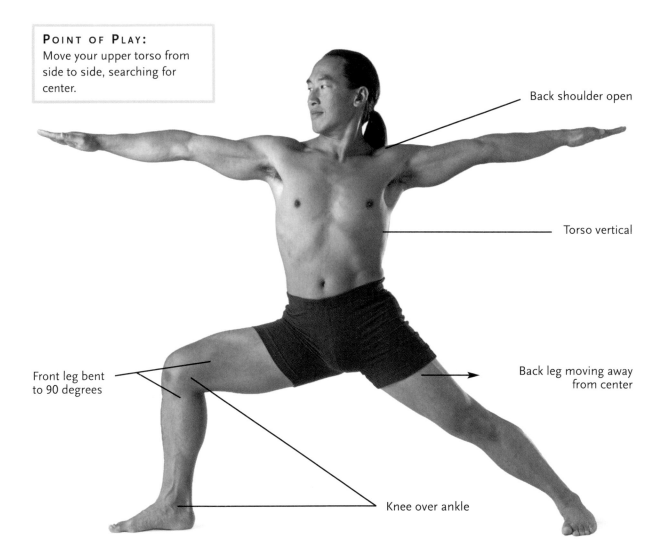

Back shoulder open

Torso vertical

Front leg bent to 90 degrees

Back leg moving away from center

Knee over ankle

EXTENDED SIDE ANGLE POSE

Extended Side Angle Pose is a complex pose that requires extensive hip opening, leg strength, integration of your arms, and deep mental focus to achieve the elongation of your side body.

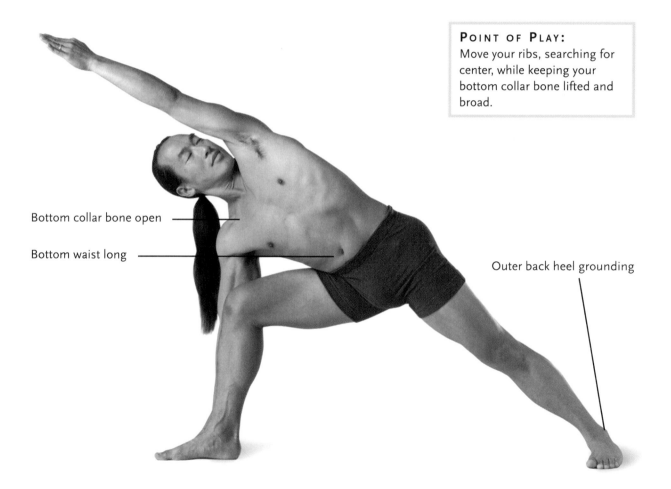

POINT OF PLAY:
Move your ribs, searching for center, while keeping your bottom collar bone lifted and broad.

Bottom collar bone open

Bottom waist long

Outer back heel grounding

TREE POSE

Tree Pose is a simple balance pose in which you can investigate the relationship among determination, ease of breath, and your emotional responses to balancing and falling.

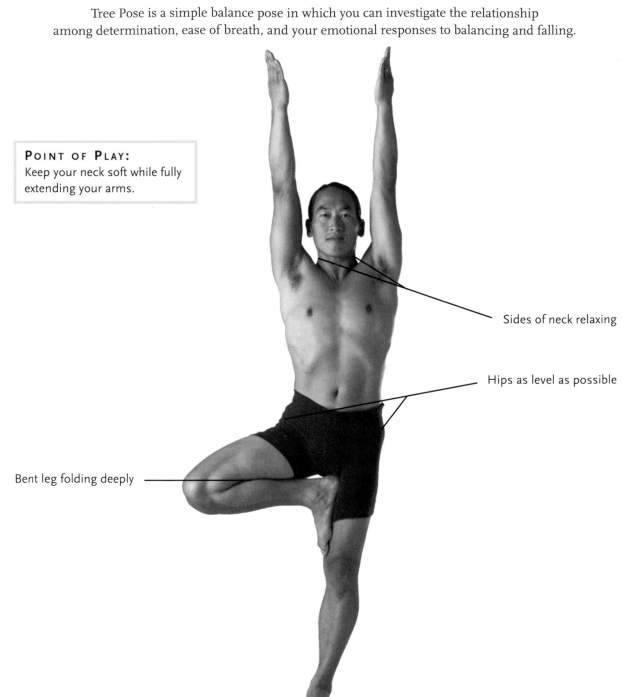

POINT OF PLAY:
Keep your neck soft while fully extending your arms.

Sides of neck relaxing

Hips as level as possible

Bent leg folding deeply

WARRIOR 1 POSE

Warrior 1 Pose is one of the most vigorous standing poses, which requires refined alignment and effort to enliven your entire spine with the integration of your arms and legs.

POINT OF PLAY:
Keep your back lower ribs broad and lifted.

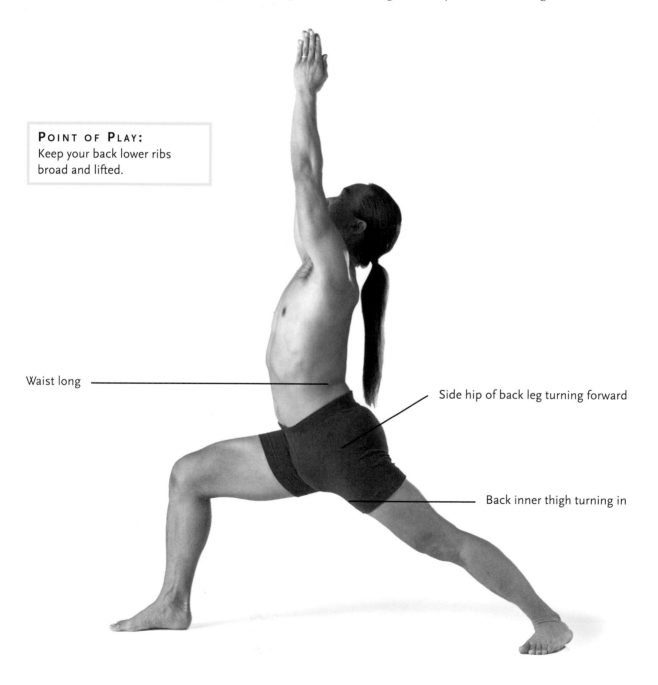

Waist long

Side hip of back leg turning forward

Back inner thigh turning in

HALF MOON POSE

Half Moon Pose addresses your fear of falling and asks that you balance
while opening into vulnerability and alignment.

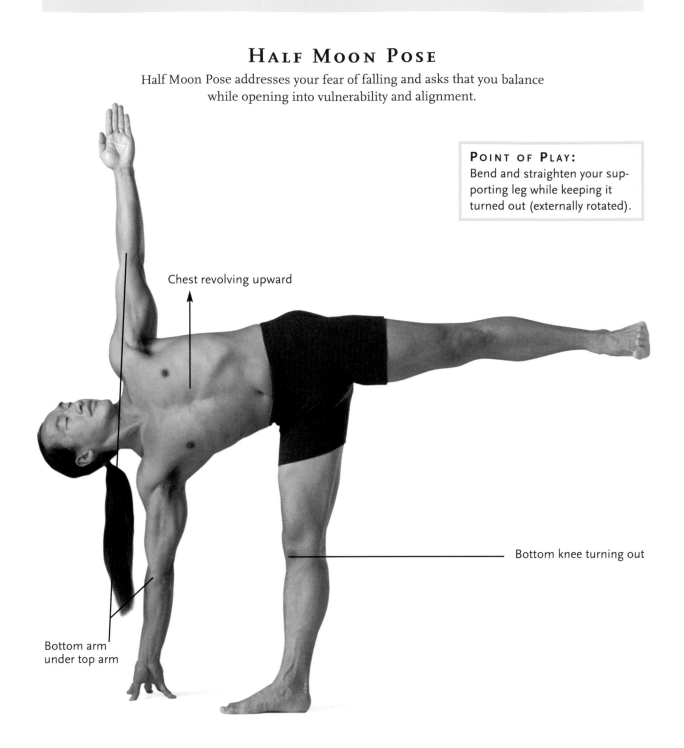

POINT OF PLAY:
Bend and straighten your supporting leg while keeping it turned out (externally rotated).

Chest revolving upward

Bottom knee turning out

Bottom arm
under top arm

PYRAMID POSE

Pyramid Pose demonstrates the cooling effect of forward bends,
even in the midst of a challenging balance.

POINT OF PLAY:
Lift your torso and extend your
front body, then release into a
rounded spine.

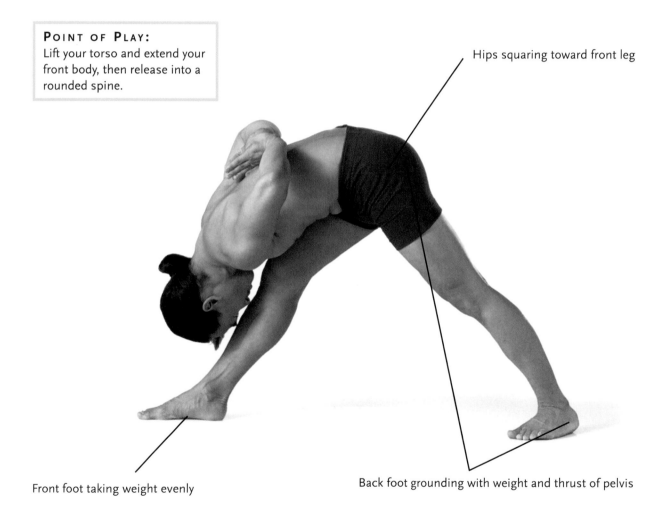

Hips squaring toward front leg

Front foot taking weight evenly

Back foot grounding with weight and thrust of pelvis

LEGS UP THE WALL POSE

Legs Up the Wall Pose rejuvenates your body as it evens out your breath
and softens the determination of your mind.

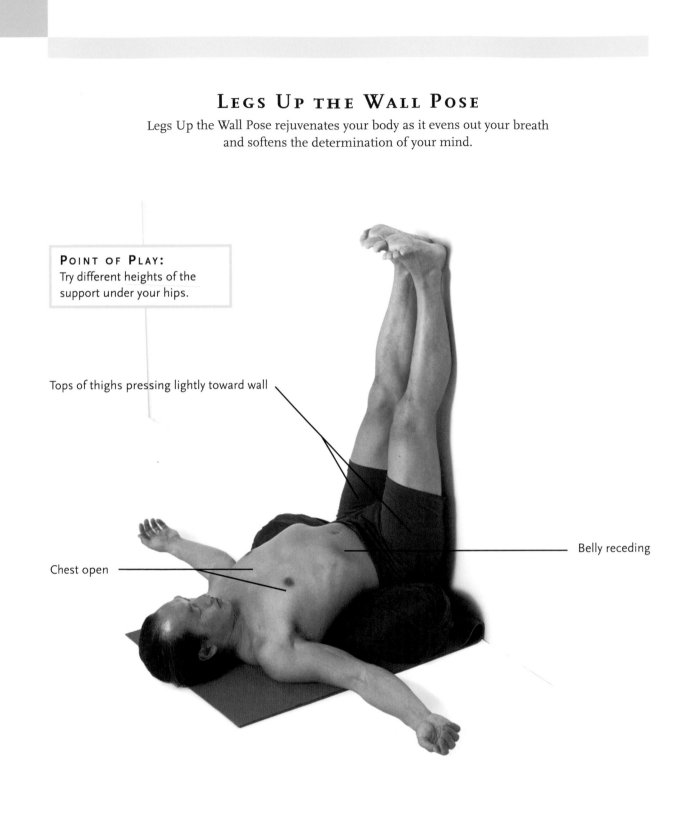

POINT OF PLAY:
Try different heights of the
support under your hips.

Tops of thighs pressing lightly toward wall

Belly receding

Chest open

RELAXATION POSE

Relaxation Pose allows you to witness your aliveness
and a synthesis between your mind, body, and breath as it restores your body.

Spine elongating, with natural curves

Legs about 8 inches apart

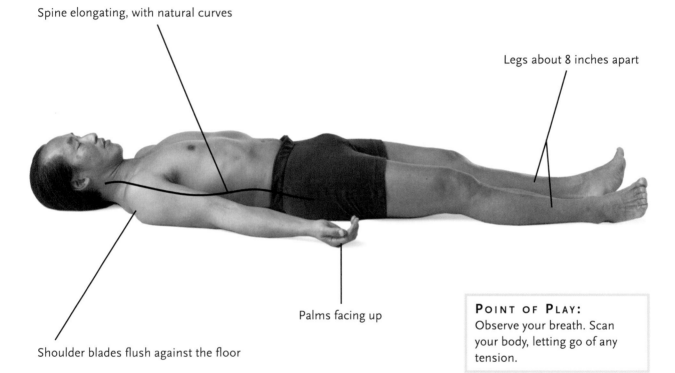

Palms facing up

Shoulder blades flush against the floor

POINT OF PLAY:
Observe your breath. Scan your body, letting go of any tension.

HERO POSE

Hero Pose rejuvenates and balances your legs
and creates a wonderful sense of grounding.

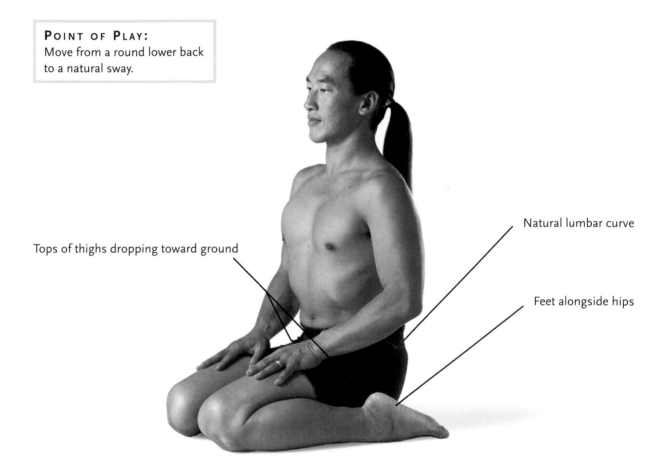

POINT OF PLAY:
Move from a round lower back
to a natural sway.

Natural lumbar curve

Tops of thighs dropping toward ground

Feet alongside hips

THE RECOMMENDATION OF A REGULAR YOGA
PRACTICE FOLLOWS THE PRINCIPAL THAT THROUGH
PRACTICE WE CAN LEARN TO STAY PRESENT IN EVERY
MOMENT, AND THEREBY ACHIEVE MUCH THAT WE
WERE PREVIOUSLY INCAPABLE OF.

—T. K. V. DESIKACHAR, *THE HEART OF YOGA*

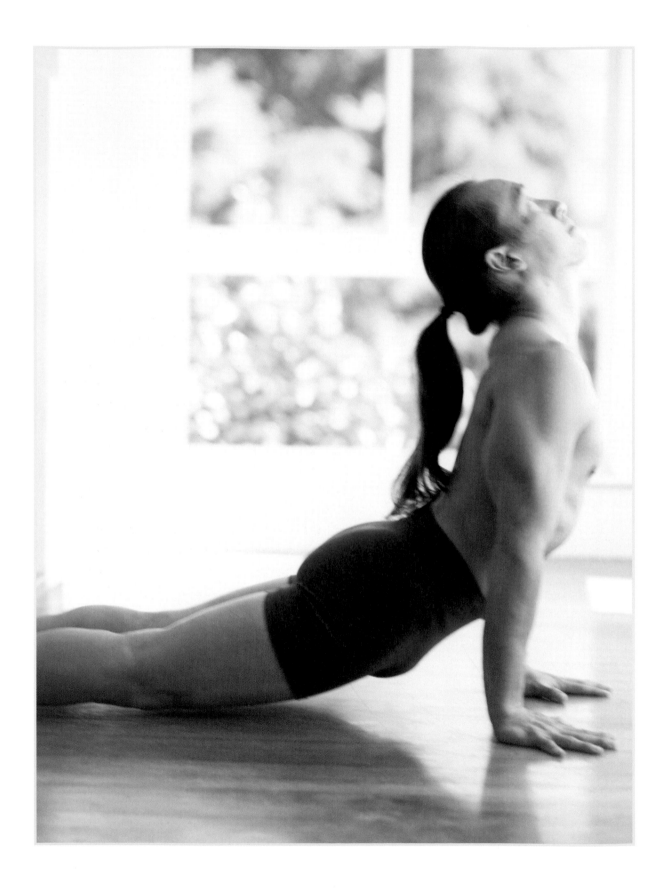

YOGA IS A SANSKRIT WORD THAT LITERALLY MEANS "YOKE." THE PRACTICE OF YOGA IS THE PRACTICE OF YOKING TOGETHER OR UNIFYING BODY AND MIND, WHICH REALLY MEANS PENETRATING INTO THE EXPERIENCE OF THEM NOT BEING SEPARATE IN THE FIRST PLACE. YOU CAN ALSO THINK OF IT AS EXPERIENCING THAT UNITY OR CONNECTEDNESS BETWEEN THE INDIVIDUAL AND THE UNIVERSE AS A WHOLE.
—JON KABAT-ZINN, *FULL CATASTROPHE LIVING*

WEEK 2:

Awakening Connection

IT'S IRONIC THAT IN AN AGE WHERE SO MUCH COMMUNICATION AND CONNECTION CAN HAPPEN ALMOST instantaneously through electronic mechanisms, most of us feel isolated and disconnected. However, as you practice yoga, you may begin to realize that it is not the lack of real connection that causes this feeling, but the *illusion* of isolation. For example, stop and consider a simple food like an apple. How many connections were made in various parts of the world just to bring that food to your table? But because you did not grow the food or water it with your own hands, it may not be easy to perceive the direct connection of the food to the earth to your body.

Some of this disconnect may come from the speed at which you are living. If you do not give an experience time to be digested or allow the flavor of the experience to sink deeply into your body—whether it is the taste of fruit in your mouth or a heart connection to your partner—you become alienated from innate connection. By taking the time to do a yoga practice, you give yourself the opportunity to digest your experiences and therefore awaken your consciousness of connection. The practice of yoga is intended to unveil the illusion of your separateness. Connecting two yoga poses together, connecting your inhalation with your exhalation, and relaxing your consciousness to merge with a collective consciousness are all ways to break down your sense of alienation.

When you first start yoga, it is typical to think first about learning the individual poses and then later move on to understanding the relationship between the poses. This is the same way many people think about the night sky. First they consider the individual stars and then move on to understanding the relationships between stars, creating "pictures" of constellations. This week I want you to start off by just trying to get a general feeling of looking at the night sky with all the stars. This chapter introduces you to the Sun Salutation, a movement practice in which you need not be so concerned about nailing down each individual pose. As you learn the Sun Salutation, suspend your need for exactitude and imagine that you are a child imitating an entire dance, focusing more on the overall movement than on the individual poses.

ABOUT SUN SALUTATIONS

This traditional movement practice—the Sun Salutation—connects balancing, forward-bending, back-bending, and centering poses. It can also be used as a general grid for connecting all the yoga postures. The Sun Salutation links together poses through movement and breath. Focusing on your breath joins your mind and your body; your inhalation draws the external world into the internal and your exhalation releases the internal world back into the external.

When you begin learning the Sun Salutation, imagine you are learning a single pose. Try to see the gross connections of the forms on a muscular, skeletal level. Ask yourself which muscles have to work; which muscles have to release; if your legs are bending, straightening, turning out, turning in; if your spine is flexing or extending; if your body is opening or closing. As you feel the shapes your body is taking, begin to watch the natural rise and fall of your breath as you move in and out of the poses. Your mind will be engaged both in the architecture of the posture and your breath. After you experience this sense of general connection, you can begin to move with more accuracy to create nuance and subtlety.

EMOTIONS. Because of the movement they require, Sun Salutations energize your emotional body and can even reverse a tendency toward lethargy or depression. The poses and the counterposes that are included in the Sun Salutation give your body an immediate sense of balance. And if you integrate your mind with your body by listening to your breath as a guide for your movement, you innately drop into the present moment. On a physical level, your circulation is enhanced, which can shift your state of being on an emotional level.

FOCUS OF YOUR MIND. In Sun Salutations, focus on the core of your body: your belly. Moving in and out of center, extending away from center, and drawing back into center connects you to your core. Awakening both strength and fluidity in your abdominal muscles and your pelvic muscles draws your mind and breath into your vital center. No matter how complex or esoteric your practice becomes, it is crucial to return to your vital center throughout your practice.

BALANCING. Balancing in movement differs from balancing in static poses. As you practice Sun Salutations, experiment with shifting your balance intricately. Play also with your balance in the transitions between poses so that balancing is not just an end result, but a constant, fluid response in any given moment in time.

BREATH. This week, as always, you should not hold or force your breath. Allow your breath to move quickly or slowly as you respond naturally to whatever your body needs. Let go of any predetermined ideas about how your breath should be and allow the movement of your body to follow your breath, rather than tailoring your breath to your movement.

LOWER RIBS. Your diaphragm is attached to your lower ribs. When you hinge your body in this area, you usually decrease the ability of your diaphragm to work easily. And because the diaphragm is your main breathing muscle, any inhibition of the diaphragm will inhibit your breath. Therefore, your first step toward freeing your breath is to keep your lower ribs supple and even. This practice can be a central focus for your work this week.

NECK AND HEAD. Letting your neck and head follow the movement of your torso allows your neck and head to be supported by their foundation. Too often we move our necks and heads separately and create a disconnection between our brains and bodies. As you feel the integrated movement of your head, neck, and torso, you will discern the connection between your mind and body.

SHOULDER JOINTS. This very loose joint connects the shoulder blade, the collarbone, and the upper arm. As you move through your poses this week, focus periodically on the articulation, movement, and feeling of the shoulder joint. Ideally, your shoulder joint should be strongly connected to your rib cage so there is harmonious movement between the two. Think of your arms as starting from your heart, so that the interconnectedness of your shoulder joints and rib cage stays at the forefront of any work that you do with the shoulder.

ANATOMY LESSON

1. Shoulder blades, collarbones, and upper arm bones (shoulder girdle)

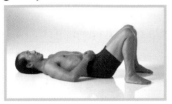

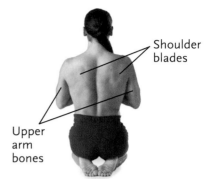

Shoulder blades

Upper arm bones

To learn about your shoulder blades, lie on the ground in Constructive Rest Pose and move your arms around so you can feel your shoulder blades and the way they articulate with your arms and rib cage.

To learn about your collarbones, touch your left collarbone with your right hand as you move your left arm around. Notice how your collarbone articulates with your upper arm and your shoulder blade.

To learn about your upper arms, move them in all directions with different rotations.

2. Lower ribs (diaphragm attachment) and upper chest

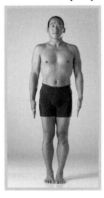

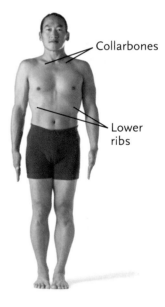

Collarbones

Lower ribs

To learn about your lower ribs, stand in Mountain Pose and touch your lower ribs, all the way around from the bottom of the breastbone to the middle of the spine (your back). As you move your lower ribs, see if you can centralize them so that the skin and muscles around the lower ribs are at ease and your breathing feels even inside your torso.

To learn about your upper chest, practice Constructive Rest Pose, while placing your hands on your upper chest. Notice any movements in your upper chest that reflect the breath.

3. Back of your neck and position of your head

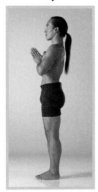

To learn about the back of your neck and the position of your head, stand in Mountain Pose and feel the back of your neck with your fingers as you move your head in all directions. During this movement, try to find the most neutral position where your head is directly over your heart.

Day 1: Learning the Variations

When you learn the variations of the poses for Sun Salutation, you will use props to experience the proper feeling and alignment of each pose. However, when you move through the Sun Salutation in its entirety, it is not practical to use props. Therefore, as you are learning the variations, deeply register the feelings that the props create so when you do the Sun Salutation without props, you can approximate the movement and integration. When you are actually moving through the Sun Salutations, experiment to determine which version of a pose you are able to do with ease without props. If needed, put your hands on your legs or on your hips or bend your legs to approximate the effects of a prop.

As you learn the variations, remember to move in and out of these poses with your breath and to link the poses with each other. I encourage you to choose the pose version that is the easiest for you because the transitions make the poses more difficult, requiring extra maneuvering and adjusting as you link the poses together.

Moving in and out of the Poses within a Salutation

Some transitions within Sun Salutations are a little tricky. Please be mindful of where you *initiate* the transition. For example, when moving from Lunge to Standing Forward Bend, focus on shifting your pelvis over your front foot. Here are suggestions for making each transition, but feel free to experiment in order to discover what works best for you.

Note that the transitions in Sun Salutations are often difficult because your mind runs ahead of your breath and of where your body is moving in space. Our minds have a tendency to fixate on the postures themselves, rather than feeling the transitions between. The reason I love Sun Salutations is that they make it very clear that there are no stagnant poses and that in some sense a pose is always in transition.

FROM MOUNTAIN POSE TO VOLCANO POSE. As you begin the Sun Salutation, center yourself in Mountain Pose. When you raise your arms over your head, there is already a tendency for you to break that center, especially in the lower rib area, and to come forward on your toes. Focus on continually centering your body.

FROM VOLCANO POSE TO STANDING FORWARD BEND.
Initiate the movement into Standing Forward Bend by moving your pelvis over your legs. Use any of these arm positions as you bend forward.

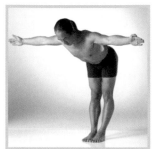

As you bend forward, support your lower back with the wide muscles of your lower spine and with the strength of your legs as they connect both to the ground and to your spine. Use your belly as well to support your lower back by drawing it back toward the front of your spine and up into your abdominal cavity. Ground your thighbones toward your hamstrings and allow your belly to rise from that action.

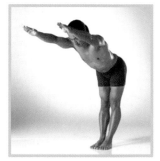

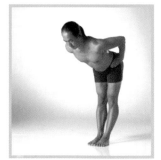

FROM STANDING FORWARD BEND TO EXTENDED STANDING FORWARD BEND.
Initiate your movement into Extended Standing Forward Bend from the grounding of your heels and the length of your belly. Let this action open your heart and create an equal sense of work throughout your spine. Look forward from your heels, not your neck muscles.

FROM EXTENDED STANDING FORWARD BEND TO PLANK POSE. As you step back to Plank Pose, initiate the movement from your legs and feet.

FROM PLANK POSE TO PUSH-UP POSE. As you move into Push-Up Pose, initiate the transition by moving the tops of your forearms back as your chest moves forward. Feel the full length of your torso and legs as one unit, and bend your arms only as far as you can while maintaining the integrity of that unit.

FROM PUSH-UP POSE TO UPWARD-FACING DOG POSE. As you move to Upward-Facing Dog Pose, initiate the transition by changing the position of your feet and allowing that movement to surge through your legs into your spine. Make a smooth, slow, mindful transition to maintain the strength of your legs and the suppleness of your spine. Support your lower back by grounding your legs and using your arms to move your rib cage away from your legs. In Upward-Facing Dog, find the appropriate distance between your feet and your hands that allows your arms to be perpendicular to the floor as you draw your pelvis through your arms. Keep your legs continually spiraling inward to get the full lift of your upper chest.

FROM UPWARD-FACING DOG TO DOWNWARD-FACING DOG. Experiment with this transition to find which is easiest for your sacrum and lower back. Some people move their heads first, contracting their abdominal muscles to support the lower back as they begin the transition. I prefer to initiate the movement from the tops of my thighs, scooping my belly up into my spine to support my lower back.

FROM DOWNWARD-FACING DOG TO LUNGE. As you move to Lunge, initiate the transition by shifting the weight of your pelvis over your front leg at the bottom of your exhalation. To get your foot between your hands, you may have to lean slightly to one side and come up on your fingertips. Or you may need to take very small steps forward into Standing Forward Bend. Although it may look easy, this transition can be the most difficult in the Sun Salutation. Use whatever method you can do without gripping and holding your breath.

FROM LUNGE TO EXTENDED STANDING FORWARD BEND. As you walk forward into Extended Standing Forward Bend, initiate the movement by shifting the weight of your pelvis over your front foot.

FROM EXTENDED STANDING FORWARD BEND TO STANDING FORWARD BEND. As you release into Standing Forward Bend, initiate the movement by grounding your heels and lifting your sitting bones.

FROM STANDING FORWARD BEND TO POWERFUL POSE. As you move from Standing Forward Bend to Powerful Pose, initiate the transition from the movement of your legs under your torso. Keep a strong focus on the balance between the elongation of the sides of your waist, the reach and the extension of your arms, and the relaxation of your neck.

FROM POWERFUL POSE TO VOLCANO POSE. As you move into Volcano Pose, initiate the movement by grounding your legs, and allow that grounding to help lengthen your waist as you raise your arms. As you move into the backbend, some of you will feel inclined to take a much deeper backbend while others will want to come to a more vertical standing position, depending on how your spine feels and what seems most integrated.

FROM VOLCANO POSE TO MOUNTAIN POSE. As you return to Mountain Pose from Volcano Pose, bring your attention to centering yourself from the front of your heels to the crown of your head.

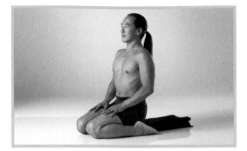

1. Practice **HERO POSE** for 1 minute. Feel the interconnect-edness of your entire body, allowing it to be a large channel for your breath.

2. Try all three versions of **CAT POSE** *(Chakravakasana)* for 15 seconds in each version. Then transi-tion from version 1 to version 2 to version 1 to version 3, with your breath. You can move right through the poses or stay in them for several breaths, using your inhalations to move into version 2 and your ex-halations to move into version 3.

VERSION 1: Neutral spine

Feel the extension of your spine, from the base of your pelvis to the crown of your head, while at the same time allowing yourself to feel the natural sway of your lower back, the natural hunch of your upper back, and the natural sway of your neck. Observe the balance between your two shins and your two hands. Move your shoulder blades down your back, broaden your collarbones, and insert your upper arm bones into their sockets.

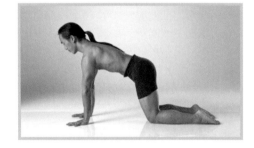

VERSION 2: Arching your back into a backbend

Initiate your movement into a backbend on your inhalation. As you work subtly with this pose, continue to breathe with ease. Lift your sitting bones and feel the full arc of your spine, the elonga-tion of your waist, and the vigor of your arms and legs supporting your spine. Challenge yourself to make every part of your spine contribute to your backbend. As your lower ribs contribute to the backbend, feel this area as a congruous aspect of the entire back-bend, rather than as a hinge.

VERSION 3: Rounding your back into a hunch

Initiate your movement into a hunch on an exhalation, continuing to breathe with ease. Tuck your tailbone, feeling as if it is meeting the crown of your head. Hollow your belly into your back to broaden your lower back. Press your feet and hands into the ground to round your spine even more. Again the challenge is to find the evenness of the entire rounding of your spine. Feel your neck and head integrated into the harmonious curve of the rest of your spine.

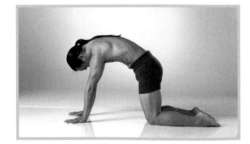

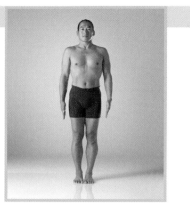

3. Practice **MOUNTAIN POSE** for 1 minute. Focus on your spine and feel how your breath moves it.

4. Try all three versions of **VOLCANO POSE** *(Urdhva Hastasana)* for 15 seconds for each version.

VERSION 1: Arms shoulder-width apart

This version allows you to extend your inner elbows as completely as possible and feel the lines of your body from your legs up through your waist and arm. Elongate your waist into the reach of your arms, without pushing your lower ribs forward. Move your shoulder blades down your back and firm them into your rib cage to support the lift and broadness of your collarbones. Move your upper arms gently into their sockets to create a conscious relationship with your shoulder blades and collarbones.

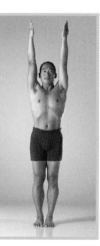

VERSION 2: Full pose, with hands together and elbows straight

This version challenges you to find a soft neck and jaw and an ease of breath without pushing your lower ribs forward. Feel the broad base of your feet moving into the strength of your legs, into the length of your waist, and all the way up into your fingers as they press together from the reach of your inner arms. Continue to move your head more and more over the center of your chest. Relax your lower ribs as you lift your upper chest.

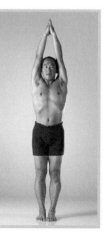

VERSION 3: Standing backbend

This version opens your upper chest into a slight backbend with the help of your legs and arms. Move your head and neck in tandem for if your head falls back too quickly, your neck will get jammed. Move your chest more upward than backward, so as you begin to bend your spine, you emphasize extension rather than bending. Feel your entire spine arcing up and back, from the tailbone to the crown of your head, and out to your fingertips.

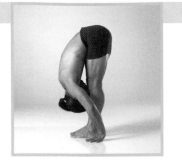

5. Practice **STANDING FORWARD BEND** for 30 seconds. Adjust the support and placement of your shoulder girdle so that the base of your neck can be as easy as possible.

6. Try all three versions of **EXTENDED STANDING FORWARD BEND** *(Uttanasana)* for 30 seconds in each version.

VERSION 1: Hands on your thighs (just above your knees)

This version provides you with enough height to keep a sway in your back and to move your chest forward from that sway. This helps you realize that you can find an opening in your hamstrings without rounding your spine. Your entire spine should be in an even backbend, from the lift of your sitting bones to the lift of your head, so there is no pinching in any part of your spine. With your spine this extended, you can easily place your shoulder blades, collarbones, and upper arm bones so they help support the lift and movement of your upper chest.

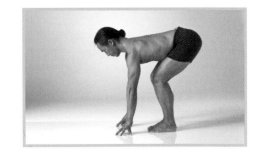

VERSION 2: Knees bent, fingertips on the floor

This version allows you to bring both your hands and feet in good contact with the ground. Bending your legs eliminates the resistance in your hamstrings. You will feel a deep folding inside your hip creases that allows you to lift your chest and head. Continue to maintain good contact and balance through your heels. Play with the placement of your lower ribs to find a good flow from your belly to your upper chest.

VERSION 3: Full pose, with knees straight, fingertips on the floor

This version is for those of you who are very flexible in the backs of your legs and can keep your legs straight while maintaining an arch in your lower back that moves into the lift of your chest and head. The challenge is to keep your fingertips in contact with the floor while your arms are fully engaged into their sockets, broadening your chest and bringing it forward. Make sure the lift of your chest allows you to have a relaxed neck and that the position of your head flows from the lift of your chest.

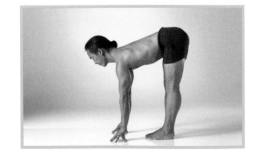

7. Try all three versions of LUNGE for 10 seconds on the right side only (left leg back, right leg forward).

VERSION 1: Knee of your back leg on the ground

This version allows your chest and spine to be more vertical and liberated. Use the grounding of your front foot and the press of your arms to elongate your waist, lift your chest, and look forward. The challenge is to maintain some activity in your back leg, reaching it in the direction of your foot, even though your leg is bent. Be on your fingertips so your upper arms, shoulder blades, and collarbones can be as close to Mountain Pose as possible.

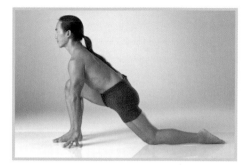

VERSION 2: Hips high and completely square, back leg straight

This version teaches you to feel the grounding of your legs and the lightness of your hips. Holding your hips high diminishes the resistance of your leg muscles, so you can keep your hips square and your spine symmetrical. Keep your back leg strong and your front foot pressing as you square your hips and extend your chest from your pelvis. Be careful not to break the energy at your lower ribs or to overuse your lower back muscles. Look forward.

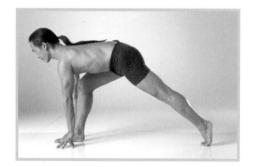

VERSION 3: Full pose, back leg lifting strongly

The challenge of the full pose is to find the flexibility in your hips to take a deep lunge with a strong, firm back leg, as you bend your front knee to 90 degrees. Release deeply in your front leg while keeping your pelvis square, lengthening both sides of your waist, moving your chest forward, and looking up. Imagine your neck starts at the base of your pelvis so you don't pinch your neck as you lift your head.

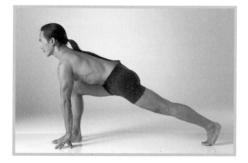

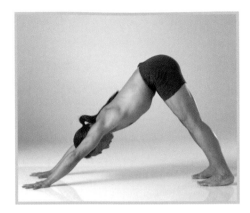

8. Practice **DOWNWARD-FACING DOG** for 1 minute. Soften the back of your neck as you reach your arms from the bottom of your rib cage.

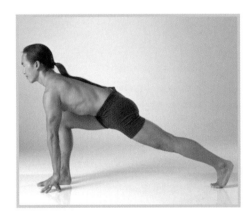

9. Try all three versions of **LUNGE** for 10 seconds on the left side only (right leg back, left leg forward).

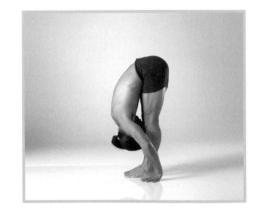

10. Practice **STANDING FORWARD BEND** for 1 minute. Feel the effects of all the other poses that have come between this and the last forward bend.

11. Try all three versions of **POWERFUL POSE** *(Utkatansa)* for 15 seconds in each version.

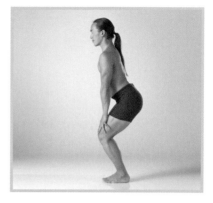

VERSION 1: Hands on thighs, just above your knees

By placing your hands just above your knees, you can use your arms to help lighten your pelvis and extend your spine. Press your thighs down and root your feet strongly from that pressing. The challenge is to allow your shinbones to slant forward over your feet, stretching your calves from your grounded heels. With your arms in this easy position, you can pay attention to the placement of your upper chest as it is supported by the work of your shoulder blades and the engagement of your upper arms.

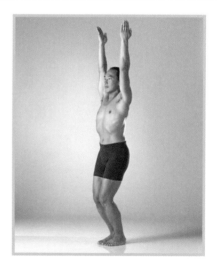

VERSION 2: Arms over your head, torso vertical

With your arms over your head, the pose becomes much more vigorous. But keeping your back vertical makes the weight of your arms and torso much easier on your legs, allowing your breath and determination to be more at ease. Challenge yourself to find the connection between the power of your legs and arms converging to lift your chest and elongate your waist. With your torso vertical, it will be easier to feel the integration of your lower ribs with your upper chest and arms.

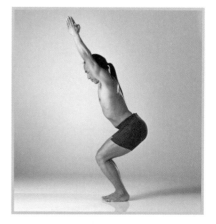

VERSION 3: Full pose, with arms vertical and torso extending forward

As your legs bend deeply and your torso comes in front of its vertical axis, your legs, back, and shoulder muscles have to work more intensely. Maintain a dialogue between the intensity of the pose and your internal surrender and ease. Grapple with the relationship between your shoulder blades, collarbones, and upper arms. Lift your head only to a position where your neck and head feel like they flow continuously from the rest of your spine.

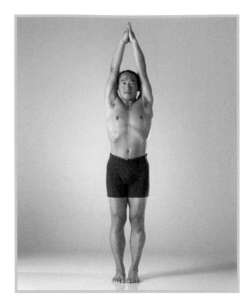

12. Practice **VOLCANO POSE** for 15 seconds. Feel the long, extended line from your heels to your fingertips.

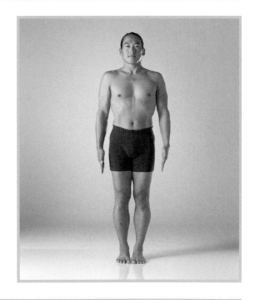

13. Practice **MOUNTAIN POSE** for 30 seconds. Feel the channel from your inner legs through your pelvis up the front of your spine.

14. Try one mini **SUN SALUTATION,** taking 2 breaths in each pose. Initiate your movements from your core (your belly) instead of your neck and head.

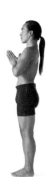 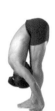 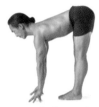

1. Mountain Pose

2. Volcano Pose

3. Standing Forward Bend

4. Extended Standing Forward Bend

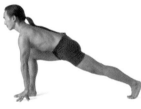 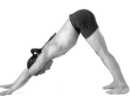 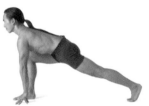

5. Lunge

6. Downward-Facing Dog

7. Lunge (alternate side)

 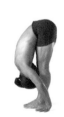 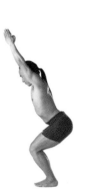 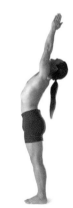 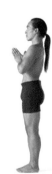

8. Extended Standing Forward Bend

9. Standing Forward Bend

10. Powerful Pose

11. Volcano Pose

12. Mountain Pose

15. Try all three versions of **PLANK POSE,** for 2 breaths in each version. Repeat the series twice.

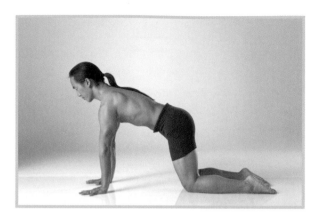

VERSION 1: Neutral cat (version 1 of Cat Pose)

This version takes a lot of weight off your arms, but imagine your arms taking the weight of your pelvis and upper body by pressing firmly into the ground, especially at the root of your index finger and the base of your thumb. To prevent your chest from being concave, engage your shoulder blades into your back, broadening your chest and moving your collarbones forward. Look forward.

VERSION 2: One knee bent, other leg extended straight back

By straightening one leg, you begin to feel the shape of the pose and the line of energy from the reach of your straight leg into your torso. You will discover that the strength moving through your legs into your body enlivens your arms. The coordination of your entire body serves as a foundation for the strength of your arms. The challenge is to continue to find the alignment from the heel of your straight leg all the way into the lift of your collarbones, while continuing to press your arms firmly into the ground. (Do this pose twice, once on the right and once on the left.) Try not to break the energy flow at your lower ribs.

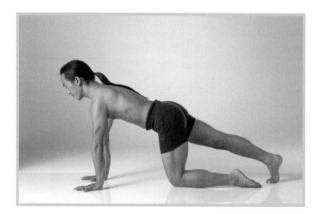

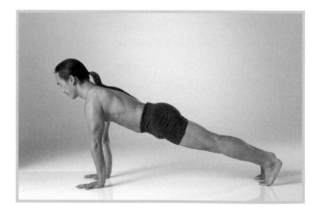

VERSION 3: Full pose, with both legs extended

The placement of your pelvis in line with your legs and torso—with the support of your abdominal muscles moving upward into your lower back—allows you to find Mountain Pose alignment. With your arms straight, use the weight of your body to align your arm bones over the heels of your hands. The challenge is to keep your pelvis in line with your neutral lower ribs while you find the lift of your upper chest and head.

16. Try all three versions of **PUSH-UP POSE** *(Chaturanga Dandasana)* for 1 breath for each version.

VERSION 1: On your belly, legs extended, hands in place, pressing

This version allows you to experience the basic position of your legs, pelvis, and torso in Push-Up Pose. By engaging your shoulder blades and moving your chest and head forward, you can begin to get an accurate view of the position of your arms and chest. Extend your body vigorously as you press your hands firmly into the ground. Challenge yourself to press strongly while keeping your face and breath relaxed. Broaden your collarbones as you press your upper arms into your side ribs.

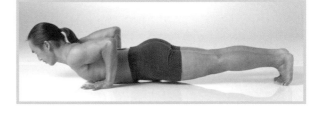

VERSION 2: Knees bent, chest scooping through, hands pressing

By having some weight on your knees, you can begin to scoop your chest forward and keep it lifted off the ground. The position of your pelvis and the action of your legs in this version differ from what you do in the full pose, but the action of your arms mimics the full Push-Up Pose. Bring your elbows closer to your side body, press the insides of your hands, and broaden your collarbones. Firm your shoulder blades into your rib cage and down toward your pelvis, as you restrain your lower ribs from falling too far toward the ground. Work your arms strongly while allowing your breath to be as easy as possible.

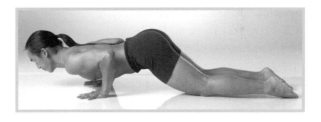

VERSION 3: Full pose, with legs extended, hands pushing you from the ground

This version is a challenging pose for everyone, especially while keeping your chest open and your pelvis aligned. Rely as much as possible on the use of your legs as they extend through your heels and lift away from the ground. Keep your buttocks from lifting upward and maintain a Mountain Pose position. Place your pelvis in line with your legs and your lower ribs in line with your pelvis as you propel your chest and then look forward.

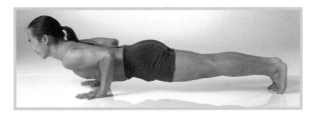

17. Try all three versions of **UPWARD-FACING DOG POSE** (*Urdhva Mukha Svanasana*) for 3 breaths for each version.

VERSION 1: Cobra pose

Keeping your legs on the ground allows you to move and adjust your spine until it is even and balanced. The challenge is to extend your legs strongly away from your hips into your elongated toes as your pelvis slides forward into your lifting chest. Don't force, but move and play to articulate and find the even arch of your spine. Straighten your arms to the point where you feel your shoulder blades, collarbones, and upper arm bones enhancing the lift of your upper chest and the ease of your neck.

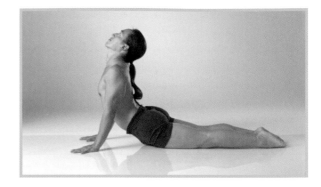

VERSION 2: Blanket roll under tops of your thighs

By placing the blanket roll under your thighs, you bring your legs into the Upward-Facing Dog position. You can let the blanket roll help you move your thighbones upward into your hamstrings. From this placement of your thighs, draw your pelvis toward a more vertical position, as the foundation for your rising spine. From this foundation you can fully liberate your spine in a magnificent backbend. Try to integrate your spine evenly so that you don't overuse the part of your spine where your lower ribs are attached.

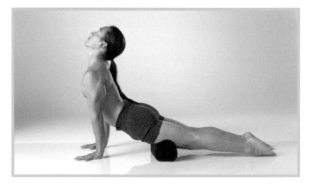

VERSION 3: Full pose, legs lifting

The full pose should be exhilarating from the full support of your arms and legs moving into your lifted, open chest. The back of your pelvis should feel suspended and your lower back elongated from this traction. This pose wakes up your entire body and shows you how your arms and legs can fully support your spine in a backbend. Work on supporting the lift of your chest without overextending or overworking your neck.

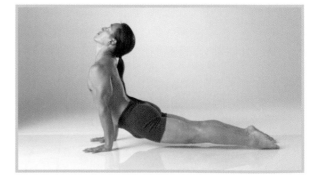

18. Try one full **SUN SALUTATION,** taking 2 breaths in each pose. Let your body be as graceful as possible in making the transitions, letting it do what it needs to make this flow of poses feel as fluid as possible. You will do this sequence many times in the coming eight weeks, and with practice, you will become familiar and at ease with this sequence. Throughout the salutation, focus your awareness on the movement in your lower ribs.

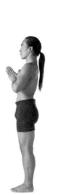 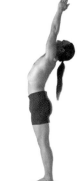 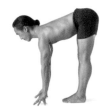 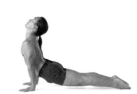 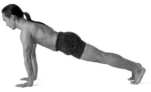

1. Mountain Pose   **2.** Volcano Pose   **3.** Standing Forward Bend   **4.** Extended Standing Forward Bend   **5.** Plank Pose

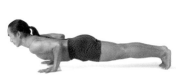 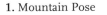 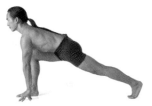

6. Push-Up Pose   **7.** Upward-Facing Dog   **8.** Downward-Facing Dog   **9.** Lunge (both sides)

 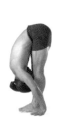 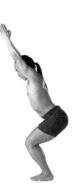 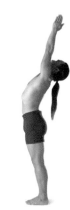 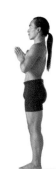

10. Extended Standing Forward Bend   **11.** Standing Forward Bend   **12.** Powerful Pose   **13.** Volcano Pose   **14.** Mountain Pose

19. Try all three versions of **STAFF POSE** *(Dandasana)* for 30 seconds for each version.

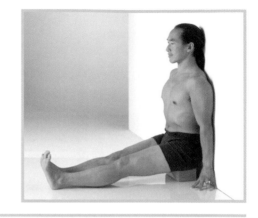

VERSION 1: Against a wall, with hips on a block

Using a block allows those who have tight hamstrings to sit up-right. With your back against the wall, you will feel the relation-ships between your shoulder blades, sacrum, and spine. Keep your legs strong, and try to feel the top of your pelvis move away from the wall. Firm your shoulder blades into your back as you lean your upper back against the wall, and raise the back of your skull up the wall. Broaden your collarbones and let your upper arms help lift your side chest.

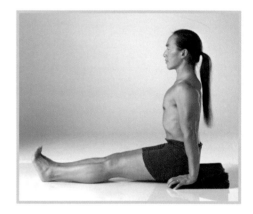

VERSION 2: In the middle of the room, with hips on a folded blanket, fingertips touching the floor

Using the blanket creates a greater angle so your hamstrings will not pull your pelvis into a rounded back. With your fingertips touching the floor beside you, you will understand how your arms aid the elongation of your waist and the lift of your chest. The challenge is to keep your spine elongated in this pose without overusing your back muscles. Engage your arms and legs as you broaden and breathe into your back body. Sit your pelvis as up-right as possible and let your lower ribs come to a neutral posi-tion.

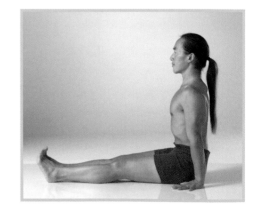

VERSION 3: Full pose, with hips on the ground, hands alongside them

When your legs are in full contact with the ground, you can fully activate them, providing the foundation for this pose. Your hands can also come into more contact with the ground. From the earth-iness of your legs and the vibrant contact of your hands, learn how to lengthen your arms and lift your chest. The challenge is to work your arms and legs vigorously without making them rigid, while at the same time keeping your torso receptive to your breath. As you work your arms, press your lower arms down into your hands. Use your upper arms to help lift your shoulder girdle and chest so that your neck is not strained and your head is floating and balanced over your chest.

20. Try all three versions of **COBBLER'S POSE** *(Baddha Konasana)* for 30 seconds for each version.

VERSION 1: Against the wall, with hips on a folded blanket or bolster

The wall gives you feedback on the position of your pelvis, spine, and head, while sitting on a bolster allows you the freedom to sit upright if you are tight in the hips. When you are supported by the wall, you can learn which muscles to contract to keep your spine erect and to create support for your torso from the power of your legs and arms. Having this much support should not distract you from investigating which muscles you need to work to create support without the wall. Keep your upper chest lifted from the action of your shoulder blades, collarbones, and upper arms.

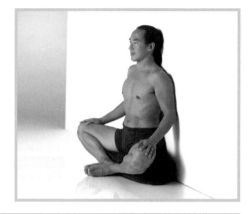

VERSION 2: In the middle of the room, with hips on a folded blanket and fingertips touching the floor behind you

With your hands behind you, you can lean slightly backward to get the full extension of your spine. By moving your torso back and forth, you learn which position of your pelvis allows your legs to fall toward the ground and how you can continue this release as you begin to sit more upright. Search for the verticality of your pelvis with wide, supple back muscles. Also try to find the natural curve of your lower back, so you lift your upper chest from your pelvis and legs, not your middle back.

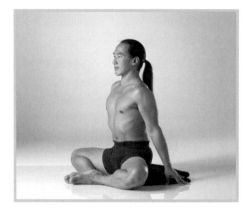

VERSION 3: Full pose without props, hands holding ankles

Sitting directly on the floor allows you to feel a very strong sense of grounding, although it will be much more challenging to keep your pelvis upright. Keenly observe where you have to release inside your hips so you can consciously let go of the binding that throws your pelvis backward. Pull lightly to keep your waist long and chest open. Learn how to engage your shoulder blades down your back—your arms moving into their sockets and your collarbones broad and lifted—without straining your neck. Feel as if your head is floating on your relaxed neck that is balanced over your chest.

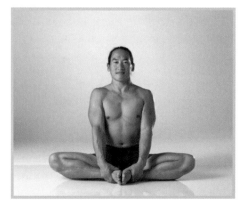

21. Try all three versions of **RECLINED COBBLER'S POSE** *(Supta Baddha Konasana)* for 2 minutes in each version.

VERSION 1: Block, bolster, or folded blanket under your feet, support under your knees

With your feet lifted, your lower back is fully supported and flush against the ground. This allows you to soften all the muscles of your waist and lower abdomen. Feeling the support of the floor, your spine relaxes deeply. Keep your focus on letting go deep inside your hip sockets as you play with slightly different positions of your knees and feet. As you lie down on the bolster, consciously drag your shoulder blades down toward your pelvis, opening your collarbones and slightly drawing your upper arms back into their sockets.

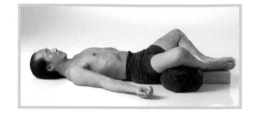

VERSION 2: Blocks or folded blankets under your knees, body flat on the ground

With your legs supported, your hip sockets feel safe to let go completely. With your feet on the ground, there will be a natural curve in your lower back, which allows your breath to move with ease into the floor of your pelvis and the front of your body. Notice the gentle movement of your spine and your belly with the rise and fall of your breath. Lengthen your lower ribs away from your buttocks and relax them as much as possible toward the floor.

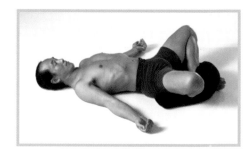

VERSION 3: Full supported version, with bolster or folded blankets under your spine and support under your knees and head

With your head higher than your chest and your chest higher than your pelvis, your body will sense its natural configuration and allow your breath to spill in easily and fill your body completely. The challenge here is to feel your immense vulnerability linked with supported comfort, and then to consciously let go. Pay special attention to relaxing your head and neck.

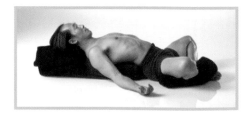

22. Try all three versions of **CONSTRUCTIVE REST POSE** for 1 minute in each version.

VERSION 1: Strap around your thighs, feet apart

This version allows for complete relaxation because you do not have to hold up your legs. The position of your legs broadens your lower back muscles and rests your lower back completely on the ground. The internal rotation of your legs softens your lower belly and allows your breath to move more easily into the base of your pelvis. Keep following the ease of your breath in the rise and fall of your belly. As you lie down, consciously drag your shoulder blades toward your pelvis, opening your collarbones and slightly drawing your upper arms back into their sockets.

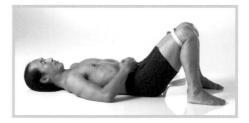

VERSION 2: Folded blanket (into a thin rectangle) under your sacrum

This version creates a slight inversion, while your body is still in a relaxation pose, providing even more ease in your nervous system. It also gives a slight traction to your lower back, which further releases any binding in your lower torso. Observe how your breath moves—this is a good indication of the direction and feeling of an unobstructed breath. Feel the relaxation that comes with the extra contact of your lower ribs on the ground.

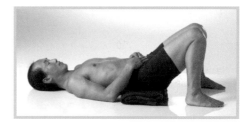

VERSION 3: Full pose, without props, knees falling toward each other

This version is a wonderful restorative pose for those times when you need the support of the earth. Without using any props, see if you can allow your body to fall into the shape of version 1 and also feel the internal release of version 2. Can you imagine that your body could move into that pattern by just surrendering? Place a folded blanket or pillow under your head so your head does not feel like it is falling back. Feel the deep release of any tension in your neck and head.

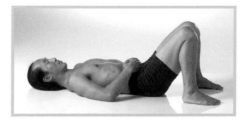

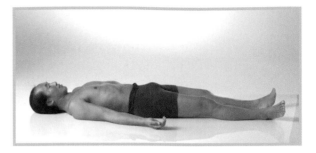

23. For 5 minutes, lie in **RELAXATION POSE.**

24. For 3 minutes, lie in **CONSTRUCTIVE REST POSE** and observe your breath as you exhale smoothly.

25. Try all three versions of **SEATED CROSSED-LEGS POSE** *(Sukhasana)* for 1 minute in each version.

VERSION 1: At the wall, sitting on a folded blanket, rolled towel or sticky mat underneath your ankles

This version creates a very supported foundation that is good for those whose hips are not very open and whose knees are high from the ground in Seated Crossed-Legs Pose. The wall gives you feedback about the placement of your spine and the work of your back muscles, while the blanket under your hips allows your pelvis to sit more upright. The support under your ankles keeps your ankles from taking a sickle shape and from jamming against the ground. Use this support to encourage your entire torso to elongate up the wall, as you broaden your back muscles away from your spine. Feel your shoulder blades move down the wall as you keep your collarbones broad and upper arms supportive.

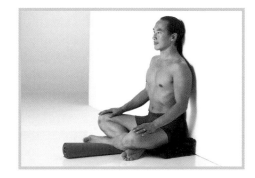

VERSION 2: In the middle of the room, your hips on a folded blanket

Sitting in the middle of the room without the wall enables you to breathe more easily into your back body and gives you a chance to feel a floating sensation in your entire upper body, neck, and head. Without the feedback of the wall, the tactile input to your nervous system is reduced, which allows your mind to quiet down. The challenge here is to keep your torso from collapsing without the extra reminder of the wall. Be mindful, however, not to overuse your lower ribs to lift your torso because this will inhibit your breath.

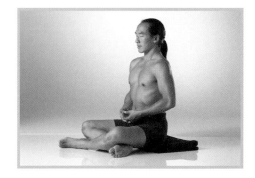

VERSION 3: In the middle of the room, with no props

This version adds to your feeling of being grounded as you are in direct contact with the floor. It is much more difficult to find the natural position of your pelvis, so you have to let go of whatever is binding in your hips and legs that pulls you out of your natural lift. Because the foundation of this pose is difficult, you will tend to lift from your neck, head, and lower ribs. Avoid this tendency and keep returning to work on your foundation.

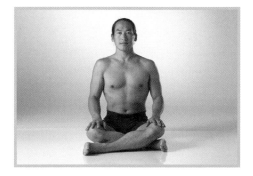

26. For 5 to 10 minutes, sit in **SEATED CROSSED-LEGS POSE.** Meditate on the energy and aliveness of your legs and feet connecting into your pelvis and vibrating up your spine.

This sequence provides many different ways to practice Downward-Facing Dog. As you repeat the Sun Salutation in this practice, you may notice that you are more able to do version 3 of Downward-Facing Dog. Eventually Downward-Facing Dog will become a great pose to do almost any time and in between other poses because it helps bring your spine, legs, and arms back to neutral. Downward-Facing Dog often comes at the very beginning of a sequence because it both opens and energizes your body, preparing you for any other posture.

FOCUS FOR THIS PRACTICE:

- In Downward-Facing Dog, play with the relationship between centering your lower ribs and opening your chest.

- In the standing poses, move your shoulder blades down toward your pelvis, firm them into your back, and widen them from your spine.

- In Standing Forward Bend and the restorative poses, relax the back of your neck and play with the position of your head.

1. Practice the mini **Sun Salutation** four times—right, left, right, and left—with an emphasis on exploring Downward-Facing Dog. Stay in all the poses except Downward-Facing Dog for 1 breath. Stay in Downward-Facing Dog for 5 breaths. Let your breath be natural between the poses.

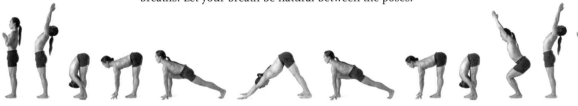

First Downward Dog: Practice with bent legs, emphasizing the lift of your sitting bones and the extension of your waist into your arms.

Second Downward Dog: Practice with your feet wide and turned in, emphasizing a deep internal rotation of your legs.

Third Downward Dog: Practice with your feet hips-distance apart, moving from internal rotation of the legs to parallel position.

Fourth Downward Dog: Practice lengthening the backs of your legs down to your heels. As your heels reach down toward the floor, lift your sitting bones and feel the full length of the backs of your legs.

2. Practice the full **Sun Salutation** two times—right, then left—with an emphasis on exploring Downward-Facing Dog. Stay in all the poses except Downward-Facing Dog for 1 breath. Stay in Downward-Facing Dog for 5 breaths. Let your breath be natural between the poses.

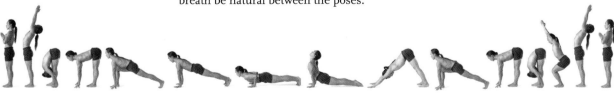
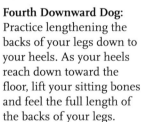

First Downward Dog: Move toward Plank Pose, with your elbow creases facing forward, and broaden your shoulder blades. As you move back into Downward-Facing Dog, keep that same broadening action of your shoulder blades.

Second Downward Dog: Extend your torso from your tailbone through your side waist into the length of your inner arms, lengthening down into the press of your index finger and thumb. Keep your forearms lifted, and your side chest and head toward the ground.

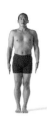 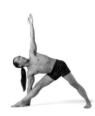

3. Practice **Mountain Pose** for 30 seconds.

4. Practice **Triangle Pose** for 45 seconds on each side.

5. Practice **Standing Forward Bend** for 1 minute.

6. Practice **Extended Side Angle Pose** for 45 seconds on each side.

7. Practice **Standing Forward Bend** for 30 seconds.

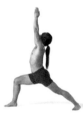 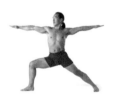

8. Practice **Warrior 1 Pose** for 30 seconds on each side.

9. Practice **Standing Forward Bend** for 30 seconds.

10. Practice **Warrior 2 Pose** for 45 seconds on each side.

11. Practice **Standing Forward Bend** for 30 seconds.

 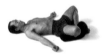 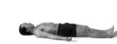

12. Lie in **Constructive Rest Pose** for 3 minutes.

13. Lie in version 2 of **Reclined Cobbler's Pose** for 1½ minutes.

14. Relaxation and Breath Awareness. For 5 minutes, lie in **Relaxation Pose** and observe the quality of your inhalation after exhaling smoothly.

15. Meditation. For 5 to 10 minutes, sit against the wall in **Seated Crossed-Legs Pose**, meditating on the length of your waist. Sit on a block or folded blanket if needed.

Push-Up Pose is one of the most challenging poses in the Sun Salutation, not to mention in this book. It takes considerable arm strength to be in this position with your chest open and your body in one long line. Most people break the line of the body so they can have the illusion of going farther down toward the ground or they close the chest to brace themselves in the shoulders. However, it is much better to maintain good alignment and not go so close to the ground, gradually building strength while keeping your alignment and ease of breath.

In the following sequence, you practice Mountain Pose and then Plank Pose to learn the proper body alignment. If you transpose this alignment into Push-Up Pose and bend your arms to the point where you can maintain your Mountain Pose alignment, your Sun Salutations will flourish. The standing poses that I have selected for this practice—Warrior 2 and Warrior 1—

open your chest from the strength of your legs. As you practice Push-Up Pose, return your attention to the strength of your legs integrating with your torso and arms, which you learned in Warrior 2 and Warrior 1. The Reclined Cobbler's Pose and Supported Relaxation Pose at the end reopen your upper chest after you have used your upper chest muscles so strongly in the Push-Up Poses. Link together the openness of your chest with both the Sun Salutation and the standing poses.

FOCUS FOR THIS PRACTICE:

- In Push-Up Pose, keep your collarbones wide.

- In the standing poses, keep your head in line with your spine as you relax your neck.

- In the Sun Salutation, relax your lower ribs and diaphragm so your breath moves easily.

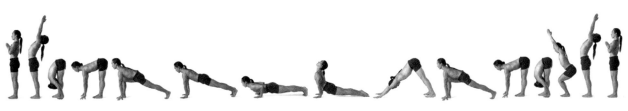

1. Practice two mini **Sun Salutations,** taking 1 breath in each pose and holding Downward-Facing Dog for 5 breaths.

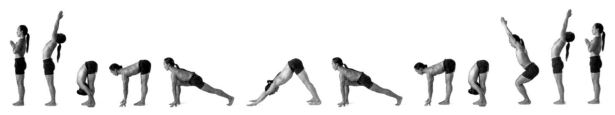

2. Practice three full **Sun Salutations,** taking 1 breath in each pose. Explore Push-Up Pose as follows:

First Salutation:
Practice **Plank Pose**
for 15 seconds.

Second Salutation:
Do version 1 of
Push-Up Pose.

Third Salutation:
Do version 2 of
Push-Up Pose.

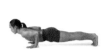

3. Practice **Push-Up Pose** with your feet against the wall for 2 seconds, repeating several times.

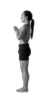

4. Practice two more full **Sun Salutations** with version 3 of Push-Up Pose, if possible. Stay in each pose for 1 breath and breathe naturally between the poses.

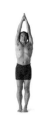

5. Practice **Mountain Pose** for 30 seconds.

6. Practice **Volcano Pose** for 30 seconds.

7. Practice **Warrior 2 Pose** for 45 seconds on each side.

8. Practice **Standing Forward Bend** for 1 minute.

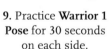

9. Practice **Warrior 1 Pose** for 30 seconds on each side.

10. Practice **Standing Forward Bend** for 30 seconds.

11. Practice **Pyramid Pose** for 1 minute on each side.

12. Practice **Standing Forward Bend** for 30 seconds.

13. Practice version 3 of **Reclined Cobbler's Pose** for 2 minutes.

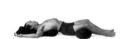

14. Relaxation and Breath Awareness. For 5 minutes, practice version 1 of **Supported Relaxation Pose** (page 268). Allow both your inhalation and your exhalation to be smooth by relaxing more completely.

15. Meditation. For 5 to 10 minutes, sit against the wall in **Seated Crossed-Legs Pose.** Sit on a block or folded blanket if necessary. Place pillows under your arms, and work your arms against the wall so your chest is open. Meditate on your heart, both your phys-ical heart and your heart's emotional center. Take this direction of meditating on your heart as a very literal meditation, and try to feel your heart organ. Take it also as a metaphorical direction, and meditate on your emotional center.

DAY 4: LEARNING UPWARD-FACING DOG POSE

Upward-Facing Dog Pose relies on your leg strength and the same leg action you learned in Downward-Facing Dog and Push-Up Pose. Your legs are the foundation for the backbending of your spine, teaching you to do the pose without straining your lower back. Your arm placement is also important so your wrists don't get strained. To properly align your arms, position your upper arms and forearms directly above the heels of your hands. To ensure that your arms and wrists are correctly aligned, you may have to readjust the placement of your feet.

Today's sequence begins with Cat Pose and version 1 of Upward-Facing Bow Pose (Cobra Pose) to bring awareness of how your entire spine aids the general arching of your back. You then practice moving from Downward-Facing Dog to Upward-Facing Dog, which teaches how to make the transition in the Sun Salutations. After working on all the Upward-Facing Dog variations, you move to the standing poses to bring your spine more toward its natural center. Cobbler's Pose and Reclined Cobbler's Pose balance and support your lower back and help bring your spine back to neutral.

FOCUS FOR THIS PRACTICE:

- In Upward-Facing Dog, don't strain your neck. Let the movement of your head emerge from the lift of your chest.

- In the standing poses, extend your arms while also drawing them into the sockets.

- In the restorative poses, bring extra awareness to your lower ribs and diaphragm.

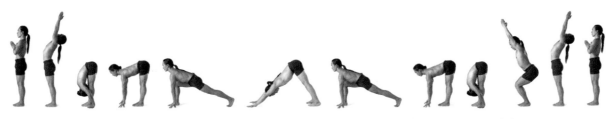

1. Practice two mini **Sun Salutations**, staying in each pose for 1 breath and breathing naturally between poses.

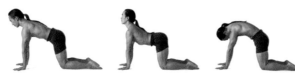

2. Practice **Cat Pose** four times in each position.

3. Practice version 1 of **Upward-Facing Dog (Cobra Pose)** two times. Move slowly in and out of the pose, but do not hold it. Breathe normally.

4. Practice **Downward-Facing Dog** for 1 minute.

5. Practice version 2 of **Upward-Facing Dog** for 5 to 10 seconds. Repeat two or three times.

6. Practice **Downward-Facing Dog** for 1 minute.

7. Practice version 3 of **Upward-Facing Dog** for 5 to 10 seconds. Repeat two or three times.

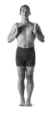

8. Practice version 2 of **Mountain Pose** for 30 seconds to 1 minute.

9. Practice four full **Sun Salutations**, with an emphasis on exploring version 3 of Upward-Facing Dog. Stay in all the poses except Upward-Facing Dog for 1 breath, breathing naturally between the poses. Stay in Upward-Facing Dog for 3 to 5 breaths.

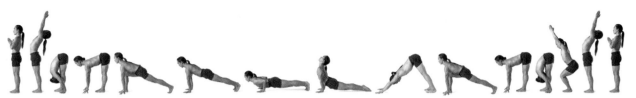

First Upward Dog: Do version 1 of Upward-Facing Dog.

Second Upward Dog: Keep your hips high and rotate your legs internally.

Third Upward Dog: Drop your tailbone between your legs while keeping your legs strong.

Fourth Upward Dog: Play with shrugging your shoulders up toward your ears and then back down again. Try to find a middle ground.

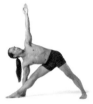

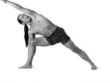

10. Practice **Triangle Pose** for 1 minute on each side.

11. Practice **Tree Pose** for 45 seconds on each side.

12. Practice **Standing Forward Bend** for 1 minute.

13. Practice **Extended Side Angle Pose** for 45 seconds on each side.

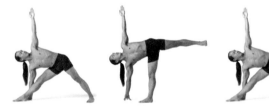

14. Practice **Triangle** to **Half Moon** to **Triangle** series, for 15 seconds, 30 seconds, and 5 seconds on each side.

15. Practice **Pyramid Pose** for 1 minute on each side.

16. Practice **Standing Forward Bend** for 30 seconds.

17. Practice **Cobbler's Pose** for 1 minute.

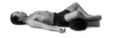

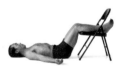

18. Practice version 1 of **Reclined Cobbler's Pose** for 3 minutes.

19. Relaxation and Breath Awareness. For 2 minutes, practice version 2 of **Supported Relaxation Pose** (see page 268). For 5 minutes, sit in a chair and observe your breath. Inhale and exhale smoothly through your nose as you are attentive to how the breath moves through your nose.

20. Meditation. For 5 to 10 minutes, sit in a chair and mentally scan your body. Start with the crown of your head and move your mind and your breath down to the soles of your feet, at an even speed. Notice all the sensations of your body, especially the alignment—your head

balancing over your chest, your chest balancing over your pelvis, your pelvis balancing over your sitting bones, and your legs actively pressing your thighs into the chair and your feet into the ground.

DAY 5: BREATHING IN SUN SALUTATIONS

Once you learn the general configuration of the Sun Salutation, it becomes an ideal sequence for learning how to follow your breath. In today's practice, I provide general directions on how to move with your breath in a Sun Salutation. However, what will actually take place when you begin to follow your breath is more subtle and refined. Because we are so conditioned to lead from our brains, it sometimes takes us years to truly follow our breath.

As you practice the Sun Salutations, explore the quality of gracefulness. When your body and mind are bridged by your breath and your body begins to move with its rhythm, you will naturally feel fluid and relaxed.

As you practice the standing poses, bring to them the same quality of gracefulness so you can feel the thread of movement that interweaves the whole prac-

tice from beginning to end. If you focus on your breath not only in all the postures but also in all the transitions, you will begin to feel your entire physical movement as a flow.

FOCUS FOR THIS PRACTICE:

- In Sun Salutation, move your neck and head from your belly. Feel the movement of your neck start from the elongation of your waist.

- In the standing poses, extend your lower ribs away from your pelvis, equally on all sides.

- In Standing Forward Bend, play with the positions of your shoulders, feeling the integration of your shoulder blades, collarbones, and upper arm bones.

1. Practice the following sequence three times, focusing on moving with your breath.

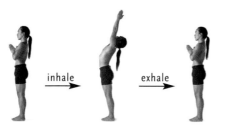

2. Practice the following sequence three times, focusing on moving with your breath.

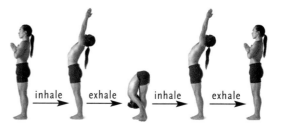

3. Practice the following sequence one time, moving with your breath.

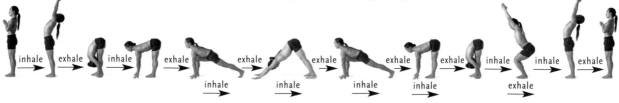

4. Practice two mini **Sun Salutations** (below), moving with your breath.

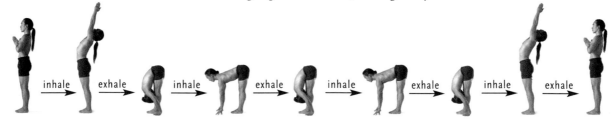

5. Practice four full **Sun Salutations** (below), focusing on moving with your breath.

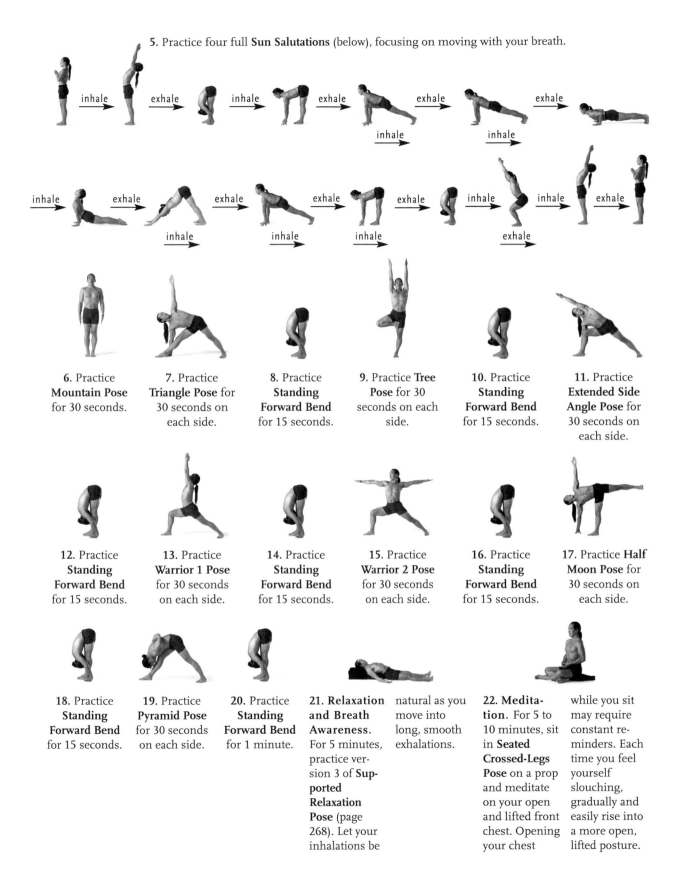

6. Practice **Mountain Pose** for 30 seconds.

7. Practice **Triangle Pose** for 30 seconds on each side.

8. Practice **Standing Forward Bend** for 15 seconds.

9. Practice **Tree Pose** for 30 seconds on each side.

10. Practice **Standing Forward Bend** for 15 seconds.

11. Practice **Extended Side Angle Pose** for 30 seconds on each side.

12. Practice **Standing Forward Bend** for 15 seconds.

13. Practice **Warrior 1 Pose** for 30 seconds on each side.

14. Practice **Standing Forward Bend** for 15 seconds.

15. Practice **Warrior 2 Pose** for 30 seconds on each side.

16. Practice **Standing Forward Bend** for 15 seconds.

17. Practice **Half Moon Pose** for 30 seconds on each side.

18. Practice **Standing Forward Bend** for 15 seconds.

19. Practice **Pyramid Pose** for 30 seconds on each side.

20. Practice **Standing Forward Bend** for 1 minute.

21. Relaxation and Breath Awareness. For 5 minutes, practice version 3 of **Supported Relaxation Pose** (page 268). Let your inhalations be natural as you move into long, smooth exhalations.

22. Meditation. For 5 to 10 minutes, sit in **Seated Crossed-Legs Pose** on a prop and meditate on your open and lifted front chest. Opening your chest while you sit may require constant reminders. Each time you feel yourself slouching, gradually and easily rise into a more open, lifted posture.

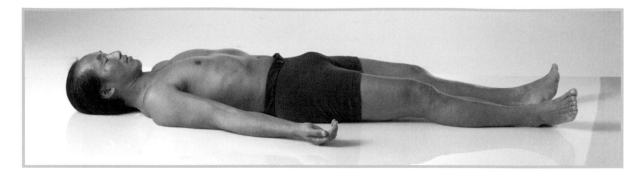

Breath Awareness

For 3 minutes, practice Relaxation Pose by scanning your body, from your feet to your head and then from your head to your feet.

Focus on relaxing your legs and arms first. Then focus on relaxing your head, neck, and torso. As you feel yourself relaxing deeply from head to toe, you have prepared yourself for the following breath awareness technique.

RECEIVING YOUR INHALATIONS. Usually when you start to think about your inhalations, you have a tendency to work your neck and facial muscles because you associate inhaling with the act of *doing*. In general, this is because you feel that to receive something, you must do something to achieve it. But for this eight-week program, I want you to experiment with the opposite approach. Consider that your inhalations are manifested by your ability to *receive*— that is, by your relaxation into receptivity. Imagine that all the doors of every cell in your body are blown open by your incoming breath, that you do not have to open the doors or windows of your body as it is their nature to swing open as the breeze of your breath is invited in.

SOFTENING YOUR EYES AND FOREHEAD. For 5 to 10 minutes, feel the backs of your eyes and the skin of your forehead soften as you inhale. When these two areas contract or tighten on your inhalation, it is from your habit of feeling that your inhalation takes place through effort. If you ask most people to take a deep breath, instead of relaxing more and letting the breath fill their body naturally, they will aggressively pull in the air. But this creates tension in your neck, brain, and sense organs. Retraining the way you take your inhalations is one of the most important exercises for relieving stress. If you continue to practice associating deep relaxation with every inhalation you take, you will find a natural balance.

While you inhale, you will notice that your belly rises. As you learned during your first week of breath awareness, focusing on the rise and fall of your belly can help you soften any pressure in your head as you inhale. Imagine your body is full of liquid, and as you inhale, the liquid flows from your brain down to your torso into the rise of your belly. As you exhale from these soft, relaxed inhalations, imagine the liquid flows from your lower abdomen toward your nose. It is important to continue the feeling of softness in your neck, head, and sense organs. As you listen to the smooth sound of your exhalation, let it soothe your nervous system as if it were a cool summer breeze moving over the surface of a quiet river. This is a good practice to do at any time during the day, whenever it comes to mind.

Meditation

For 5 to 10 minutes, sit in Seated Crossed-Legs Pose against the wall, with your hips on a block or folded blanket and your legs and ankles supported if desired. Bring your shoulder blades into contact with the wall, with your elbows lightly touching the wall. Turn your palms upward on your thighs. Use the wall to make yourself aware of when your posture begins to collapse. Gradually elongate and widen your back body along the wall. Let the back of your head touch the wall and elongate from the base of your pelvis.

ARCHITECTURE OF YOUR BODY. After taking the time to support your legs and your spine, give yourself to the sitting meditation. Unless the sensations are extreme, any physical sensations, even painful ones, that come up will probably not cause any injuries, so see if you can sit completely still for 5 minutes. Just this suggestion will probably create some resistance. Notice that resistance in your mind, body, and breath, and see if you can let it go. Begin to meditate on the general architecture of your body by scanning from the crown of your head to the soles of your feet slowly enough so you are cognizant of the shape of your body and how the breath is moving through it. Check your contact with the wall periodically to see how it has shifted and check the elongation of your waist and your sense of lifting from a strong feeling of grounding.

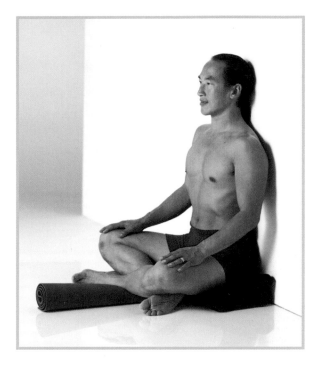

NONJUDGMENT. If you dedicate yourself to sitting 5 to 10 minutes a day, you will begin to notice from day to day the radical difference in how your mind and body respond. At first there is a tendency to judge your meditation, as in, Oh, today was quiet and yesterday I was really agitated, so I think it's improving. But I believe one of the most important reasons to meditate is to notice that meditation itself changes all the time, and there is no need to place a judgment on what has taken place.

CAT POSE

Cat Pose allows you to explore your spine, bringing
understanding and health through its full articulation.

POINT OF PLAY:
Making small movements with
your spine to feel its fluidity.

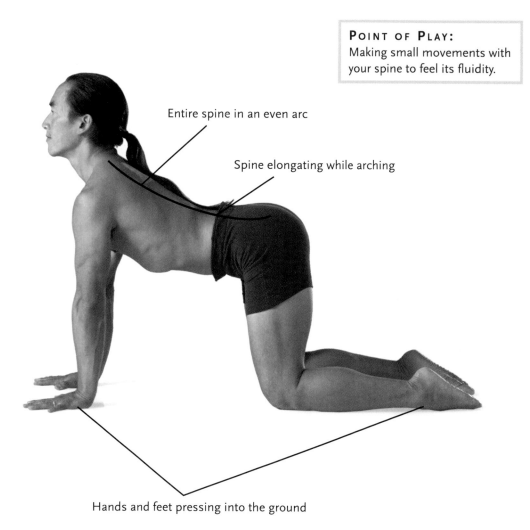

Entire spine in an even arc

Spine elongating while arching

Hands and feet pressing into the ground

VOLCANO POSE

Volcano Pose helps you find the full linear extension
of your body.

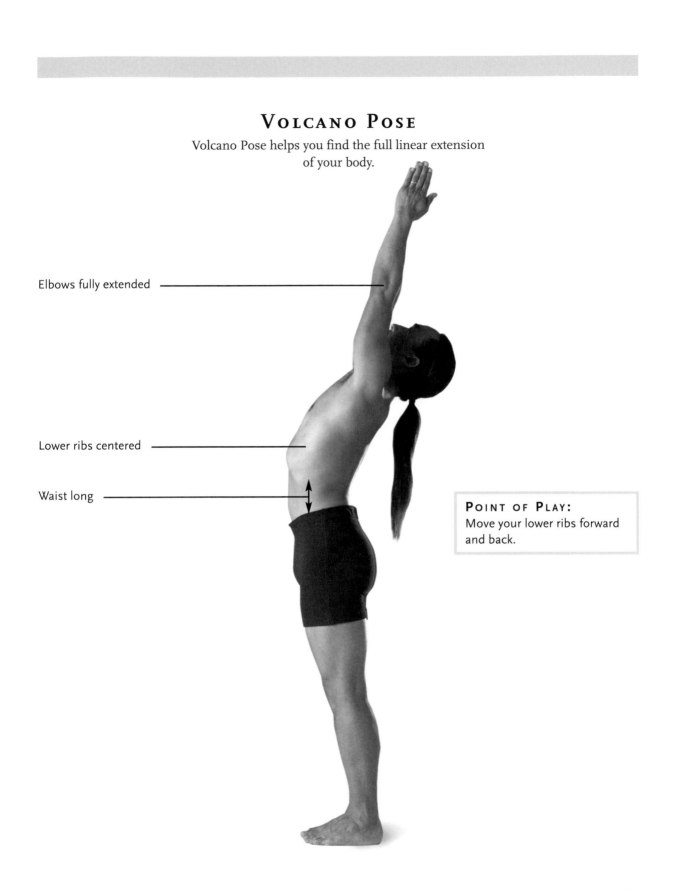

Elbows fully extended

Lower ribs centered

Waist long

POINT OF PLAY:
Move your lower ribs forward
and back.

EXTENDED STANDING FORWARD BEND

Extended Standing Forward Bend opens your chest and
extends your spine from the strength of your legs.

> **POINT OF PLAY:**
> Bend your legs, while lifting
> your chest. Straighten your
> legs, while keeping your chest
> lifted.

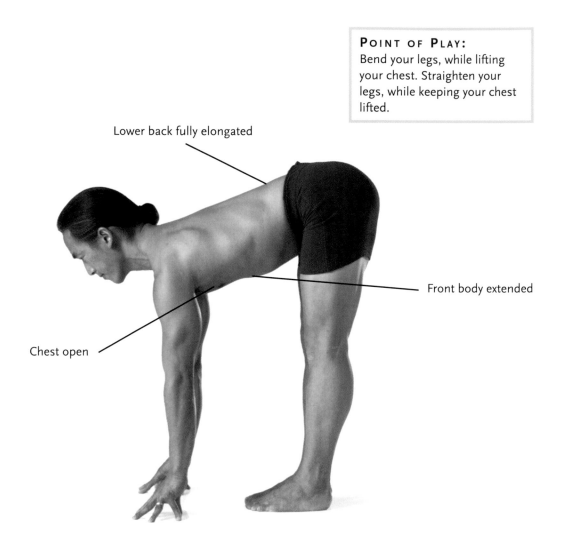

Lower back fully elongated

Front body extended

Chest open

LUNGE

Lunge gathers the force of both legs into your spine even as it
teaches you how to move them in opposition.

Chest and head moving forward

POINT OF PLAY:
Raise and lower your hips.

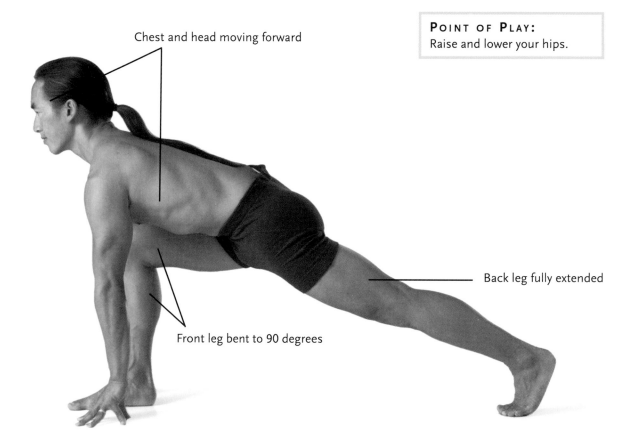

Back leg fully extended

Front leg bent to 90 degrees

POWERFUL POSE

Powerful Pose supports your spine from the
power of your legs.

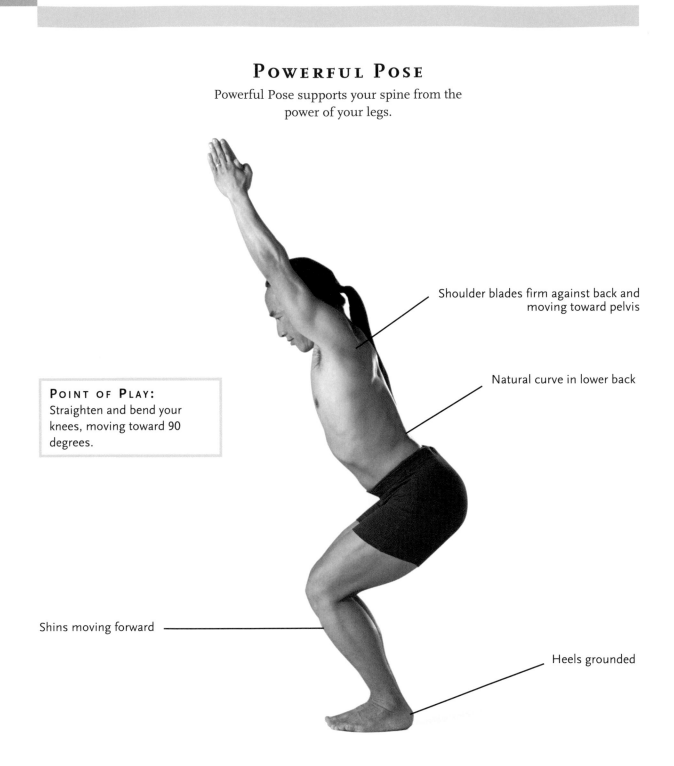

Shoulder blades firm against back and
moving toward pelvis

Natural curve in lower back

POINT OF PLAY:
Straighten and bend your
knees, moving toward 90
degrees.

Shins moving forward

Heels grounded

PLANK POSE

Plank Pose demands the integration of the strength of your
legs and arms with the length and support of your spine.

Looking forward

Chest open

POINT OF PLAY:
Lift and lower your pelvis,
searching for alignment.

Pelvis in line with legs and chest

Legs powerful, extended fully

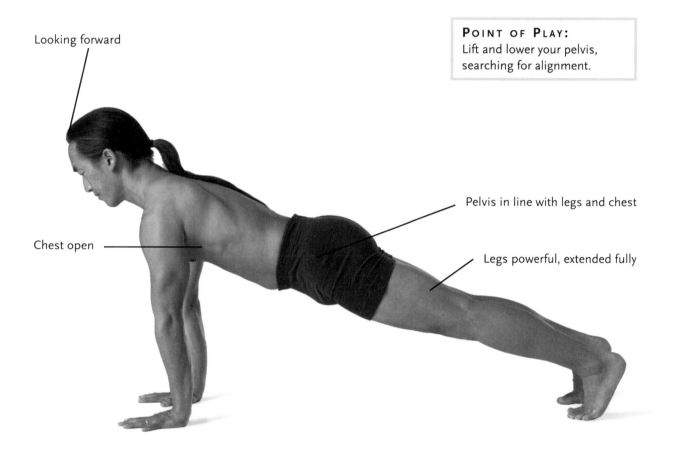

PUSH-UP POSE

Push-Up Pose integrates the strength of your legs and torso
with the strength of your arms.

POINT OF PLAY:
Extend your heels back while
moving your chest forward.

Legs strong, reaching through inner heels

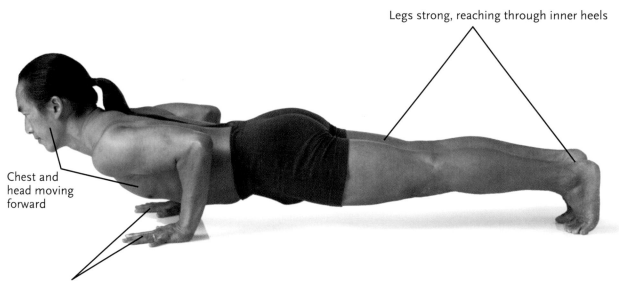

Chest and
head moving
forward

Inner hands pressing down

UPWARD-FACING DOG POSE

Upward-Facing Dog Pose integrates your legs with your entire spine, rejuvenating and revitalizing your spine.

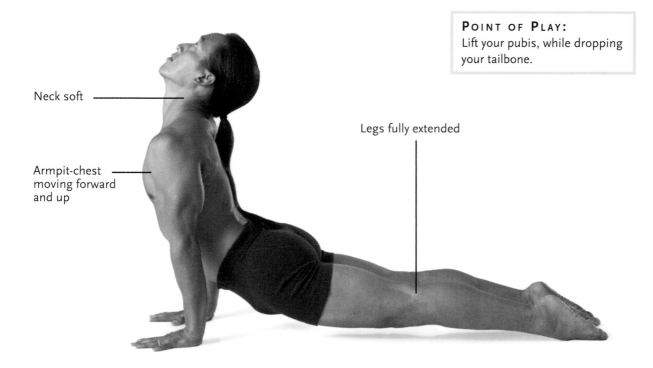

POINT OF PLAY:
Lift your pubis, while dropping your tailbone.

Neck soft

Legs fully extended

Armpit-chest moving forward and up

STAFF POSE

Staff Pose helps you connect to the earth to
elongate your spine.

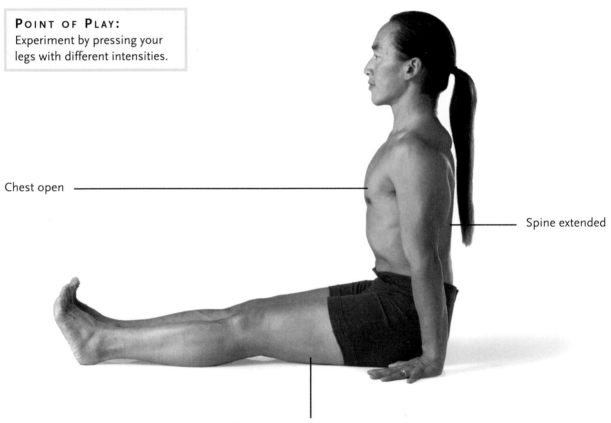

POINT OF PLAY:
Experiment by pressing your
legs with different intensities.

Chest open

Spine extended

Backs of legs pressing toward the ground

COBBLER'S POSE

Cobbler's Pose opens your hips to maximize the transfer of energy from your legs to your spine.

POINT OF PLAY:
Rock your pelvis back and forth.

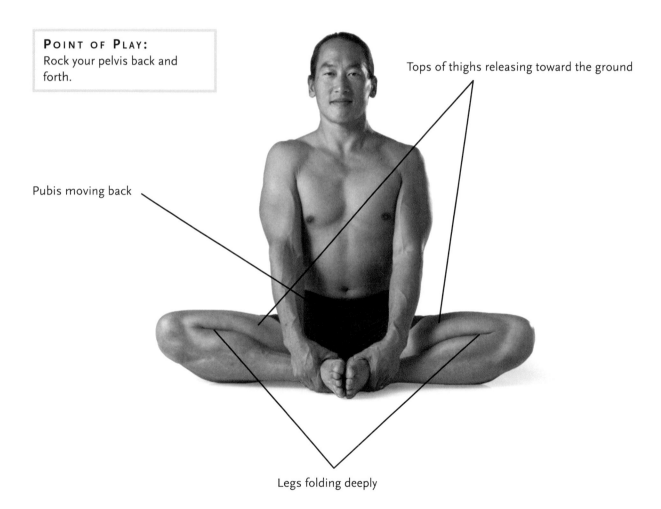

Tops of thighs releasing toward the ground

Pubis moving back

Legs folding deeply

RECLINED COBBLER'S POSE

Reclined Cobbler's Pose opens your chest and pelvis,
teaching you to relax with your vulnerability.

POINT OF PLAY:
Experiment with moving your
feet closer to and farther from
your hips.

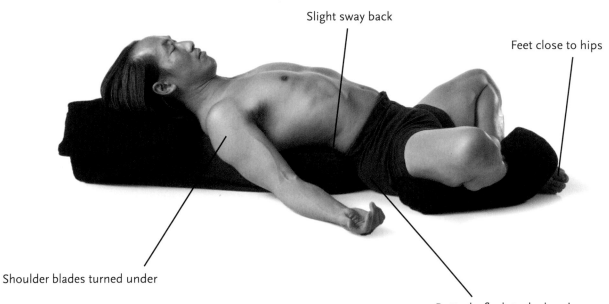

Slight sway back

Feet close to hips

Shoulder blades turned under

Buttocks flesh tucked under you

CONSTRUCTIVE REST POSE

Constructive Rest Pose allows you to exhale with ease.

POINT OF PLAY:
Practice breathing with a smooth exhalation, pausing briefly at the end of your exhalation.

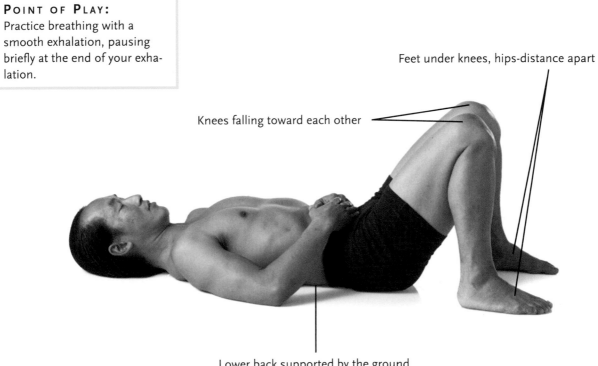

Feet under knees, hips-distance apart

Knees falling toward each other

Lower back supported by the ground

SEATED CROSSED-LEGS POSE

Seated Crossed-Legs Pose is the basic meditation pose, teaching you the relationship between posture, ease of breath, and steadiness of mind.

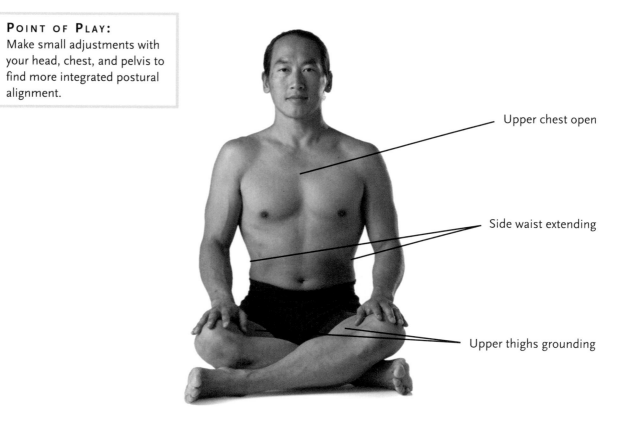

Upper chest open

Side waist extending

Upper thighs grounding

To reestablish contact with your body is to be in contact with the cosmos. Balance is restored, space is around us and that tremendous power, arising from the earth in unison with the true universal forces, will become part of us.

—Vanda Scaravelli, *Awakening the Spine*

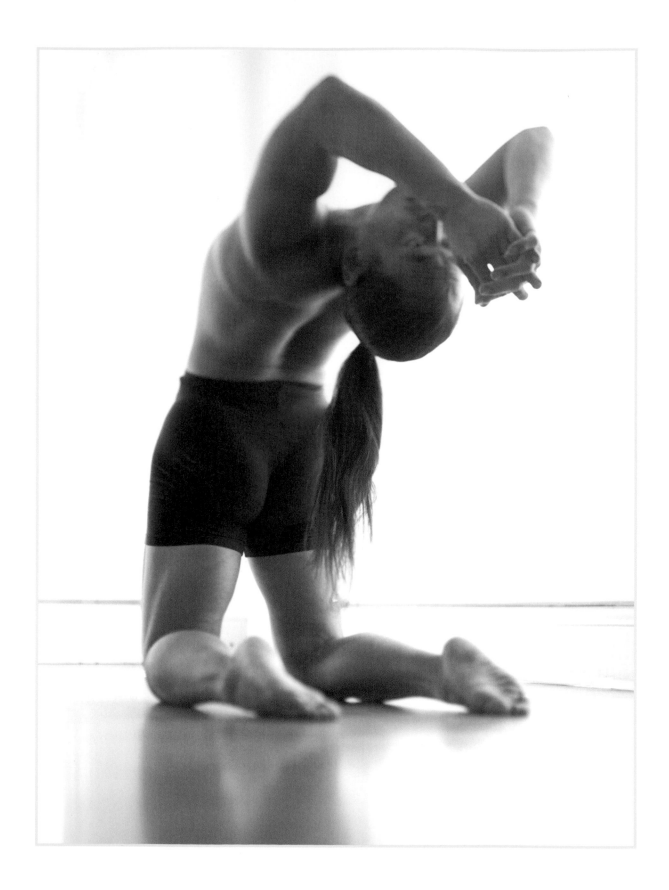

WEEK 3:

Opening into Vulnerability

AS ANIMALS, WE INSTINCTIVELY KNOW THAT WE MUST PROTECT OUR VITAL ORGANS, OUR THROAT, AND our face, so we have a natural protective response to cover our front bodies. But when you do a backbend, you take a position that is the antithesis of your natural protective posture and intentionally expose the soft parts of your body, which in an animal, when on all fours, are always protected. Therefore, while backbends will feel liberating, they will also be very difficult because your body feels so vulnerable. You may have both physical and emotional resistance to doing backbends and will need to muster up your physical and emotional strength to move in this direction.

By opening your front body, you demonstrate a willingness to be in the world, to feel, to be hurt, to be ecstatic. Backbends allow your emotional body to be receptive and responsive. As a human being, it is vital for you to feel connected to the world around you, but if your heart is always guarded, the walls become too thick to allow that connection. The fact is that we are already connected and it's an illusion to think that you can hide or protect yourself so much that you will be completely safe. In fact, the more vulnerable you allow yourself to be, the more connected you are, which enables you to listen and respond to what is occurring in the present moment. But if you hide in the illusion that you can be safe and protected, you end up responding and reacting only to what's in your head. And that lack of awareness and connection can create a dangerous situation. For instance, if you become frozen with fear and shut down, there is no way you can respond appropriately to a given situation.

The act of being able to feel—to *truly feel*—is important for balance, whether physical, mental, or emotional. A lot of people are doing yoga with a sense of performance but with no sense of vulnerability. What is needed instead is a willingness to fall in balance poses, to lose control in backbends, to feel unprotected on a physical level, and to challenge the survival mechanisms of your body. Because you tend to protect your body, your body will become physically unbalanced if you never move toward openness and vulnerability. Also, when you walk (your most common way of moving through the world), you are basically falling forward and catching yourself. So it is unfamiliar to feel your head move behind your chest and your chest move behind your pelvis. Most people have a tendency to lean forward all the time and they feel secure in that position. So to open up in backbends creates a sense of losing control, of being vulnerable, and of being out of "normal" balance. But, in fact, backbends will bring you back into center and into a more neutral state.

About Backbends

Our natural tendency to protect our heart and lungs, both physically and emotionally, closes and binds the muscles in our shoulders, arms, upper chest, and lower back. In fact, the habitual posture for most of us is somewhat bent forward from our everyday work and from our emotional and physical protecting. However, although this habitual posture may feel natural to you, it is also quite detrimental to your body's functioning and to the vulnerability and receptivity of your heart. Therefore, backbends are the yoga poses that will rebalance your spine, shoulders, neck, and pelvis.

The sequences this week will teach you many ways to challenge your habit of protecting yourself. To practice standing in the center between front and back requires you to retool your awareness and confront your fears. The active backbends are vigorous poses, requiring at first much determination and effort. Eventually the opening will become less effortful and more subtle, but it is always profound. Passive backbends between active backbends help you rest your back muscles while still opening your front body, to help you avoid overusing your back muscles.

EMOTIONS. The backbends open the door to your heart *chakra*, which is the emotional center of your entire body. Your "emotional body," where you experience both joy and grief, is centered in this chest cavity. Opening the door to your heart *chakra* means having both a willingness to connect to your emotional center—to feel intense movements of joy and happiness as well as despair and grief—and a willingness to connect to the outside world from your emotional body. I believe your heart and lungs are so

sensitive that regardless of whether or not you put walls around them, they will continue to feel the emotional landscape of the present moment, just as when parents think they are protecting a child from feeling a certain situation—a divorce or a death of a family member—the child feels it anyway. By opening your chest with backbends, you will become more conscious of your feelings and the emotional atmosphere of your environment.

FOCUS OF YOUR MIND. In backbends focus your mind on bringing your spine into an even arc, so that every part of your spine, shoulders, and hips open evenly and no single point is stressed. While doing a backbend, most of you will have a great deal of movement in a few places, such as in your lower back or at the point where your lower ribs meet your lower back. Because of the natural mobility in these areas, it is easy to rely on *only* these areas to perform the backbends. As you strive for evenness, become acutely aware of where your bindings and weaknesses are, so you can intelligently open up your bindings and build up strength in your weak areas.

ELONGATION. It is important not to compress your spine or your shoulder or hip joints while doing a backbend. Therefore, you must learn to elongate out of your joints while you are bending your back. Your ability to elongate depends on how you integrate the use of your legs and arms in the backbend. Learn how to use the strength of your legs to create support for the length of your spine and how to use your arms to help lift and support your chest without creating

ANATOMY LESSON

1. Top of your sacrum, tailbone, and shoulder blades

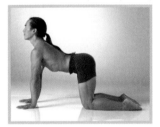 To learn about the relationship between the top of your sacrum, your tailbone, and your shoulder blades, practice Constructive Rest Pose and play with tucking and untucking your tailbone. Observe the effect this action has on your entire sacrum. As you feel your sacrum come into its most neutral position—with the top of the sacrum slightly off the ground—move your shoulder blades to observe their relationship with the sacrum. Firm the bottom tips of your shoulder blades into your back as your shoulder blades themselves move down toward your pelvis and broaden from the spine.

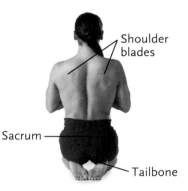

2. Spine

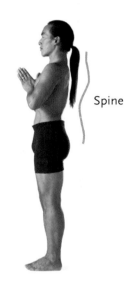 To learn about your spine, practice Cat Pose and move your spine in every possible way. Undulate your entire spine, from the tip of your tailbone to the base of your skull.

3. Hip flexors

To learn about your hip flexors, practice version 2 or 3 of Supported Bridge Pose and use your hands to feel how the fronts of your thighs connect with the front of your pelvis. Don't be scared to dig into your belly with your fingers to feel some of the deeper muscles that connect the front of your spine with the fronts of your legs. As you touch this area, try bending and straightening the leg on the side you are touching.

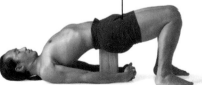

compression or dislocation in your shoulder joints or your upper spine. Finding this integration takes more than effort and determination; it takes inquiry, playfulness, and observation.

BREATH. Initially most of you will feel that you have to push full out even to begin to get the movements and strength required to lift into some of the backbends. When you use so much determination and effort, you may find yourself holding your breath and gripping your neck and facial muscles. If so, focus on learning to breathe while you're working your arms and legs and back muscles vigorously. Using a little less muscular effort and keeping a continuous breath while you are in the backbends will help you build these poses much more quickly and maybe even allow them to be delightful.

SHOULDERS. Backbends teach you how to integrate your shoulder blades, upper arms, and collarbones to create much more efficiency in your shoulder joints. This in turn teaches you how to move your shoulder joints to return to good posture. In ad-

dition, the placement of your shoulders—including your shoulder blades, upper arms, and collar bones—is key to relaxing your neck, one of the most important areas to relax in order to reduce stress.

SPINE. Your spine, made up of 26 vertebrae and 27 joints, is capable of much strength, fluidity, and possibility of movement. It is a shame that most of us rarely articulate our spines at all, which is one reason our spines deteriorate. Using backbends to play with your spine and begin to feel movement up and down its entirety can be a source of much joy and health.

PELVIS. Sitting for prolonged periods of time and most sports (running, tennis, soccer, basketball) tighten the fronts of your pelvis and thighs. Backbends open up the fronts of your hip joints to bring them back to balance. After doing backbends, it feels great to let your legs hang from your pelvis so that as you stand upright you don't feel like you are fighting against major restrictions. The leg muscles that run through your pelvis can be supple and strong, like the body of a cat, instead of constricted and bound.

DAY 1: LEARNING THE VARIATIONS

When you try all the backbend variations, move gradually into the poses. By working slowly, you can feel how your whole spine articulates with your legs and arms. You will learn so much about your shoulders, your spine, and your pelvis doing these poses. Although deepening your backbends is fun and exhilarating, there is much greater benefit in integrating your backbends so you have a sense of ease and breath. If you push to your maximum, you may shut off your ability to observe and breathe, which is not the optimum way to move toward understanding.

MOVING IN AND OUT OF BACKBENDS

When you move into a backbend, you have an innate tendency to prepare for struggle. But if you can clear your mind by focusing it on the ease of your breath and the foundation of the pose, you can then move into the backbend from a place of receptivity and presence. While in a backbend, continually adjust the distance between your hands and feet to find the maximum traction and elongation of your spine. As you come out of a backbend, continue the action of the backbend so that as you begin to come out, your sense of elongation and support will carry on as you slowly lower down. After you have come fully out of the pose, spend time scanning your body, feeling not only the effects of the pose, but noticing where you have created any difficulty or jamming so that the next time you can make the pose more even. In the beginning it is much better to repeat the backbends more often than to hold them for a long period of time. This will let your body warm up sufficiently, without making your muscles lock or harden around your spine to protect it.

In general, move into and out of backbends gradually and mindfully.

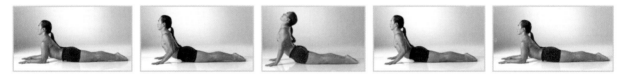

This photo sequence illustrates moving in and out of Cobra Pose.

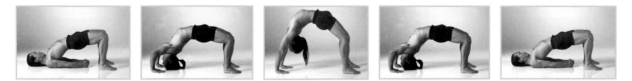

This photo sequence illustrates moving in and out of Upward Bow Pose.

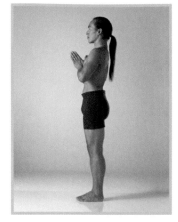

1. Practice two mini **SUN SALUTATIONS** (page 87), taking
   5 breaths in Downward-Facing Dog. Focus on the fluidity
   of your spine coming from the strength of your legs.

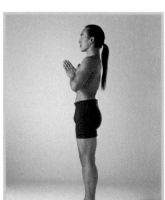
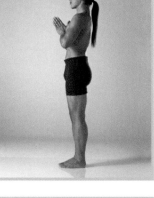

2. Practice two full **SUN SALUTATIONS** (page 91), taking
   5 breaths in the second Downward-Facing Dog. Integrate
   the strength of your arms with the elongation of your waist
   and the openness of your chest.

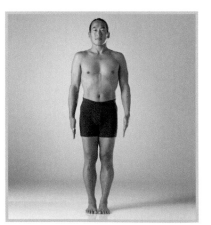

3. Practice **MOUNTAIN POSE** for 15 seconds. Feel the lift of
   your armpit-chest.

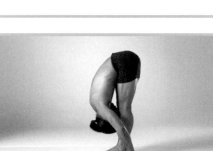

4. Practice **TRIANGLE POSE** for 30 seconds on each side. Notice the natural curves of your lower back.

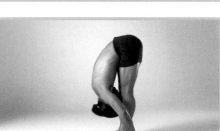

5. PRACTICE STANDING FORWARD BEND for 15 seconds. Broaden all the muscles of your lower back.

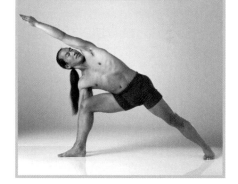

6. Practice **EXTENDED SIDE ANGLE POSE** for 30 seconds on each side. Elongate your back lower ribs away from your pelvis.

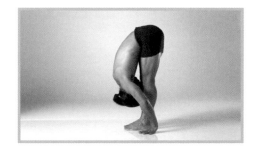

7. Practice **STANDING FORWARD BEND** for 15 seconds. Allow your neck to be soft.

8. Try all three versions of **COBRA POSE** *(Bhujangasana)* for 10 seconds in each version.

VERSION 1: Elbows bent, forearms on the ground

In this version, you can focus on elongating as well as arching your back. With your forearms on the ground and your elbows directly below your shoulders, pull your chest forward strongly. Reach your legs away from your torso, separating your pelvis from your legs and beginning its journey toward vertical. This action will lengthen your waist and gradually create an even arc of your spine. Drop the top of your sacrum into your body, feeling its muscular connection with the bottom tips of your shoulder blades, and draw your tailbone toward your pubis.

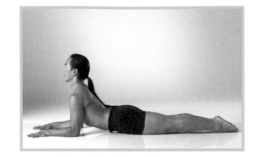

VERSION 2: Arms bent, hands on the ground

This version allows you to find an ease of breath and an even fluidity of your spine because you can adjust your chest to any height by bending your arms more or less. Harness your elbows close to your torso, gradually extending your arms to a position where you can lift your chest fully without compressing your lower back. Plant the insides of your hands firmly and strengthen your legs. Be playful and explore the traction of your spine as you move deeper into the backbend. The challenge is to use the appropriate push of your arms while your spine opens up gracefully.

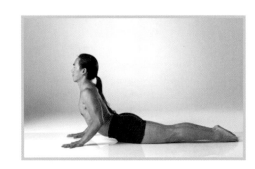

VERSION 3: Full pose, with straight arms

In the full pose, the movement of your hips toward verticality allows you to soften your effort but requires flexibility. To keep your legs on the ground while you fully extend your arms, you must open the fronts of your legs and pelvis. To open the energetic channels from the base of your pelvis into your torso, spiral your legs inward so that your knees move toward each other and your heels move away from each other. Open your spine evenly so the skin on your chest feels as round as a wheel and yet porous and receptive.

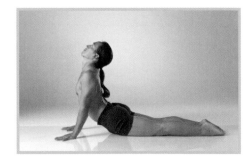

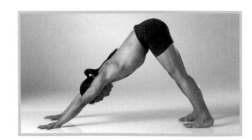

9. Practice **DOWNWARD-FACING DOG** for 15 seconds. Elongate your back waist by moving the back of your pelvis away from your lower back ribs.

10. Try all three versions of **UPWARD-FACING DOG** (*Urdhva Mukha Svanasana*) for 10 seconds in each version.

VERSION 1: Hands on the seat of a chair

This version creates an amazing lift of your chest without requiring extreme flexibility—you feel the upward movement that arises from the strength of your legs and the press of your arms. Do not overextend the sides of your neck, but focus on lifting the sides of your chest and on keeping your legs strong. Let the top of your sacrum fall deeper into your body and firm the bottoms of your shoulder blades into your back. Connecting the movement of your sacrum and shoulder blades, release your tailbone between your legs.

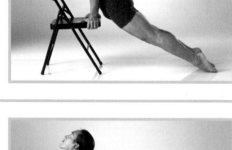

VERSION 2: Hands on same-size blocks

This version reduces the height under your hands, so lifting your chest requires more flexibility and more work from your legs. Reach your legs strongly all the way through your toes, and lift your thighbones upward into your hamstrings. Drop your sacrum and tailbone forward toward your pelvic organs, and draw your belly back to meet them, supporting your lower back and adding elongation. Feel your entire supple spine contribute to the backbending of the pose.

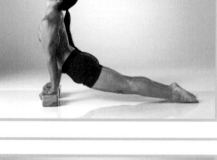

VERSION 3: Full pose, with hands on the ground

It is exhilarating to thrust your upper chest from the even grounding of your feet and hands. To prevent compromising your wrists, keep your arms as vertical as possible and do not move them forward over your fingertips. To lift your legs fully while your spine and pelvis extend vertically, focus on finding an opening between the front of your pelvis and the front of your legs.

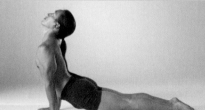

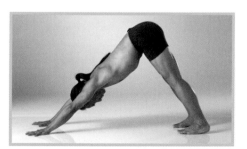

11. Practice **DOWNWARD-FACING DOG** for 15 seconds. Elongate your back waist by moving the back of your pelvis away from your lower back.

12. Try all three versions of **SUPPORTED BRIDGE POSE** *(Setu Bandha Sarvangasana)* for 30 seconds in each version.

VERSION 1: Lowest height of the block (block flat on the ground)

With the block at its lowest height, most of you will feel a delightful comfort. This version allows you to begin the movement of lifting your pelvis while keeping your lower belly supple, your sacrum supported, and your thighs parallel. In this version you can feel all the actions and movements of the pose in their proper form and direction. The challenge is to learn how to engage—and keep engaging—the muscles that support this pose without the block: rolling your upper arms under your chest, pressing your arms into the ground, and using your hamstrings to draw your thigh bones toward the ground as your pelvis lifts. Release your pubis downward toward the block to allow the top of your sacrum to go deeper into your body and connect that movement with the firming of the bottom tips of your shoulder blades. Lengthen your tailbone and move it upward toward your pubis.

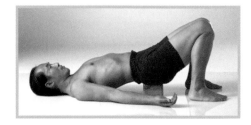

VERSION 2: Middle height of the block (standing on its side)

For some of you, this version will challenge the opening of your hip flexors while you keep your thighs spiraling internally, your knees dropping toward each other, and your heels moving away from each other. With the block at its middle height, you are moving closer to the true configuration of Bridge Pose, where your pelvis will eventually become the highest part of the pose. Explore which muscles you need to relax while discovering which muscles you use to lift your pelvis without externally rotating your thighs or thickening and hardening your belly. Feel the fluidity of your spine as it makes a gentle, complete arc from your sacrum to your upper chest.

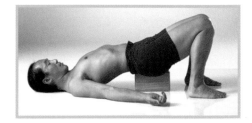

VERSION 3: Full height of the block (standing on its end)

This version provides you with a full opening of your chest, while you also receive the effects of an inverted, supported backbend. When you lift your pelvis this high, you tend to exert all your leg, pelvis, and lower back muscles. Instead, learn to determine which parts of your body to relax, such as your neck, throat, belly, and face, while your hip flexors slowly release and open. Discover how to pattern the actions of your legs so you can push strongly while rotating your thighbones internally. (Note that if you are tall or very flexible, you may need to use more than one block to get a sufficient height.)

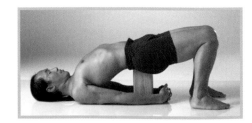

13. Try all three versions of **RECLINED HERO POSE** (*Supta Virasana*) for 30 seconds in each version.

VERSION 1: Blanket between lower leg and hips, blanket on edge of chair, head on backrest of chair

Using the chair as a support for your upper back and head allows you to feel the direction of movement and the opening of the pose without any strain and without having to hold up your body in a seemingly awkward position. The opening of your legs provided by this pose is necessary for the ongoing vitality and health of your lower body, but it is also an extremely foreign movement for most adults. Using the chair allows you to approach this difficulty without injuring yourself or being overly determined. Approach this pose with a sense of ease and make yourself as comfortable as possible. Play with the seesaw action of allowing the top of your sacrum to go deeper into a backbend and then tucking your tailbone toward your pubis. Keep engaging your shoulder blades as you search for ease.

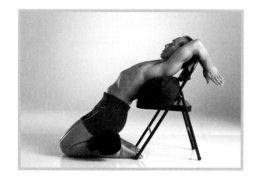

VERSION 2: Leaning back onto a high bolster, arms down along the ground

In this version, lifting your chest helps your breathing and your digestion. Even if you are flexible enough to do the full pose, still practice with a bolster occasionally. Do this pose frequently and challenge yourself to develop by gradually lowering your spine closer and closer to the ground and discovering exactly where your fear and holding exist. Keep elongating your entire spine.

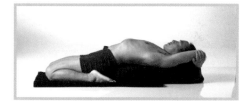

VERSION 3: Full pose, without props, arms extended overhead

This version opens the channels between your torso, pelvis, and legs, and helps rejuvenate the deep muscles of the abdomen and legs. Your hip flexors will be very challenged. See if you can soften them and feel their elongation along the bone. By doing this pose without props, you will learn where your body compensates for any tightness. Maybe your knees will lift off the ground or maybe you'll have a deep sway in your lower back. Be concerned only if the pose causes pain. Create as much length as possible, dropping your thighs toward the ground and drawing your buttocks flesh and tailbone toward the backs of your knees.

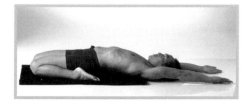

14. Try all three versions of **BOW POSE** *(Dhanurasana)* for 10 seconds in each version.

VERSION 1: On your belly, knees bent, shins up the wall, pushing up with your arms

For those of you who cannot hold your ankles comfortably, this version allows you to take the basic shape of the pose while you lift your chest to any height. In this version, you can begin to build your strength and flexibility with ease. If you feel an acute sensation in any area of your spine or pelvis, try to even out your spine and create as much equality as possible within the pose. Focus on the interplay between the top of your sacrum, shoulder blades, and tailbone.

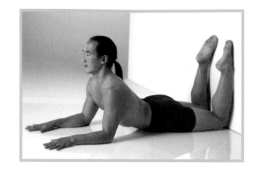

VERSION 2: Holding your feet, but not lifting your legs off the ground; looking forward, not up

This version allows you to elongate the pose first, gradually using the strength of your legs while maintaining their internal spiral. This action keeps the channel of your pelvis open so your legs and spine can be directly connected. Start lifting your chest by moving it forward, and firm your shoulder blades into your back to rotate your armpit-chest circularly into the lift of your collarbones. Not lifting your legs gives you the chance to play with the absorption of your breath and the relaxation of your sense organs. This softness will allow your actions to arise from observation. Run your mind up and down your entire spine, searching for equality.

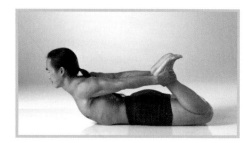

VERSION 3: Full pose, with legs lifted and head facing upward

In any backbend, your alignment is the essential foundation for the liberation of your spine. By lifting your legs, you will begin to understand the vital relationship between your thighbones and your sacrum—your thighbones must lift higher than your sacrum to allow for deep backbending without overusing the lower back. It is essential to concentrate on releasing your body at the hip flexors while stabilizing your lower back. Continue to look for evenness in your backbend so that your legs, pelvis, and spine all contribute to a beautiful arc.

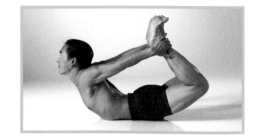

15. Try all three versions of **PASSIVE BACKBEND** *(Matsayasana, modified)* for 1 minute in each version.

VERSION 1: Over a rolled blanket, head on a folded blanket, strap around your upper arms

This version gives a basic lift to your chest and offers the possibility of separating your upper chest from your middle and lower chest. Lifting your head to the same level as your chest keeps your neck from feeling compromised, so your body can relax and surrender its habitual restrictions. Use your breath as a subtle but powerful tool to open all the restrictions in your rib cage. As you keep your legs strong, learn how to stay fluid and responsive in your sacrum, tailbone, and shoulder blades.

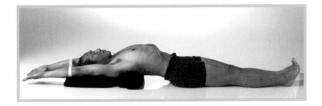

VERSION 2: Over a rolled blanket, head on the ground, strap around upper arms

In this version your neck is allowed to join in and follow the gentle arc of your spine. Once you get past the unusual feeling of having your head lower than your chest, you can visualize—and enjoy—your spine as one graceful, languid arc, from your tailbone to the base of your skull. Let your entire spine be moved and enticed by the motion of your breath. (If this pose creates any strain, do not try the next version.)

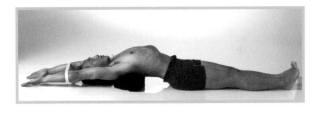

VERSION 3: Over a block positioned under your shoulder blades, strap around upper arms

Against the block's hardness, your back muscles are asked to surrender more completely. The edges of the block will be like the firm and specific press of a masseuse, bringing your mind into very specific places to let go. Often your upper back is nearly frozen. Receiving this direct information from the pressure of the block helps you understand exactly where to free yourself. As your legs extend along the ground and your pelvis rises from your legs, feel your hip flexors relax and open.

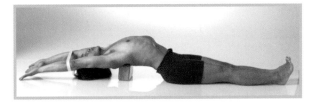

16. Try all three versions of **CAMEL POSE** *(Ustrasana)* for 10 seconds in each version.

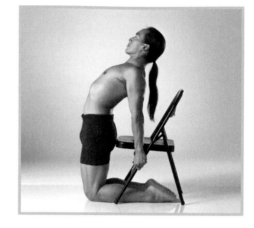

VERSION 1: Hands on the front legs of a chair

This version gives you the necessary height and support to feel the general shape of the pose—your thighs perpendicular to the floor as your shins press into the ground, your sacrum deepening toward your belly, and your chest rising from the foundation of your legs and the support of your arms. As you arch your back, continue to reestablish the length of your spine from the lift of your chest. Continue to find the connection between your firm shoulder blades, the natural arch of your sacrum, and the tucking of your tailbone.

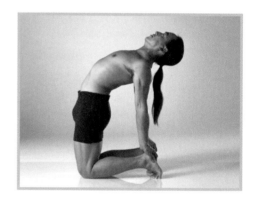

VERSION 2: Feet flexed, hands on your heels

This version adds height and gives you the direct contact of touching your hands to your feet. This connection brings the satisfaction of a feeling of completion and connects a circuit that enlivens the entire pose. Lift your chest first before you fully release your head backward. Focus on descending your shins and ankles downward as you press your sacrum forward and raise your chest higher and higher. (If this is difficult, do not try the next version.) Move through your spine mindfully and feel each successive vertebrae lift off the vertebrae before it.

VERSION 3: Full pose, with tops of feet flat on the floor

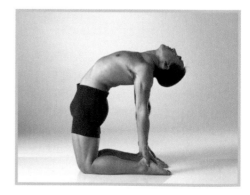

Having your shins flush on the ground and your hands flush against your feet allows you to access the full strength of both your legs and your arms to open your chest as you arch your spine from your tailbone to the crown of your head. Keeping your thighs vertical while having full contact with your hands on your feet will require a firm foundation—press your shins into the ground and press your sacrum toward your belly as your thighbones press into your hamstrings. These actions maximize the opening of your hip flexors.

17. Try all three versions of UPWARD BOW POSE *(Urdhva Dhanurasana)* for 10 seconds (if possible) in each version.

VERSION 1: Bridge Pose without support

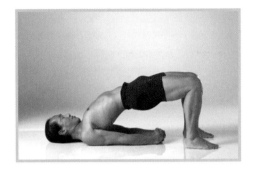

In this version you can focus solely on the lower half of your body moving into your spine. You can learn how to use your legs to lift your pelvis straight up without pushing your weight toward your arms and head. When you try the next two versions, return to this focus—letting your legs initiate the lift of your pelvis—and you will have the beginnings of an integrated pose. Continue to articulate the relationship between the top of your sacrum, your tailbone, and the bottom tips of your shoulder blades.

VERSION 2: On the top of your head

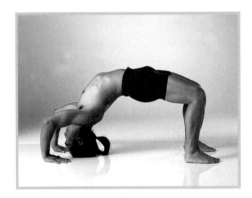

By coming onto the top of your head, you integrate your entire spine. Using this as a midway point before pushing up into the full pose allows you to make necessary adjustments in your arms, legs, and spine before you engage the muscular effort to take the full backbend. As you rest lightly on your head, draw your shoulder blades toward your pelvis and firm them against your back, move your arms into their sockets, and keep the internal spiral of your legs. Taking these actions, you begin to understand the direction of movement necessary to keep the channels of your breath free and the channels of your arms and legs moving into your spine.

VERSION 3: Full pose, with straight arms (if possible)

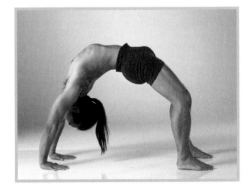

This pose takes a concerted integration of coordination, strength, and flexibility. For most of you there will be limited flexibility in your hips, part of your spine, or your shoulders, which will make you work far too aggressively just to "get up." However, if you come to this pose consistently, with both observation and persistence, your body will open up. The exhilaration and excitement that comes from the expanse of this posture is unparalleled. We all have a tendency in this pose to work everything. Learning to distinguish between what you need to work and what you need to surrender is an ongoing process that will lead you to a balanced pose of ease and steadiness.

18. Try all three versions of **RECLINED LEG STRETCH POSE** *(Supta Padangusthasana)* for 1 minute in each version, on each side.

VERSION 1: Bottom foot against wall, strap around top foot

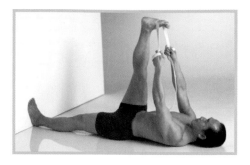

Placing your foot on the wall reminds you to give attention to your bottom leg, the anchor of this pose. The strap allows you to maintain the alignment of your spine and shoulders and the openness of your chest. Challenge yourself to find the full extension of your knees, the broadness of your chest, and the grounding of your bottom leg. Even in this reclined pose, feel the top of your sacrum move toward a backbend as your shoulder blades engage with it and your tailbone finds its natural tuck.

VERSION 2: In the middle of the room, strap around top foot

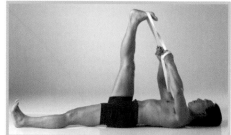

With your foot off the wall, be especially attentive to the alignment and grounding of your bottom leg. Feel how the activity of your feet and legs surges through your pelvis into the elongation of your torso and the opening of your upper chest. It is so tempting to pull strongly on your top leg; instead, see if you can awaken your entire body evenly. Feel the undulation and suppleness of your entire spine.

VERSION 3: Holding your big toe

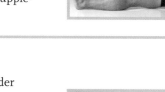

If you can keep your bottom leg grounded and your shoulder blade on the floor while doing so, try holding your big toe instead of using a strap. Use this direct circuitry to go even deeper into your breath and into the subtle alignment qualities of the pose. However, if holding your big toe distorts your top foot, rotate your bottom leg (which should rotate internally); if it contorts the shoulder of the arm that is holding your foot, go back to version 2 until your hip flexors can drop back into your body and not be challenged.

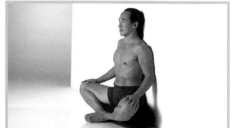

19. Practice version 1 of **COBBLER'S POSE** for 2 minutes. Feel the release of your inner thighs and the elongation of your waist.

20. Try all three versions of **HAPPY BABY POSE** for 30 seconds in each version.

VERSION 1: Shins crossed, hands holding your feet or knees

In this version your lower back is able to relax deeply into the floor, which provides amazing relief from backbend practices. Your breath flows very naturally into your lower back and your nervous system can let go. Keep breathing into your back body and feel yourself resting more completely on the floor. Let your sacrum and shoulder blades relax toward the floor.

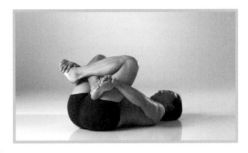

VERSION 2: Strap around your feet

By using the strap around your feet, you can isolate your hip sockets, while keeping your spine elongated and your back body resting easily on the floor. Use as much strap as is necessary to allow your spine and shoulders to be at ease, while your hip sockets open gradually. Keep releasing your entire spine so it is supported by the floor.

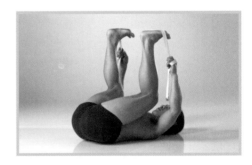

VERSION 3: Holding your feet, with hips and sacrum dropping toward the floor

In this version you are isolating your hip sockets and moving them further into their resistance. Actively deepen your groins and move your sacrum back toward its natural arch while keeping your knees close to your armpits and down toward the floor. These actions allow you to fully fold your thighs toward your armpits. Relax the deep muscles of your abdomen that line the front of your spine.

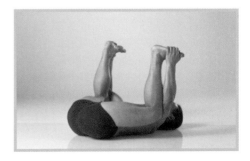

21. Try all three versions of **WALL HANG** *(Uttanasana, variation)* for 1 minute in each version.

VERSION 1: Head and arms on a chair seat

The chair supports much of the weight of your torso and is therefore helpful if you are less flexible and have a pelvis that does not spill easily over your thighs. This version will not stress your lower back. It is a good intermediary pose for cooling down after backbends, allowing you to slowly release your back body rather than going from one extreme—a deep backbend—to another, a deep forward bend. Use the wall to increase your tactile knowledge of moving your sitting bones up (away from your heels) and spreading them wide away from each other. Even in this forward bend, keep a light, conscious interplay between the top of your sacrum, your tailbone, and your shoulder blades.

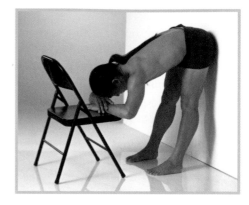

VERSION 2: Hands on the floor, forehead resting on a block

With your head on a block, your nervous system will release its subtle tendency to grip. Whenever the weight of your head is supported, your breath tends to flow more easily because your neck muscles can relax more completely. Having your hands on the floor can also help support some of the weight of your torso. As your lower back and waist release slowly, you can use your arms less. Feel your whole spine flow down from your pelvis like a waterfall.

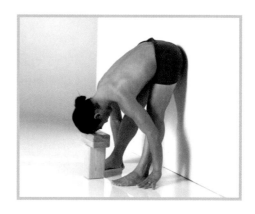

VERSION 3: Holding your elbows

Holding your elbows creates traction on your lower back and waist by hanging the full weight of your torso, head, and arms from the height of your sitting bones. Leaning against the wall gives your body a sense of support and orientation, as well as the mechanical advantage of allowing your pelvis to counterbalance the pull of your chest and head. Let your nervous system and body continue to unwind into a complete exhalation, with a full release of your entire back body and the backs of your legs. Hollow your belly and feel a deep relaxation and emptiness in your hip flexors.

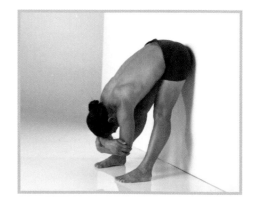

22. Try all three versions of **CHILD'S POSE** *(Balasana)* for 1 minute in each version.

VERSION 1: Bolster under your torso, head turned to the side

Supporting your front body with a bolster provides a sense of great comfort. The bolster support tells your body that it is safe and protected. Lifting your torso and head encourages the deep folding of your legs and the falling of your weight back on your pelvis toward your heels. Find the completion of your exhalation and keep letting go. In this restorative pose, find the connection of the top of your sacrum, your shoulder blades, and your tailbone with your mind and breath.

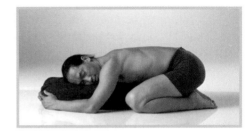

VERSION 2: Thin roll (half a sticky mat) between your lower belly and your upper thighs

Using a support between your upper thighs and your belly encourages your thighs to fall deeper toward your heels and at the same time hollows your belly to support your lower back. The prop also encourages a deeper release of your lower back muscles, creating a tucking of your tailbone and a gentle roundness of your entire spine. On the completion of your exhalations, continue to search for a complete drop of your legs and a hollowness of your belly.

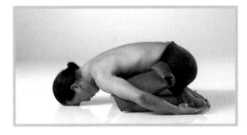

VERSION 3: Full pose, belly against thighs

Feeling your body in contact with the skin of your thighs and your sitting bones in contact with your heels encourages you to feel safe, turning inward while fully connected to your body and to the earth. Allow your hips to drop deeper and deeper, letting go of the tension in your calves, knees, the fronts of your shins, the tops of your thighs, and your lower back. Allow your hip flexors, which have been elongated and stretched, to soften into your body to restore their natural length.

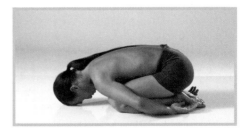

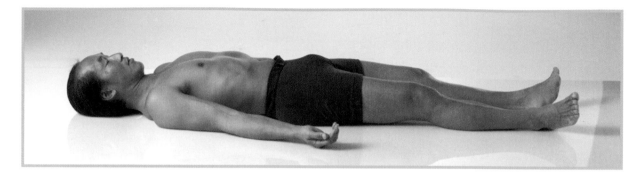

23. For 5 minutes, practice Relaxation Pose. Observe your breath as you relax your eyes and the skin of your face. Your tendency on your inhalation will be to make an effort whether you are conscious of it or not. Your tendency on the exhalation will be to drop so deeply that there is no observation. So consciously relax your eyes and the skin of your face on your inhalation and continue that relaxation on your exhalation. Be vigilant with your observation and you will discover depths of release and relaxation that you haven't felt for a long time.

24. For 5 to 10 minutes, sit in Seated Crossed-Legs Pose against the wall. Meditate on the broadness and lift of your collarbones—the openness of your chest. Let this lift come from the slight backbend at the top of your sacrum along with the tuck of your tailbone.

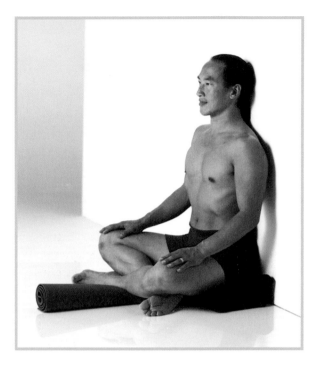

DAY 2: LEARNING COBRA POSE AND UPWARD-FACING DOG

In these two backbends, you will feel at first as if gravity is working against you because you have to lift your head and your upper chest up from the ground. However, you can use gravity to your advantage by dropping your sacrum and your tailbone deeper into your body, which allows you to feel the traction of your spine. In both poses, feel the connection of your legs to your spine and the movement of energy between them. Reaching your legs strongly sets the anchor from which your pelvis and spine can rise. These two postures strengthen the muscles of your back body but it is important to learn how to engage these muscles strongly while simultaneously widening them from the center of your spine.

In Cobra Pose, you can gradually increase the opening of your spine by slowly lifting your upper body and head farther and farther from the ground. It is a wonderful pose for learning how to lengthen your spine from the strength of your legs. However, you may forget how important your legs are, so try to remember to energize and lengthen them while they are on the ground.

In Upward-Facing Dog, your legs are forced to be more energetic but there is a tendency to jam your lower back or your wrists. By shifting the distance between your hands and feet and utilizing your entire spine in the backbend, you can eliminate any jamming or hardness from your spine and your wrists in this uplifting backbend.

In this practice, you repeat both Cobra Pose and Upward-Facing Dog, which gives you a chance to see the effects of these backbends on standing poses as well as the effects of the standing poses on the backbends. You may notice that an element of backbending exists in all the standing poses. The last part of the practice provides poses that safely bring your spine back to neutral.

FOCUS FOR THIS PRACTICE:

- In the Sun Salutations and standing poses, play with your spine, searching for ease and relaxation in the position of your neck.

- In Cobra Pose and Upward-Facing Dog Pose, open and elongate your hip flexors as much as possible.

- In every reclined pose, move your shoulder blades down your back. Move the top of your sacrum a bit off the ground as you feel a slight tucking action in your tailbone.

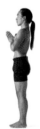 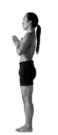 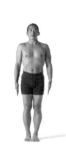 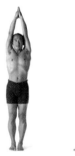 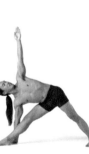 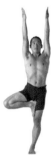

1. Practice two mini **Sun Salutations**, with 5 breaths in Downward-Facing Dog. Breathe into your back body.

2. Practice two full **Sun Salutations**, with 3 breaths in Upward-Facing Dog and 5 breaths in the second Downward-Facing Dog.

3. Practice **Mountain Pose** for 30 seconds.

4. Practice **Volcano Pose** for 30 seconds.

5. Practice **Triangle Pose** for 30 to 45 seconds on each side.

6. Practice **Tree Pose** for 30 to 45 seconds on each side.

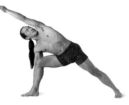 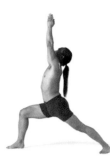 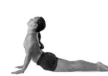 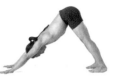

7. Practice **Extended Side Angle Pose** for 30 to 45 seconds on each side.

8. Practice **Standing Forward Bend** for 30 to 45 seconds.

9. Practice **Warrior 1 Pose** for 30 to 45 seconds on each side.

10. Practice **Cobra Pose** for 30 seconds.

11. Practice **Downward-Facing Dog** for 30 seconds.

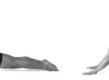 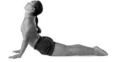 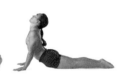 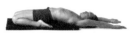

12. Practice **Upward-Facing Dog** for 15 seconds.

13. Practice **Downward-Facing Dog** for 15 seconds.

14. Practice **Bow Pose** for 10 to 15 seconds.

15. Practice **Cobra Pose** for 15 seconds.

16. Practice **Reclined Hero Pose** for 1 minute.

 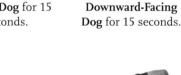 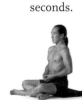 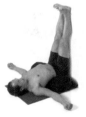

17. Practice **Upward-Facing Dog** for 15 seconds.

18. Practice **Supported Bridge Pose** for 1 minute.

19. Practice **Upward-Facing Dog** for 15 seconds.

20. Practice **Passive Backbend** for 1 minute.

21. Practice **Cobra Pose** for 15 seconds.

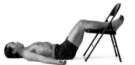 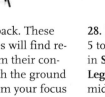 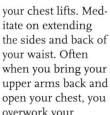

22. Practice **Reclined Leg Stretch Pose** for 45 seconds on each side.

23. Practice **Cobbler's Pose** for 30 seconds.

24. Practice **Happy Baby Pose** for 30 seconds.

25. Practice **Wall Hang Pose** for 30 seconds.

26. Practice **Legs Up the Wall Pose** for 2 minutes.

27. Relaxation and Breath Awareness. For 5 minutes, practice version 2 of **Supported Relaxation Pose** (see page 268). Inhale into your lower back ribs and

lower back. These muscles will find relief from their contact with the ground and from your focus of consciously breathing into them.

28. Meditation. For 5 to 10 minutes, sit in **Seated Crossed-Legs Pose** in the middle of the room. Bring your upper arms back so your shoulders open and

your chest lifts. Meditate on extending the sides and back of your waist. Often when you bring your upper arms back and open your chest, you overwork your

middle back muscles. By focusing on breathing into your lower back ribs and extending the sides of your waist, you will circumvent this difficulty.

Day 3: Learning Bow Pose and Supported Bridge Pose

Examining both Bow Pose and Supported Bridge pose within this practice is revealing because these two poses are the same basic shape with different relationships to gravity, one being completely active and the other supported.

Bow Pose is a very active pose for the entire body; some people will have a resistance to practicing it because of the amount of effort it requires. The muscles of your back and legs work strongly in this pose. The challenge is to get as much opening from the fronts of your legs and hips as you do from your entire spine. Initially many of you will take the entire backbend in your lower back and end up compressing and overbending in this one area. Therefore, I suggest not going to your maximum height but creating instead an evenness to the opening of your entire front body, feeling your legs, spine, arms, and chest all contribute evenly to the backbend. When you lift up like this against gravity, the muscles of your back tend to overwork and pinch inward toward your spine. Attempt to keep the muscles of your back as broad as possible as they are activated.

On the other hand, Supported Bridge Pose uses gravity to open up your front body. Because the block supports you, you can easily try different actions with your legs and arms to create evenness throughout your spine in this backbend. This supported posture emphasizes the opening of the fronts of your hips and thighs, which is where your backbends should eventually become most fluid. To achieve this takes both mental concentration and playfulness.

Today's sequence focuses on opening up your hip flexors so you can initiate your movement into the backbends from the fronts of your hips and thighs. Lunge and Hero Pose begin this opening. The Powerful Pose, Downward-Facing Dog, and Warrior 1 follow to open your spine. Supported Bridge Pose, Hero Pose, and Reclined Hero Pose continue to open up your hip flexors. Bow Pose adds both the spinal opening and hip flexor opening, and is the culmination of the practice. Reclined Leg Stretch Pose and Happy Baby Pose return you to neutral.

Focus for this practice:

- In the sun salutations, firm your shoulder blades into your back and move them down away from your neck.

- In Bow Pose, elongate your spine as you backbend.

- In Supported Bridge Pose, release and elongate your hip flexors.

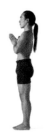 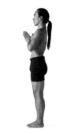 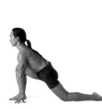 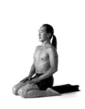 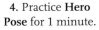 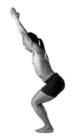

1. Practice two mini **Sun Salutations**, staying in Extended Standing Forward Bend for 5 breaths and Downward-Facing Dog for 5 breaths.

2. Practice two full **Sun Salutations**, staying in Upward-Facing Dog for 3 breaths and the second Downward-Facing Dog for 5 breaths.

3. Practice version 1 of **Lunge** for 30 seconds on each side.

4. Practice **Hero Pose** for 1 minute.

5. Practice **Powerful Pose** for 15 seconds.

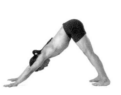 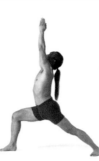

6. Practice **Standing Forward Bend** for 30 seconds.

7. Practice **Downward-Facing Dog** for 30 seconds.

8. Practice **Warrior 1 Pose** for 30 seconds on each side.

9. Practice **Supported Bridge Pose** for 1 minute.

10. Practice **Hero Pose** for 15 seconds.

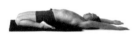 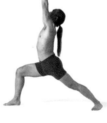 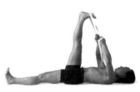

11. Practice **Reclined Hero Pose** for 1 to 2 minutes.

12. Practice **Bow Pose** for 15 seconds.

13. Repeat Steps 8 through 12.

14. Practice **Reclined Leg Stretch Pose** for 1 minute on each side.

 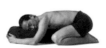 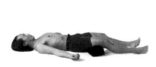 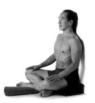

15. Practice **Happy Baby Pose** for 1 minute.

16. Practice version 1 of **Child's Pose** for 2 minutes.

17. Relaxation and Breath Awareness. For 5 minutes, practice version 2 of **Relaxation Pose**. Breathe into your middle back and middle ribs.

18. Meditation. For 5 to 10 minutes, sit in **Seated Crossed-Legs Pose** against the wall. Meditate on the natural curves of your spine.

DAY 4: LEARNING CAMEL POSE AND RECLINED HERO POSE

This practice centers around Camel Pose and Reclined Hero Pose, two poses that focus strongly on the hip flexors. Camel Pose teaches you how the strength of your legs translates into the lift of your chest and the extension of your spine. Because your shins are on the ground, you get a good foundation from which you can lift up strongly. With this much power in your foundation, be careful that the strong movement doesn't get jammed into your lower back. It is also very important to maintain the internal rotation of your thighs so that your belly doesn't get thrust forward and the main channel of your pelvis and abdomen stays clear for your legs to lift your chest. Some of you may be confused about where to place your head and neck in this pose. Ideally, your chest lifts so fully from the press of your shins and the grounding of your thighs that your head and neck can spill backward with ease, giving some traction to your neck. Until you can find this much lift of your chest, keep your head more vertical or in a congruous line with the rest of your spine. In Reclined Hero Pose, as you become more and more open in the fronts of your thighs and pelvis, the natural curves of your spine begin to elongate along the ground. The opening of the fronts of your legs and pelvis that you find in Reclined Hero Pose is exactly the channel that needs to be opened for a fully realized Camel Pose.

Today's sequence begins with Sun Salutations and standing poses to heat up your body and use your hip flexors. You then move on to Supported Bridge Pose and Reclined Hero Pose, which release and open your hip flexors. This opening is utilized next in Bow Pose and Camel Pose. After these backbends, you return to Reclined Hero Pose to observe their effects. You then practice Camel Pose two more times to learn how repetition can help deepen your understanding and your opening. Cobbler's Pose begins your return to neutral and Reclined Leg Stretch Pose and Wall Hang balance you completely from all the backbending.

FOCUS FOR THIS PRACTICE:

- In the Sun Salutations and standing poses, focus on the elongation and suppleness of your spine.

- In Camel Pose, keep your thighs as perpendicular to the floor as possible as you press your pelvis forward and up to open your hip flexors.

- In Reclined Hero Pose, let your sacrum take its natural curve as you move your tailbone down toward your knees.

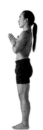 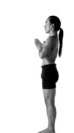 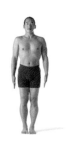 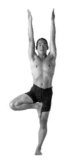 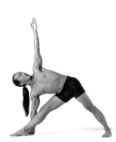

1. Practice two mini **Sun Salutations** with 5 breaths in Downward-Facing Dog Pose.

2. Practice two full **Sun Salutations** with 3 breaths in Upward-Facing Dog Pose and 5 breaths in the second Downward-Facing Dog Pose.

3. Practice **Mountain Pose** for 15 seconds.

4. Practice **Tree Pose** for 30 seconds on each side.

5. Practice **Triangle Pose** for 30 seconds on each side.

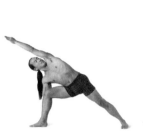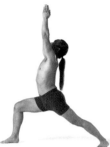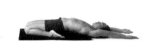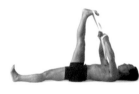

6. Practice **Extended Side Angle Pose** for 30 seconds on each side.

7. Practice **Warrior 1 Pose** for 30 seconds on each side.

8. Practice **Supported Bridge Pose** for 2 minutes.

9. Practice **Reclined Hero Pose** for 1 to 2 minutes.

10. Practice **Bow Pose** for 15 seconds.

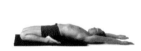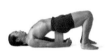

11. Practice **Camel Pose** for 15 seconds.

12. Practice **Reclined Hero Pose** for 1 minute.

13. Practice **Camel Pose** for 15 to 30 seconds.

14. Practice **Supported Bridge Pose** for 1 minute.

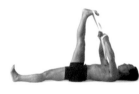

15. Practice **Camel Pose** for 30 seconds.

16. Practice **Cobbler's Pose** for 1 minute.

17. Practice **Reclined Leg Stretch Pose** for 1 minute on each side.

18. Practice **Wall Hang** for 1 minute.

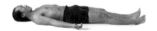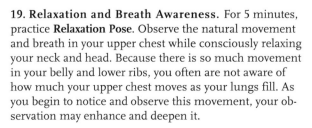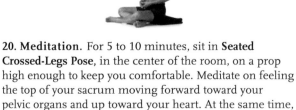

19. Relaxation and Breath Awareness. For 5 minutes, practice **Relaxation Pose**. Observe the natural movement and breath in your upper chest while consciously relaxing your neck and head. Because there is so much movement in your belly and lower ribs, you often are not aware of how much your upper chest moves as your lungs fill. As you begin to notice and observe this movement, your observation may enhance and deepen it.

20. Meditation. For 5 to 10 minutes, sit in **Seated Crossed-Legs Pose,** in the center of the room, on a prop high enough to keep you comfortable. Meditate on feeling the top of your sacrum moving forward toward your pelvic organs and up toward your heart. At the same time, broaden and breathe into your back lower ribs.

DAY 5: LEARNING PASSIVE BACKBEND AND UPWARD-FACING BOW POSE

When you practice a demanding pose like Upward Bow, one of the most difficult distinctions you need to make is between what you need to activate and what you need to let go. When you need so much effort just to begin to do a pose, you tend to activate everything. But this basically leads to paralysis, with all your muscles contracting. Combining Passive Backbend with Upward Bow Pose in today's practice provides you with room and time for observation and play. Observing your breath makes you realize that while backbends are intended to allow us to breathe more freely, in many of the more demanding backbends you end up holding your breath. When you initially start practicing, this is an unavoidable fact, but eventually you begin to realize that it is not beneficial to work strongly without the aid of your breath and without room for observation. When doing Passive Backbend, your body has time to soak in different muscular skeletal patterns and shapes so that new habits, both in your posture and in your muscular coordination, begin to form. When you do Passive Backbend, it is important to continue to find the actions of extension and support, though they might not be as obviously necessary.

Today's sequence begins with Sun Salutations to awaken and coordinate your body, mind, and breath. This is followed by Passive Backbend and Supported Bridge Pose to open your body without effort. Next, Cobra Pose opens up your front body even further, with the engagement of your back muscles, arms, and legs. Downward-Facing Dog brings neutrality to your spine while emphasizing the opening of your shoulders. Warrior 1 utilizes the chest opening of the Passive Backbends and the spine and shoulder opening from Downward-Facing Dog to bring you into a powerful backbend. You then return to Passive Backbends to help let go of the bindings in your front body. The active backbends that follow teach you how to activate your back body and let go of the front body simultaneously. This knowledge of what to release and what to activate makes Upward Bow Pose easier. The sequence ends with Reclined Leg Stretch Pose and Cobbler's Pose to ease your spine back to neutral.

FOCUS FOR THIS PRACTICE:

- In the Sun Salutations, press your thighbones toward your hamstrings. Lift your pelvis from your legs as you slightly tuck your tailbone to open your hip flexors.

- In the backbends leading up to Upward Bow Pose, focus on finding an even opening of your entire spine. If there is compression in one part of your spine, reduce your backbending to the point where there is more equality of work throughout your spine.

- In Upward Bow Pose, press your shoulder blades forward and deepen your sacrum into your body as you tuck your tailbone.

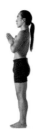 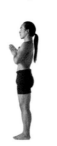 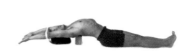 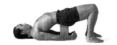

1. Practice two mini **Sun Salutations,** with 5 breaths in Downward-Facing Dog Pose.

2. Practice two full **Sun Salutations,** with 3 breaths in Upward-Facing Dog Pose and 5 breaths in the second Downward-Facing Dog Pose.

3. Practice **Passive Backbend** for 2 minutes.

4. Practice **Supported Bridge Pose** for 2 minutes.

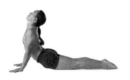

5. Practice **Cobra Pose** for 15 seconds.

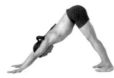

6. Practice **Downward-Facing Dog** for 30 seconds.

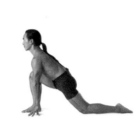

7. Practice version 1 of **Lunge** for 15 seconds on each side.

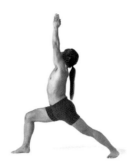

8. Practice **Warrior 1 Pose** for 30 seconds on each side.

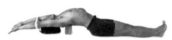

9. Practice **Passive Backbend** for 1 minute.

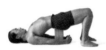

10. Practice **Supported Bridge Pose** for 1 minute.

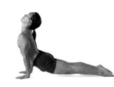

11. Practice **Upward-Facing Dog Pose** for 15 seconds.

12. Practice **Camel Pose** for 15 seconds.

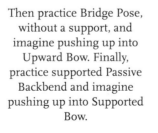

13. Practice **Upward Bow Pose,** three times if possible, for any length of time. If you cannot get into this pose, try imagining it: Lie in Constructive Rest Pose and imagine pushing up into Upward Bow.

Then practice Bridge Pose, without a support, and imagine pushing up into Upward Bow. Finally, practice supported Passive Backbend and imagine pushing up into Supported Bow.

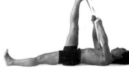

14. Practice **Reclined Leg Stretch Pose** for 1 minute on each side.

15. Practice **Cobbler's Pose** for 1 minute.

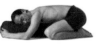

16. Practice version 1 of **Child's Pose** for 1 minute.

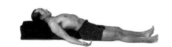

17. Relaxation and Breath Awareness. For 5 minutes, practice version 3 of **Supported Relaxation Pose** (page 268). Notice how your breath opens your entire rib cage—back, sides and front, top to bottom. Be careful not to force your breath to do this, but observe how it is already taking place, especially after the sequence of backbends.

18. Meditation. For 5 to 15 minutes, sit in **Seated Crossed-Legs Pose,** on your awkward side. Meditate on finding the length in your lower back and a broadness and lift to your collarbones.

Meditation

For 5 to 10 minutes, sit in Seated Crossed-Legs pose against the wall with your legs crossed on your awkward side. Fold your hands on your lap, with your right fingers over your left and your thumbs together, creating an open chest with circular arms.

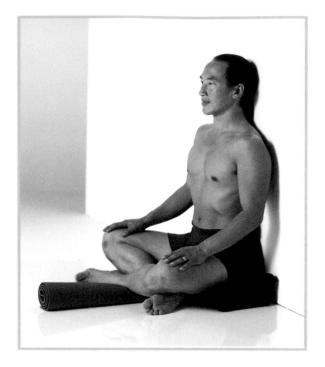

FOCUSING ON YOUR BREATH. When you meditate on your breath, you will realize how connected your breath is to the ease and lift of your posture. If you overwork in your sitting posture, your breath will be stifled. Likewise, if you collapse and become habitual with your sitting posture, your breath will be minimized. Continue to explore the relationship between effort and surrender, and try to maximize the amount of lift in your posture with the least amount of effort. This will be reflected in your breath. Your breath will move easily and will be deeply absorbed throughout your body when your posture moves into better alignment.

STAYING PRESENT. Focusing on your breath will also keep your mind present; it is one of the greatest seeds of meditation. At first, focusing on your breath doesn't seem enticing enough to harness the wild horses of your mind, but with practice, focusing on your breath is actually the most powerful technique for observing your mind and your body. You may be frustrated with your ability to concentrate.

However, there is no need to compare yourself with who you were yesterday or with someone else who seems to be sitting peacefully and quietly. It is like being in a dream. In a dream, you have no idea how long an event lasts, and a full-length movie can take place in 5 seconds. When you are meditating, some of your daydreams might last only a split second. It's hard to tell, and it doesn't matter. Just bring yourself back to focusing on the breath.

Breath Awareness

For 5 to 10 minutes, sit in any comfortable seated position. Breathe with smooth inhalations and exhalations, emphasizing the ease of your breath as you slightly elongate your breaths.

SITTING. Sitting up for this breath awareness means that you are taking a leap into a much more difficult experiment. As you stay seated 5 to 10 minutes, you may feel a lot of uneasiness in your body. If this is going to disrupt your ability to focus on your breath, lie down in any comfortable version of Relaxation Pose.

ELONGATING YOUR BREATH. Now, slightly elongate your inhalations and exhalations, emphasizing the smoothness and ease of your breath. You may find it helpful to close your throat slightly so you can hear the sound of your breath. This sound will help you concentrate on bringing your mind back to the rise and fall of your breath, and will also help you regulate the smoothness of your inhalation and exhalation. I specifically tell you here to take only a *slightly* elongated breath because you will have a tendency to force a deep breath, which will undo what you learned during the first week (to take an easy, smooth, soft inhalation). I have you slightly elongate your breath here because your habitual breath is often unnaturally restricted. By intentionally elongating and smoothing out your inhalations and exhalations, you will move beyond your habit. If smoothing out your inhalations and exhalations and taking slightly elongated breaths creates any agitation in your sense organs or any strain in your head or neck, discontinue this technique and return to scanning your body, to realigning your posture, and practicing the release of all tension. If necessary, return to any comfortable version of Relaxation Pose.

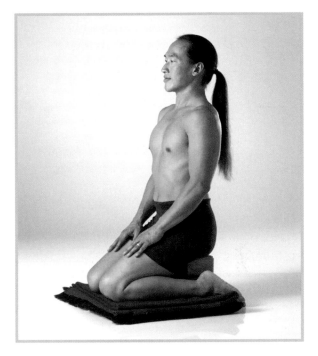

Meditation

For 2 minutes, return to meditation, focusing on your posture.

Relaxation

For 3 to 5 minutes, return to Relaxation Pose to let go completely of any tension you may have become aware of or that may have resulted from the breathing and/or meditating.

COBRA POSE

Cobra Pose returns your spine to its natural suppleness.

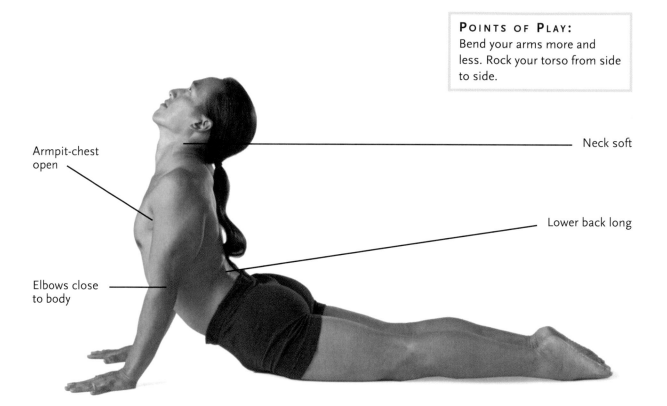

POINTS OF PLAY:
Bend your arms more and less. Rock your torso from side to side.

Neck soft

Armpit-chest open

Lower back long

Elbows close to body

UPWARD-FACING DOG POSE

Upward-Facing Dog Pose awakens your spine
from the power of your legs.

POINT OF PLAY: Lift the
tops of your thighs as you
descend your tailbone.

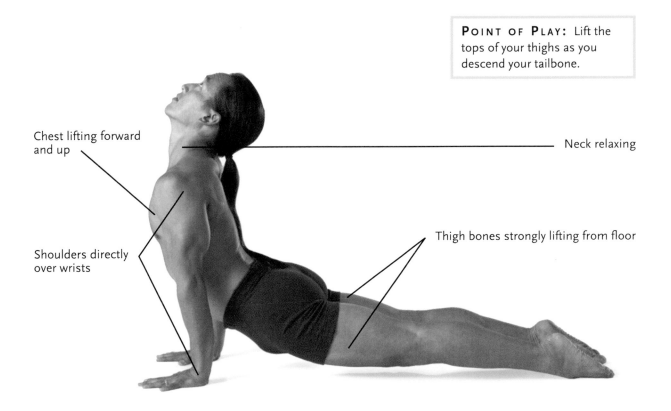

Chest lifting forward
and up

Neck relaxing

Shoulders directly
over wrists

Thigh bones strongly lifting from floor

SUPPORTED BRIDGE POSE

Supported Bridge Pose restores your body
while opening your chest and the front of your pelvis.

POINTS OF PLAY:
Draw your hip points toward
each other as you release your
groins, and then tuck your
tailbone.

Thighs turning in (internally rotated)

Block under sacrum

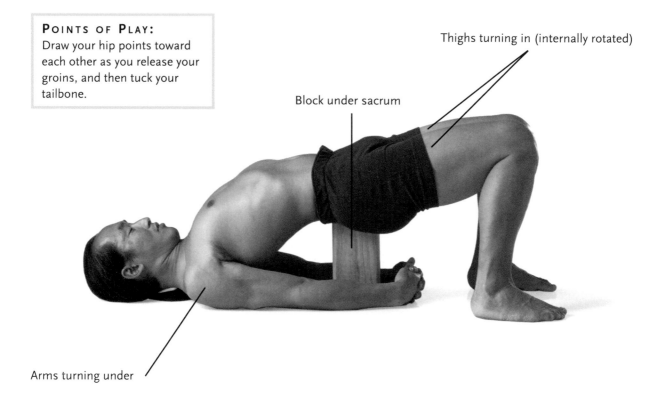

Arms turning under

RECLINED HERO POSE

Reclined Hero Pose opens your hip flexors
to integrate your legs with your spine.

POINT OF PLAY:
Move from a deeper backbend
to a flatter back.

Pubis dropping

Rib cage extending away from pelvis

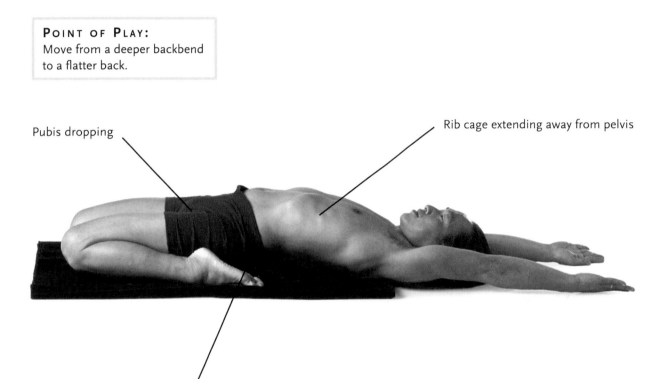

Buttocks flesh moving away
from the lower back

BOW POSE

Bow Pose opens your entire front body as it engages
and strengthens all the muscles of your back body.

POINTS OF PLAY:
Lift your thighs. Move your
chest forward.

Head looking up

Knees hips-distance apart

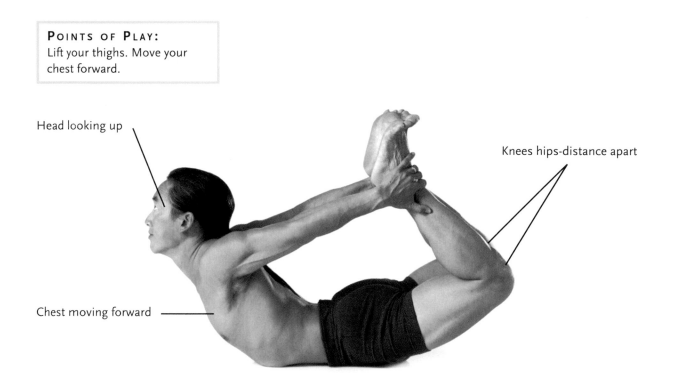

Chest moving forward

PASSIVE BACKBEND

Passive Backbend allows you to fully open your chest
by breathing into the bindings of protection.

POINT OF PLAY:
Move the blanket roll under
different parts of your back.

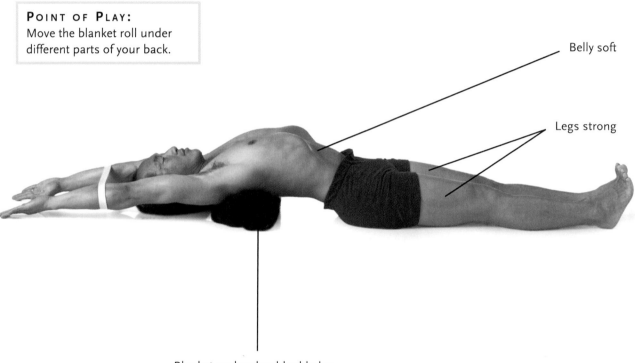

Belly soft

Legs strong

Blanket under shoulder blades

CAMEL POSE

Camel Pose sends the strength of your arms and legs
into the upward expansion of your chest.

Chest lifted ————

Sacrum forward ————
into the body

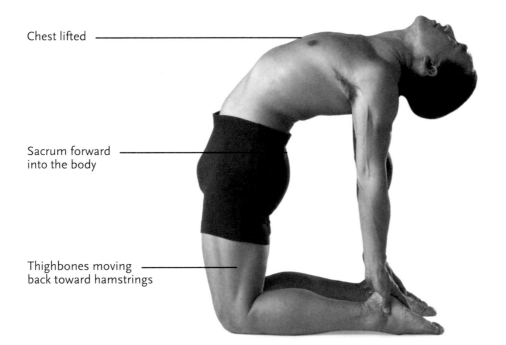

Thighbones moving ————
back toward hamstrings

POINTS OF PLAY:
Draw your hip points toward
each other as you release your
groins, and then tuck your tailbone. Move your thighs back
and deepen your sacrum.

UPWARD BOW POSE

Upward Bow Pose opens your entire front body,
creating an exhilarating emotional and physical lift.

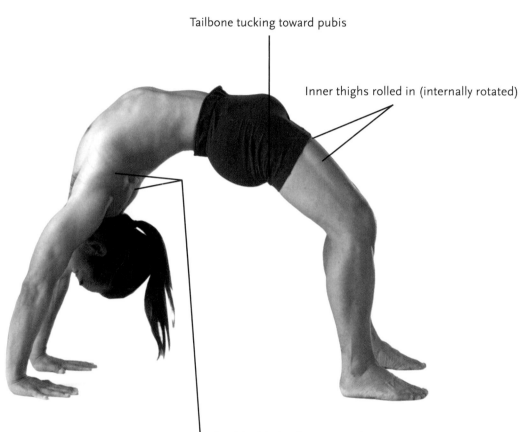

Tailbone tucking toward pubis

Inner thighs rolled in (internally rotated)

Shoulder blades firming into back and moving toward hips

POINTS OF PLAY: Rise up on your toes, then ground your heels—while keeping your lower back long.

RECLINED LEG STRETCH POSE

Reclined Leg Stretch Pose balances your spine
from the even work of your arms and legs.

POINTS OF PLAY:
Try emphasizing your bottom
leg and then your top leg.

Top leg extending fully

Shoulders on
the ground

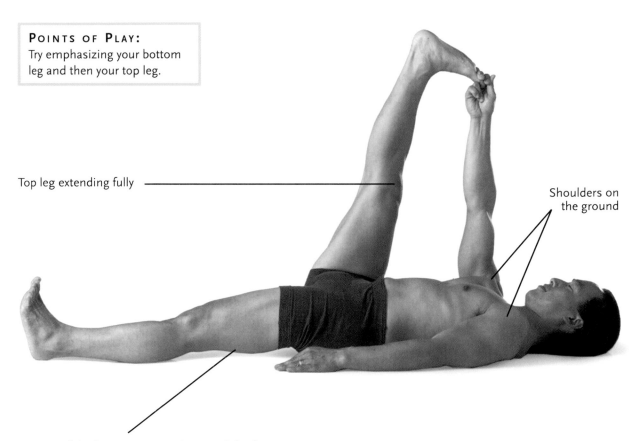

Bottom of thigh moving strongly toward the floor

HAPPY BABY POSE

Happy Baby Pose gently rounds your lower back while opening your hips,
creating a feeling of ease and playfulness.

Feet over knees

POINT OF PLAY:
Try rounding your back
different amounts.

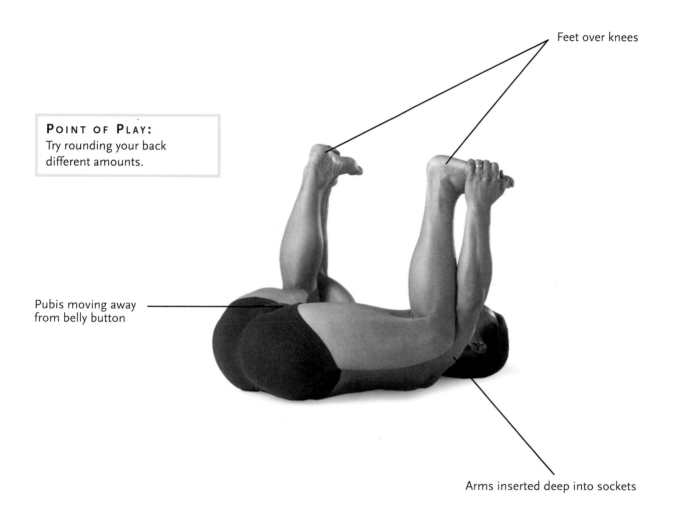

Pubis moving away
from belly button

Arms inserted deep into sockets

WALL HANG

Wall Hang opens your entire back body
as it turns your mind and senses inward.

POINT OF PLAY:
Wiggle your torso and head to
find maximum length in your
spine.

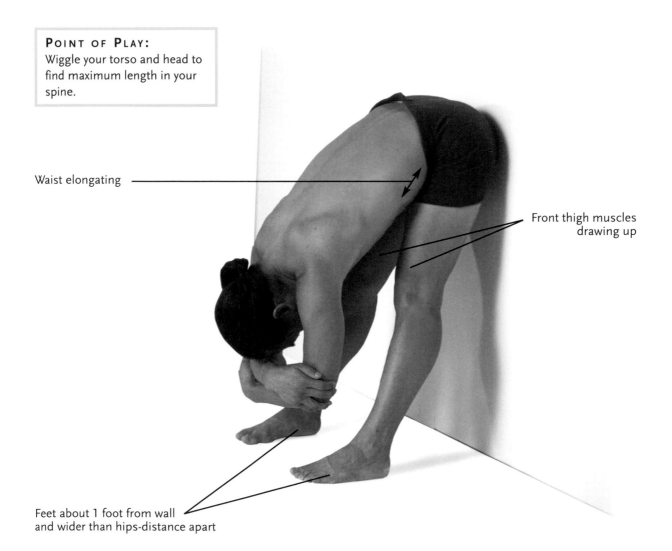

Waist elongating

Front thigh muscles
drawing up

Feet about 1 foot from wall
and wider than hips-distance apart

CHILD'S POSE

Child's Pose releases the muscles of your back away from your spine
as it comforts your body and mind.

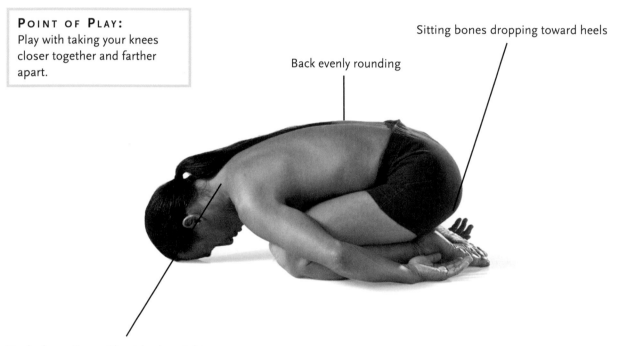

POINT OF PLAY:
Play with taking your knees
closer together and farther
apart.

Sitting bones dropping toward heels

Back evenly rounding

Neck elongating, without body weight

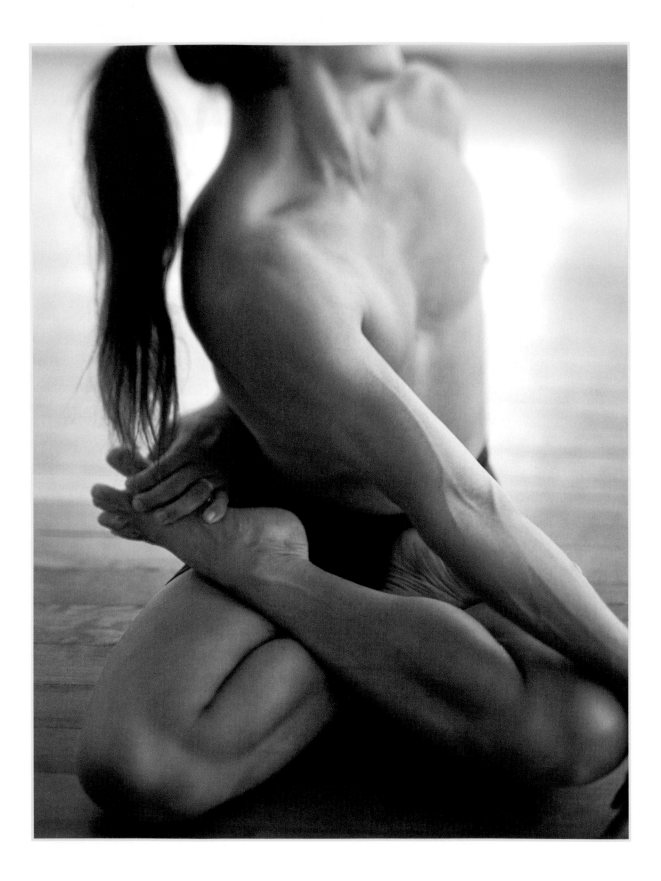

WEEK 4:

Allowing Receptivity

OFTEN WHEN WE ENCOUNTER A PROBLEM, WE TEND TO THINK THAT ALL WE HAVE TO DO IS TRY HARDER. Instead, when you come up against a barrier, it is important to back up enough to observe, breathe, and assess. It is vital to allow yourself to sit with the difficulty and confusion until some understanding comes to mind. In twists, many people come up against a wall, not only of physical tightness but also of emotional frustration. Your breath usually becomes more rapid and is sometimes even held. So relax and find spaces to inhale into and release. In twists, your physical movements should arise from first observing your breath and then moving with it. Otherwise, if your mind is determined or aggressive, the twists become abusive.

Classically, twists are considered cleansing postures. When you squeeze and then release your body, a rush of new circulation clears your digestive tract and your vital organs. This cleansing begins to leave space. Giving yourself time to evolve your twists from your internal receptivity will create an organic opening. This teaches you that balance in your body is connected to the relationship between effort and surrender. Where do you need to work and where do you need to surrender so that the twists have a sense of balance?

In this week, you are taking the vitality of the first week, the movement of the second week, and the vulnerability of the third week and combining them into the natural, organic evolution of twists. At a certain point, the act of going deeper is not to go further (or twist farther) but to integrate your mind, body, and breath on a more subtle level through receptivity.

ABOUT TWISTS

Twists affect people differently on mental, physical, and breath levels. Some of you will find twists easy and enjoyable, while others will feel resistance and agitation as you confront your limitations. However, whether you find twists easy or difficult, they always teach you how to drop into your breath, whether by learning not to hold or force your breath or learning more about how your breath is being absorbed. Mentally, when you come up against resistance, whether in twists or in other aspects of your life, what is your initial reaction? Because most people are eager to twist more deeply, many of you will forgo the observation time needed to assess how the pose needs to be balanced and how you can find breath and continual ease in the twist. As you observe how you react in your twists, you can change your habitual reaction into a mindful response.

Because many of us are sedentary, the usual twisting that comes from, for example, walking, running, and moving in the world is no longer part of our daily life. Therefore, twists are very important for your digestive system and your other vital organs because their motion improves your circulation and the health of your internal organs. As a result, your body detoxifies, so I recommend that after practicing twists, you drink plenty of water to flush out your system. And after an extensive twist practice, you may feel a bit lethargic and unclear or stirred up and irritated; but in a few hours, a feeling of clarity comes. Your body and mind begin to feel like the fresh air that comes after a good rainstorm. Your spine can also feel rejuvenated and supple.

Muscular or heavier people may find that twists feel congested and unapproachable. However, twists can be especially beneficial for you as long as you move into the twists with relaxation and steadiness and twist only to an extent that allows ease of breath and an erect spine. Often the very poses that are most difficult for us bring the most balance to our bodies and minds.

EMOTIONS. Often your muscles, organs, and minds are so full of past experiences and future expectations that you have no capacity to be receptive to the present moment. Twists squeeze and release the tension from your body, sometimes bringing up old stored emotions—whether general feelings or specific memories. Take the time to respect whatever is arising emotionally and, if need be, find another yoga pose or even another person that can help comfort you.

FOCUS OF YOUR MIND. In twists, focus on the rise and the fall of your breath and let this natural, strong internal movement move you into and out of the twist. This will ensure some gentleness and respect for the slow release of habitual tension. As you notice where your breath flows easily and where it is trapped, you will realize which parts of the body you have to wake up or to let go in order to make the twists more organic, harmonious, and deep.

GROUNDING AND LIFTING. As you move into a twist, you tend to think only about turning, so it's easy to become disconnected from the ground. It is helpful to feel that as you rise from the ground, a natural spiral takes place. When you do twists with this connection, they become much less constricted and isolated. As you twist there will be some areas that you lift strongly and some areas that you allow to collapse, such as different parts of your spine. So try to balance the front, back, and sides of your entire spine in a lifted, spiraling movement.

BREATH. As you inhale in a twist, feel your breath moving from your nose down into your pelvis, as you allow your body to feel juicy and absorbent. As you exhale, elongate and hollow your body as you deepen the twist. I find it beneficial to come out of the twist slightly on my inhalation and to deepen the twisting action on my exhalation. If you follow your breath, you will be much less aggressive and much more responsive to the natural flow of the pose.

SACRUM. In twists, the muscles around your spine become broadened. As this happens, deepen your sacrum further into your body toward your belly. Search for evenness between the left and right sides

ANATOMY LESSON

1. Groins

To learn about your groins, sit in a loose Cobbler's Pose and take the 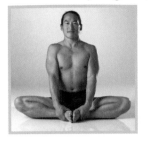 fingers of one hand inside one groin as you use your other hand to help lift that same leg. Feel the change in the depth, the width, and the sensation of the groin as you lift and release that leg.

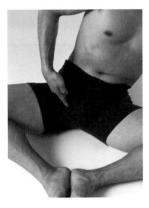

Throughout this book, when I use the phrase "deepen your groins," I mean that the creases of your groins drop deeper into your body toward your sacrum and sitting bones.

2. Sides of the waist

To learn about the sides of your waist, sit in Seated Crossed-Legs Pose and place your hands beside your hips. As you press down into the ground, gradually and evenly elongate both sides of your waist.

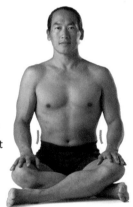

Sides of the waist

3. Broad muscles of the back

To learn about the broad muscles of your back, practice version 3 of 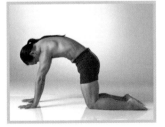 Cat Pose. As you curl your tailbone strongly and drop your head, observe how all the muscles of your back broaden from your spine.

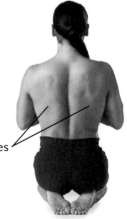

Broad muscles of back

of the sacrum, feeling the sides release evenly downward toward your tailbone. As your sacrum deepens toward the front of your belly and moves toward a natural backbend, allow your organs and belly to release toward the front of your sacrum.

ARMS AND SHOULDERS. Your arms and shoulders often contort as you attempt to go deeper into the twists. After making the initial step to twist, recenter your upper arms in their sockets so that they augment the lift of your chest and the broadness of your collarbones. Consolidate your upper arm, shoulder blade, and collarbone, broadening your chest as you do so, to help ensure the safety of your shoulders and deepen your twist.

LEGS AND FEET. Whether you are doing a straight- or bent-leg twist, remember that your legs are still your roots. Your feet should be very alive, so activate and spread your toes and the soles of your feet, while your legs pulsate in their search for connection with the ground.

DAY 1: LEARNING THE VARIATIONS

Your main movement in twists comes from your spine, so it is valuable to observe how different the twists feel when your spine is rounded and compact versus how they feel when your spine is lifted and extended. With a more extended spine, your breath will be much freer. In some twists, using props will help you find the evenness of the left and right sides of your sacrum, allowing the sacrum to feel much more centered, with less torque.

Everything will not be visually symmetrical, but from the inside you can create as much symmetry as possible in the feelings of the right and left sides of your body. This allows your twists to be more beneficial for your spine.

MOVING IN AND OUT OF TWISTS

Just learning where your body parts go in the twists can be confusing! So take your time to look at the photographs and build your posture from the ground up. For the seated twists, first organize your legs and then pause for a moment and ask yourself which way you are going to turn. Look to see if the twist is a cross-the-body twist where the opposite arm goes to the opposite knee, or if it is an open twist where the arm is going to the same-side leg. Begin to move your arms in the appropriate direction and gradually turn your spine. As you place your arms, take time to observe the general shape of the pose and determine where you're going to ground yourself and in which direction you are going to turn. Move into the twist on your exhalation and initiate the movement from the foundation of your legs up to the crown of your head. Then go inside your breath, and allow your breath to be the rhythm and flow of the twist.

Once you are in the basic shape, ask yourself how your arms and legs are contributing to the extension of your spine. Many of you will initiate the twist from your neck and head (your neck is designed in such a way that it turns very easily). However, it is better to initiate the twist from the ground up. Try to find a gradual, supported twist, in which your entire body cooperates in adding to the spiral.

Even though it is good to take your time moving in and out of the twist, it is not that beneficial to be at your maximum in the twist for an extended period of time. When you are coming out of the twist, slowly unwind and come back to a symmetrical seated position or the center of your lying-down position, and take a couple of moments to feel the effects of the twist and the recentering of your body. As you begin to take the other side, realize that it will be like a counterpose to the first side. Move even more slowly, and respect that your spine has just come from the opposite direction and that even after you have spent some time in a neutral position, there still may be an internal flow in the first direction.

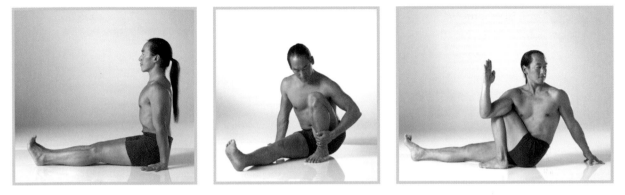

This photo sequence illustrates moving into a twist by building the posture from the ground up.

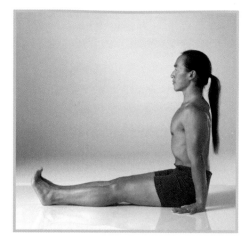

1. Practice **STAFF POSE** for 1 minute. Elongate the sides of your waist as much as possible from the grounding of your legs.

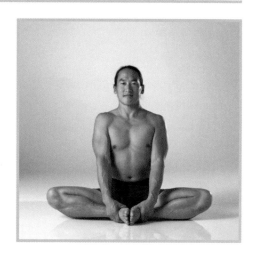

2. Practice **COBBLER'S POSE** for 2 minutes. Deepen and lengthen your groins as evenly as possible.

3. Try all three versions of **WIDE ANGLE POSE** *(Upavista Konasana)* for 1 minute in each version.

VERSION 1: Hips on a block, back against the wall

This version allows you to sit in the pose without overusing your back muscles. Those of you who are less flexible can stay in the pose longer and slowly open up the tightness in your hamstrings and the insides of your legs. Use the wall as an extra support to keep your pelvis upright while you press and extend your legs along the ground. Broaden and extend your back body along the wall.

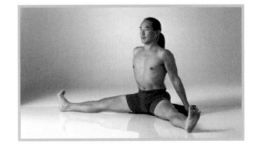

VERSION 2: On a folded blanket in the middle of the room, hands behind you

Propping up your pelvis provides the necessary height for those of you who are tight in the hamstrings and insides of the legs. Sitting with your pelvis upright and with the natural curves of your spine allows a natural breath and encourages the release of extra tension from your body. The challenge is to use the strength of your legs pressing into the ground to support your spine while you release the tension from your calves and hamstrings. Extend the sides of your waist.

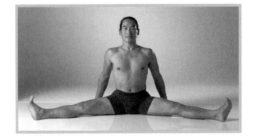

VERSION 3: On the floor, hands behind you

This version allows you to find the full grounding of the backs of your legs, providing you with a deep connection with the earth. If you are flexible enough for this variation, the charge you receive from your legs through your pelvis to your torso is gratifying. The challenge is to ground your legs with a fully natural spine, as if you were standing in Mountain Pose. To do so, continually deepen your groins to bring yourself completely on your sitting bones.

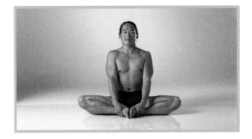

4. Practice **COBBLER'S POSE** for 1 minute. Feel the broadness of the muscles of your back.

5. Try all three versions of **HALF BOAT POSE** *(Arda Navasana)* for 15 seconds in each version.

VERSION 1: Legs bent, feet on the ground, spine rounding, sacrum on the ground, hands holding backs of knees

This version will cause the least amount of strain for those of you with lower back problems. With your hands on the backs of your knees, you can use your arms to assist your abdominal muscles to round your spine to any degree possible while you breathe freely. Because your feet are on the ground, the weight of your legs does not create extra work for your abdominal muscles. Keep your chest as broad and open as possible, and keep your arms inserted into your shoulder sockets while using them to assist the lift of your chest. Feel and breathe into the broad muscles of your back.

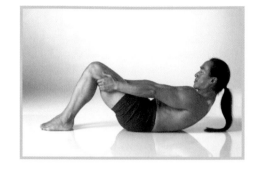

VERSION 2: Legs fully extended, spine rounded, arms extending, hands beside legs

In this version you use both your arms and legs to assist in lifting your chest as they help counterbalance the weight of your head and chest. Learn how to activate your abdominal muscles as well as the strength of your arms and legs. Focus on curling your tailbone as you deepen your groins to activate your abdominal muscles. Encourage your abdominal muscles to release down toward your spine instead of popping up away from your spine.

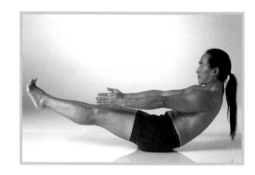

VERSION 3: Legs fully extended, hands behind the head, spine rounded, only sacrum on the ground

This version provides the extra challenge of adding the weight of your arms to that of your head and chest while you must use solely your legs and abdominal muscles to lift and round your spine. Can you take this rounded position while still hollowing your belly and broadening your chest? Even as you curl your spine, continue to find the length of the sides of your waist.

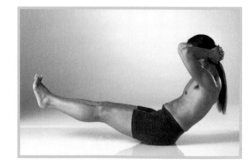

6. Practice the following CORE STRENGTHENING SERIES three times, without props.

In the transitions, make sure you do not hold or force your breath. Use your arms to help support your spine and move your legs gracefully. The first time you do the series, stay in each pose as long as necessary to understand the sequence. The second time, take 2 breaths per pose. The third time, take 1 breath per pose. Throughout the sequence, focus on the changing depth of your groins.

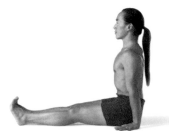

1. Staff Pose

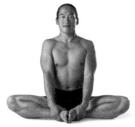

2. Cobbler's Pose

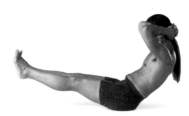

3. Half Boat Pose

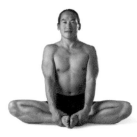

4. Cobbler's Pose

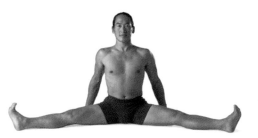

5. Wide Angle Pose

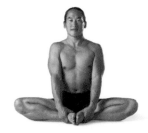

6. Cobbler's Pose

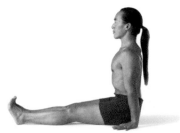

7. Staff Pose

7. Try all three versions of **ONE-LEGGED DOWNWARD-FACING DOG POSE** for 45 seconds in each version.

VERSION 1: On your back, a strap around your raised foot, arms above your head and reaching along the ground

With a strap around your foot, take the ends of the strap in each hand and pull your arms over your head until your hands are close to or on the ground with your arms straight. This version allows you to find the full extension of your bottom leg through your torso into the reach of your arms. Using that full extension as a foundation, the back of your top leg stretches and opens. Use the ground as a reference to elongate and open your entire back body. Feel the broad muscles of your back, especially at your lower ribs.

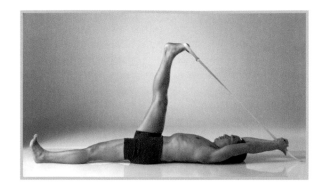

VERSION 2: Downward-Facing Dog with one leg in the air

This version allows you to intensify the opening of your supporting leg and further challenge the foundation of your shoulders and arms. Try to maintain symmetry and space inside your hip sockets, spine, and shoulders. The challenge here is to keep your foundation as balanced as possible while you take one leg up into the air, keeping your pelvis as square and as centered as possible. Keep both sides of your waist equal length.

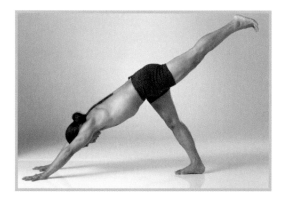

VERSION 3: Raised leg bent, torso twisting

Along with full extension of the spine, in this version you begin to find the organic spiraling that moves from your legs into your spine, opening your body even further. The challenge is to keep your waist on the side of your supporting leg open, your belly hollow, and your back extended. Continually monitor the even depth of your groins.

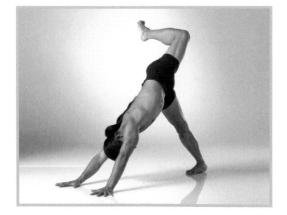

8. Try the **RECLINED LEG STRETCH SERIES** *(Supta Padagustasana)*, with timing as follows.

VERSION 1: Upper leg extended toward ceiling, back body on the ground (30 seconds)

This version opens the back of your top leg while challenging the grounding of your bottom leg. Use your arms to help lift and open your chest. As you draw your top leg closer to your chest, try to find the depth of the groin of your bottom leg. This action will keep open the channel that runs from your legs into your hips and spine. Keep as much awareness in grounding your bottom leg as you do in pulling your top leg.

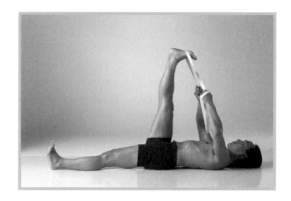

VERSION 2: Upper leg extended toward ceiling, head and upper back curling up into a sit-up (15 seconds)

This version helps bring attention to the core of your body while further opening the back of your top leg. The challenge is to keep grounding and deepening the groin of your bottom leg as well as to maintain the expanse of your chest and the hollowing of your belly. Find the length of the sides of your waist while curling your spine.

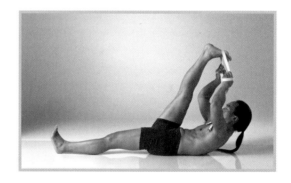

VERSION 3: Upper leg out to the side (30 seconds)

This version creates an amazing sense of broadness and openness, in both your pelvis and your upper chest. However, your top leg will tend to pull you away from the grounding of your bottom leg and the opposite side of your pelvis. Focus your concentration on using your legs and arms to anchor your body and maintain the openness of your torso, especially the broadness of your back. Lower your top leg out to the side slowly and conservatively.

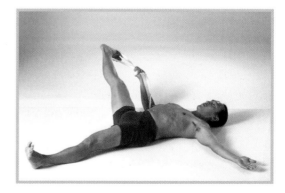

9. Try all three versions of **RECLINED TWIST** *(Jathara Parivartanasana)*, modified, for 30 seconds in each version on each side.

VERSION 1: Bolster under your bent knees

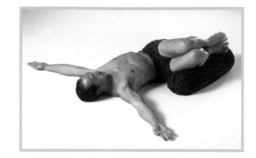

With the bolster bearing the weight of your legs you can find subtle relationships between your legs, pelvis, spine, and chest and feel how your breath is moving through the pose. The challenge is to keep your attention in your legs and feet, not allowing them to become sloppy. Recognize that your legs are still the foundation for the spiral of your spine and the openness of your chest. Which groin is deeper here, the right or the left?

VERSION 2: Knees bent and resting on the ground

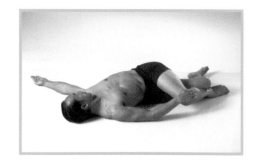

This version increases your twist, which challenges the alignment of your shoulders and lower back. Try to continue the movement of your lower back toward its natural backbend, feeling the relationship between your groins moving back, the top of your sacrum moving deeper into your body, and your chest broadening. Fully lengthen your lower back by extending the sides of your waist vigorously and yet maintain a sense of ease.

VERSION 3: Thigh crossed over thigh, rather than side by side

This version gives a deeper twist to your spine as it opens the outside hip of your top leg. The challenge is to let the twist come equally from your pelvis and your spine, feeling an equal depth to both groins and evenness on both sides of your sacrum. Because of the depth of the twist, some of your back muscles will tend to be clenched and overworked. Focus on bringing as much broadness as possible to the muscles of your back and evenness between its left and right sides.

10. Practice **HAPPY BABY POSE** for 1 minute. Try to find the depth of your groins, the length of the sides of your waist, and the broadness of the muscles of your back, all in relation to each other.

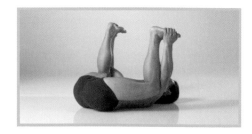

11. Try all three versions of **RECLINED STRAIGHT-LEG TWIST** *(Jathara Parivartanasana)* for 10 seconds (or less) in each version on each side.

VERSION 1: Bolster under your feet and calves

The bolster reduces the twist and carries the weight of your legs so you can adjust your spine and observe the relationship between your legs, spine, and arms. Keep your legs awake and do not rely on resting them on the bolster. Extending your legs creates a strong surge of power through your spine into the reach of your arms.

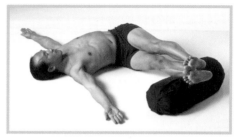

VERSION 2: Feet touching the ground

Bringing your legs to the ground increases the twist and challenges you to keep your spine extended. The side of your waist that is closer to the ground will tend to foreshorten. Extend both sides of your waist equally to align your spine and find ease of breath. Do not contort your upper chest and shoulder blades—if needed, keep your opposite arm slightly off the ground.

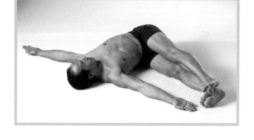

VERSION 3: Legs 2 inches off the ground

In this version, the weight and leverage of your legs is extreme and the amount of effort it takes to keep them off the ground is great, but you build strength in your back and abdominal muscles at the same time you receive a deep twist. Waking up the strength of your arms and legs in tandem with your abdominal and back muscles allows you to be in this pose without gripping your neck or breath. As your back muscles work vigorously, focus on maintaining their broadness.

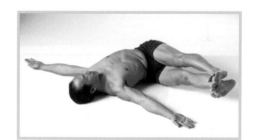

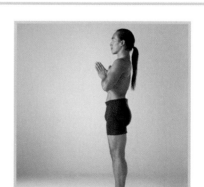

12. Practice three full **SUN SALUTATIONS,** staying in Downward-Facing Dog for 5 breaths. In the first Sun Salutation, search for the depths of your groins; in the second, search for the length of the sides of your waist; and in the third, search for the broadness of your back muscles throughout the movements of the salutations.

13. Try all three versions of **SIMPLE TWIST** *(Bharadvajasana)* for 20 seconds in each version on each side.

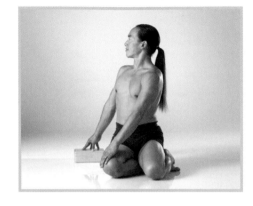

VERSION 1: Hips on a block, back hand on a block

This version enables you to maintain a symmetrical pelvis and a fully extended spine. This shows you the relationship between extension and twisting—how you can twist with ease and evenness, as you lengthen your lower back and open your upper chest. With your legs in an asymmetrical foundation, check your groins for an equal feeling of depth and emptiness. How can your legs help begin the twist and fully support your pelvis and your torso?

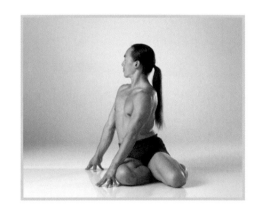

VERSION 2: Full pose, without props

In this version, your pelvis becomes asymmetrical but the pose is more organic, allowing both a spiral and a lift from the roots of your legs. Even though your body may lose some of its extension in this version, full contact with the ground enhances your feeling of connection and security. To get an equal length to both sides of your waist may be difficult, but within the difficulty try to find as much movement in that direction as possible.

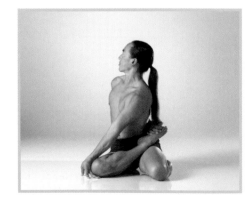

VERSION 3: Top leg in Half Lotus, arm around back, clasping big toe

The version requires much greater hip opening but also grounds the thigh of your back leg. Holding the lotus foot brings an internal connectivity and completion to a pose that naturally spirals upward. Because this version increases the twist, your back muscles begin to grab inward toward the center of the spine. Broaden your back muscles, engage your shoulder blades, and open, lift, and spiral your chest.

14. Try all three versions of **MARICHI'S TWIST 1** *(Marichyasana 1)* for 20 seconds in each version on each side.

VERSION 1: Hips on a block, back hand on block, elbow inside knee

Elevating your pelvis and back hand allows you to extend your spine fully and keep your pelvis upright, so you can twist without being hampered by the tightness of your pelvis, the resistance of the folding of your bent leg, or the tightness of the hamstrings of your straight leg. Your challenge is to keep your legs involved in both the lift of your torso and the spiral of your spine. Because the foundation of the pose is asymmetrical, there will be a tendency for one groin to be thick and swollen while the other is empty and hollow. Equalize them as best as possible.

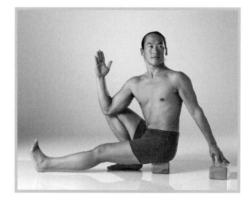

VERSION 2: Hips on the ground, elbow inside knee

Even for those of you who are flexible, your lower back will be somewhat rounded in this version. To extend your spine without clenching the muscles of your back, allow the twist to arise from the grounding of your legs and the slight rounding of your lower back, which opens your hips much more dramatically. Deepening your hip crease and the groin of your bent leg will begin to bring the sides of your waist to equal lengths. Allow your inhalation to fill your entire pose, even if you have to reduce the twist. As you complete your exhalation, find your entire body adding to the complete twist.

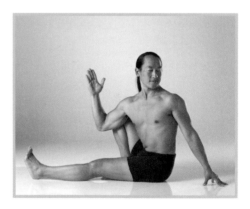

VERSION 3: Clasping your hands behind your back

This version integrates your arms and shoulders into the twist, bringing an openness and yet a challenge to the muscles of your chest and fronts of your shoulders. For most of you, when you begin to make the clasp, your front body will collapse. As a prelude to turning, re-extend from the depth of your groins to the lift of your collarbones. As you deepen the twist, your back muscles will tend to overwork; instead use your legs and the power of your arms to lift and turn your spine. Continually broaden the muscles of your back as evenly as possible.

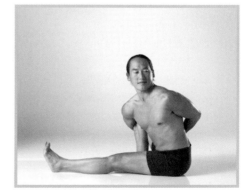

15. Try all three versions of **SEATED CROSSED-LEGS TWIST** *(Parsva Sukhasana)* for 20 seconds in each version, on each side.

VERSION 1: Hips on a block, back hand on a block

This version enables you to feel the twist with the natural curves and full extension of your spine. It is always easier on your respiratory system to have your front body fully open as you twist. To initiate the twist, energize your feet, then your legs, and then your pelvis. Because there is a natural ease to this twist, you might be too aggressive in the amount of twist that you try to achieve. Instead, continue to be gentle and observe the organic fluid spiraling of your entire body. Maintain the depth and release of both groins to increase your grounding, allowing your spine to begin its twist from your real foundation, the earth.

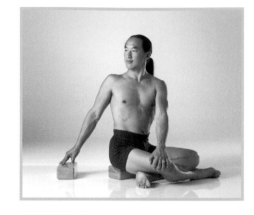

VERSION 2: Full pose, without props

This version allows for the full connection with the earth. Having your pelvis and legs in full contact brings sturdiness and consciousness to your grounding. Without sitting on the block, you will be challenged to keep your pelvis completely upright because it requires a deep hip opening. Without the full, easy uprightness of your pelvis, the length of the sides of your waist will be reduced. Search for the depth of your groins to allow for the natural length of the sides of your waist.

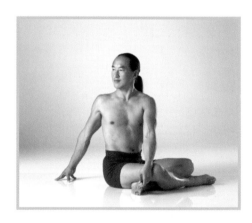

VERSION 3: Half Lotus, clasping your big toe

This version further challenges the openness of your hips, but for those of you who can clasp your big toe, this pose will complete an internal circuit of touch and breath. This version increases your twist, while giving much more internal freedom. Concentrate your mind and the movement of your breath on maintaining the broadness of your back muscles.

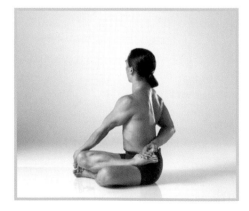

16. Try all three versions of **SIDEWAYS WIDE ANGLE POSE** *(Parsva Upavista Konasana)* for 20 seconds in each version on each side.

VERSION 1: Hips on folded blanket, hands on either side of leg toward which you are turning

This version allows you to fully extend your spine while your legs are in a fairly difficult position. It can be challenging to find the separate actions of moving your legs toward the ground and raising your spine upward. But the twist in this pose depends on that separation. Focus on reaching the leg you are turning away from and on finding the depth of both groins while you discover a regal lift and a subtle turn.

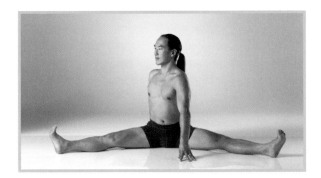

VERSION 2: Strap around foot, bending slightly forward

This version adds the beginning of a forward bend to the twist, which releases the muscles of your side lower back. Challenge yourself to keep the full grounding of both legs, although your sitting bone and the upper thigh of your back leg might slightly leave the ground. The waist of the side you are turning toward will shorten—release into the forward bend only so far as you can maintain as much length in that side as possible.

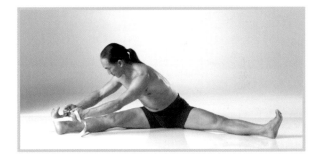

VERSION 3: Full pose, hands clasped around foot, bending forward

This version teaches you that you must begin this twist from your pelvis in order to keep the integrity in your lower back and the sides of your waist. Turn and bend forward from your pelvis to allow the full opening in the back of your front leg and your lower back. Focus on broadening the muscles of your lower back on the side to which you are turning.

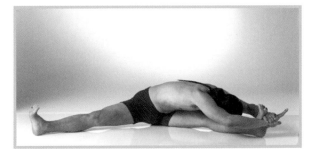

17. Try all three versions of **MARICHI'S TWIST 3** *(Marichyasana 3)* for 20 seconds in each version on each side.

VERSION 1: Hips on a block, back hand on a block, hugging your knee

By hugging your leg you keep your upper chest and shoulders in their natural openness. By sitting on a prop, you keep your spine neutral as you begin to explore this deep twist. As you maintain a neutral spine and shoulders, search for an evenness in the depths of your groins and approach the twist with steadiness and ease. Stay in the subtlety that these props allow, noticing the relationship between your breath and the twist.

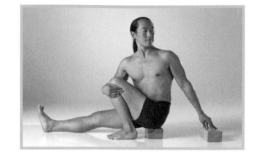

VERSION 2: Hips on the floor, armpit over your knee

This version gives you a deep turning of the abdominal cavity and massages your abdominal organs with the squeeze of the twist and a slight forward bend. However, by sitting on the ground, you lose the verticality of your pelvis as you must lean back slightly to keep the extension of your spine as it twists more deeply. To ensure the safety of the shoulder joint for the arm that is crossing your leg, draw your upper arm back into the socket as you firm your shoulder blade down your back and open your collarbone. Ground your straight leg strongly and lift your ribs on that side, so you begin to get an evenness of length in both sides of the waist.

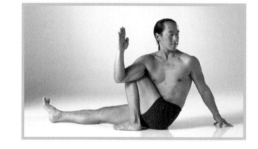

VERSION 3: Full pose, hands clasped behind your back

This version adds the complete turning and opening of your shoulders and arms, further challenging the extension of your spine and the openness and lift of both collarbones. However, once you make the clasp, the interconnectedness of your outer body brings an ease to your inner body so that even though your breath is more challenged, you will find a quietness and calmness.

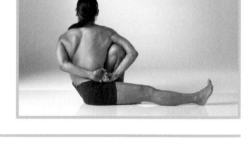

18. Practice version 2 of **COBBLER'S POSE** (with slight backbend) for 30 seconds. Lengthen both sides of your waist evenly.

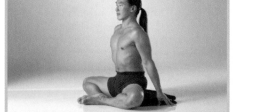

19. Try all three version of **LORD OF THE FISHES POSE** *(Arda Matsayendrasana)* for 20 seconds in each version on each side.

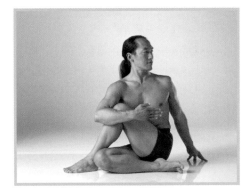

VERSION 1: Hugging your knee

This version teaches you about the foundation of the pose without overemphasizing the twist. Feel how this twist challenges the outside of your top leg and how the twist must emanate from that opening. By being able to adjust how far you go into the twist, you can focus on releasing the outside of your hip. Focus also on finding the equal depth of both groins as a way to stabilize the foundation of the pose. Use your bottom hand to stabilize you as well.

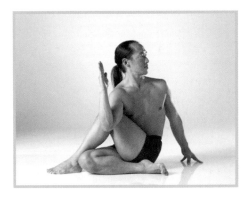

VERSION 2: Armpit over your knee

This version deepens the twist considerably, adding the full turn of your spine to the opening of your hips. When your armpit is in contact with your knee, consciously elongate and hollow your waist and belly. Slide your belly through the inside of your upper leg to find the organic turn of your spine.

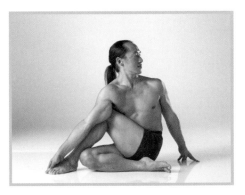

VERSION 3: Full pose, clasping your big toe

This version integrates your arms into the complete twist, allowing you to have far greater leverage in turning your spine. Clasping your toe brings an internal connection, which completes the spiral of the twist, allowing you to feel as if you have come full circle. This connection helps you to go deeper into integrating your entire body into the twist. With your legs, spine, and arms all deeply in the twist, broaden your back muscles away from your spine.

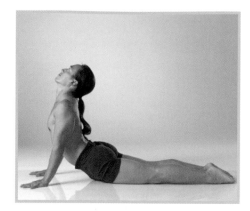

20. Practice **COBRA POSE** two or three times, for 15 seconds each time. Search for the depth and evenness of your groins.

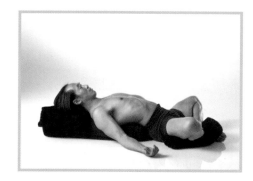

21. Practice **RECLINED COBBLER'S POSE** for 3 minutes. Search for the broadness of your back muscles.

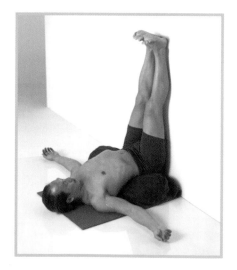

22. Practice **LEGS UP THE WALL POSE** for 2 minutes. Search for the length of the sides of your waist.

RELAXATION AND BREATH AWARENESS

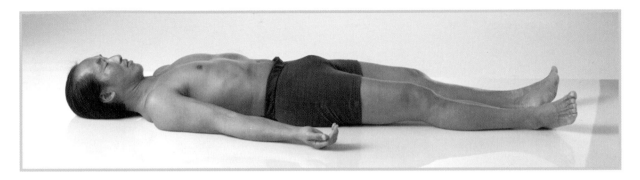

23. For 5 minutes, practice Relaxation Pose. Test which nostril breathes more freely by pinching one closed and then the other. Then see if you can notice the difference between the two nostrils with both open. Focus your mind on the breath that is moving through the entrance of your nostrils.

MEDITATION

24. For 5 to 15 minutes, sit in Seated Crossed-Legs Pose at the wall, with a blanket roll between the wall and your lower back. Meditate on using the wall as an indication of the continuation of the lift and alignment of your torso.

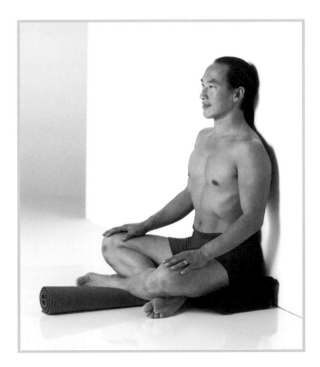

DAY 2: LEARNING SIMPLE TWIST
AND MARICHI'S TWIST 1

Both of these twists are open-body twists, which means that the foundation of the poses spirals in the same direction as the midsection of your belly and your chest, neck, and head. Because of this, your diaphragm, abdomen, and pelvic floor do not become challenged and you can hold these twists for longer periods of time with ease of breath. When setting up the foundation for Simple Twist, try to level your pelvis so that the side to which you are twisting is not uncomfortably collapsed. From here make sure that your hands can reach the ground easily, so your chest and upper back don't collapse as you twist. You may not feel like you are doing much in this twist, but this allows you to go much deeper in the subtle unwinding of your spine. Marichi's Twist 1 has the same characteristics as Simple Twist except that you can use the power of your arms more strongly. Because you'll be tempted to force the twist with the power of your arms, I encourage you to make sure that your spine and sacrum can fully receive that extra power.

Today's sequence begins with the Core Strengthening Series, a perfect prelude to twists. It centers your mind in your core and opens up your hips to create a good foundation for the twists. The Downward-Facing Dog and standing poses that follow open your hamstrings to let your legs fold more easily. And both Triangle Pose and Tree Pose mildly

twist your body. Simple Twist and Marichi's Twist 1 organically evolve from Triangle Pose and Tree Pose. The twists in this practice are interspersed with symmetrical poses, such as Standing Forward Bend, Wide Angle Forward Bend (page 264), Hero Pose, and Staff Pose, to reset the symmetry in your body. Repeating the twists toward the end of the sequence allows you to go further into them without force. You will find it more beneficial to repeat twists than to hold them for long periods of time. The sequence ends with three symmetrical poses to reset your sacrum and to move you deeper into relaxation after the opening and the cleansing that the twists provided. After the twists cleanse your organs, the restorative poses flush and release the toxins from your body.

FOCUS FOR THIS PRACTICE:

- In the Core Strengthening Series, deepen your groins and lift your chest from the strength of your legs.

- In the standing poses, lengthen the sides of your waist without overusing your back muscles.

- In Simple Twist and Marichi's Twist 1, broaden all your back muscles. Turn from the power of your legs and the suppleness of your belly.

1. Practice the **Core Strengthening Series** three times, flowing with your breath to transition between poses. Hold each pose for 1 breath. The third time, bend forward in Wide Angle Pose and Cobbler's Pose and hold each for 5 breaths.

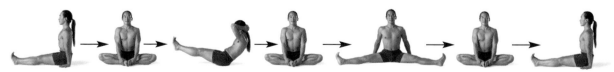

Staff Pose   Cobbler's Pose   Half Boat Pose   Cobbler's Pose   Wide Angle Pose   Cobbler's Pose   Staff Pose

Wide Angle
Forward Bend

Cobbler's
Forward Bend

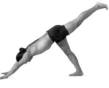   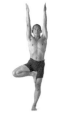 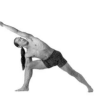

2. Practice **Downward-Facing Dog** for 1 minute.

3. Practice version 2 of **One-Legged Downward-Facing Dog** for 30 seconds on each side.

4. Practice **Standing Forward Bend** for 1 minute.

5. Practice **Triangle Pose** for 30 seconds on each side.

6. Practice **Tree Pose** for 30 seconds on each side.

7. Practice **Extended Side Angle** for 30 seconds on each side.

    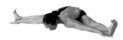

8. Practice **Simple Twist** for 30 seconds on each side.

9. Practice **Marichi's Twist 1** for 30 seconds on each side.

10. Practice **Hero Pose** for 1 minute.

11. Practice **Staff Pose** for 15 seconds.

12. Practice **Wide Angle Forward Bend** (page 264) for 30 seconds.

13. Practice **Downward-Facing Dog** for 30 seconds.

14. Practice version 1, 2, or 3 of **Simple Twist** for 30 seconds on each side.

15. Practice **Staff Pose** for 15 seconds.

16. Practice version 3 of **One-Legged Downward-Facing Dog** for 15 seconds on each side.

17. Practice **Marichi's Twist 1** for 30 seconds on each side.

18. Practice **Child's Pose** for 1 minute.

  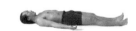 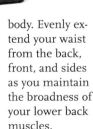

19. Practice version 3 of **Reclined Cobbler's Pose** for 3 minutes.

20. Practice **Legs Up the Wall Pose** for 3 minutes.

21. Relaxation and Breath Awareness. For 5 minutes, practice **Relaxation Pose.** Focus on the smoothness and evenness of your inhalation and exhalation.

Do not force the smoothness and evenness, but ask yourself: what is binding my breath to keep it from being smooth and even? Let go of that binding.

22. Meditation. For 5 to 10 minutes, sit in **Hero Pose,** on a prop high enough to keep you comfortable. Emphasize an equal length to both sides of your

body. Evenly extend your waist from the back, front, and sides as you maintain the broadness of your lower back muscles.

DAY 3: LEARNING THE RECLINED TWISTS

When you lie on the ground, your spine naturally elongates, providing a good orientation from which to twist. Yet with the floor support, you tend to be a bit sloppy with the work of your legs and feet, forgetting how important they are in supporting your spine. Some of you are limited in your ability to twist, so your knees and your opposite shoulder may lift off the ground. But you have the option of supporting underneath your legs, which decreases the twists and allows you to observe the subtle nuances of the pose. The advantage of twisting without this support is that your legs and arms have to stay more active. Gravity helps you twist deeper into these poses, with the weight of your legs creating a fairly strong force. If it feels like the muscles of your back and abdomen are too taxed by the weight of your legs, use support. In Reclined Straight-Leg Twist, there is so much more force and torque on your spine from the leverage of your straight legs that it helps build strength for your back and abdominal muscles. However, if you are not ready for this much work, you can easily overdo the twist, so try to find a balance between effort and surrender. Another challenge in these reclined twists is to keep your chest open. The work of your arms and the press of the shoulder blades into your back help you keep the broadness and lift of your upper chest. As you work your arms to keep your chest open, it is easy to grip your neck and throat. If releasing your neck is not possible, support your legs.

Today's sequence begins with Sun Salutations and the Core Strengthening Series to bring movement and warmth to your body, integrating your body with your mind and breath. The rest of the sequence is quite restorative, with only reclined or seated poses. Reclined Leg Stretch Series opens up the backs of your legs and allows you to feel the connections between your legs and spine and your arms and chest. The reclined twists that follow are interspersed with symmetrical poses to return the spine to neutral. In this sequence, you experience deep twisting without much exertion. Because these poses do not require much effort, you can use this whole practice to be more internal. The twists will balance and open up your back muscles to prepare you for seated meditation.

FOCUS FOR THIS PRACTICE:

- In the Sun Salutations and Core Strengthening Series, lengthen the sides of your waist by lifting your rib cage strongly from your pelvis.

- In the Reclined Twist, deepen your groins and move your sacrum into your body and up toward your open and broad chest.

- In the restorative poses, set up your foundation by broadening and lengthening your back muscles. As you lie down, release the skin of your back.

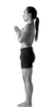

1. Practice two mini **Sun Salutations**, staying in Downward-Facing Dog for 5 breaths.

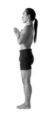

2. Practice two full **Sun Salutations**, staying in the second Downward-Facing Dog for 5 breaths.

3. Practice the **Core Strengthening Series** two times. The second time, bend forward in Wide Angle Pose and in Cobbler's Pose for 15 seconds.

  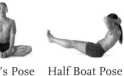

| Staff Pose (1 breath) | Cobbler's Pose (1 breath) | Half Boat Pose (1 breath) | Cobbler's Pose (1 breath) | Wide Angle Forward Bend (15 seconds) | Cobbler's Forward Bend (15 seconds) | Staff Pose (1 breath) |

  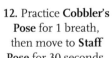

4. Practice the **Reclined Leg Stretch Series** to the front for 30 seconds, with a sit-up for 15 seconds, and to the side for 30 seconds, on both left and right sides.

5. Practice version 2 of **Reclined Twist** with knees together (not thigh over thigh) for 45 seconds on each side.

6. Practice **Happy Baby Pose** for 30 seconds.

7. Practice version 3 of **Reclined Twist** with thigh over thigh for 15 seconds on each side.

8. Practice version 2 of **Reclined Cobbler's Pose** for 30 seconds.

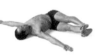 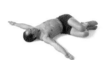 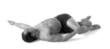 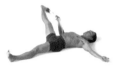

9. Practice **Reclined Straight-Leg Twist** for 15 seconds on each side.

10. Practice **Cobbler's Pose** for 1 minute.

11. Practice **Wide Angle Pose** for 1 minute.

12. Practice **Cobbler's Pose** for 1 breath, then move to **Staff Pose** for 30 seconds.

13. Practice version 1 of **Marichi's Twist 3** for 30 seconds to 1 minute on each side.

   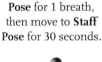 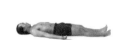

14. Practice **Reclined Hero Pose** for 1 to 2 minutes.

15. Practice version 1 of **Child's Pose** for 1 to 2 minutes.

16. Practice **Seated Crossed-Legs Twist** for 45 seconds on each side.

17. Meditation. For 5 to 15 minutes, sit in **Seated Crossed-Legs Pose**, meditating on the pathway and movement of your breath.

18. Relaxation and Breath Awareness. For 5 minutes, practice **Relaxation Pose.** For 1 minute, imagine you are breathing in the right nostril and out the left nostril, then in the left nostril and out the right nostril. Then breathe evenly in and out of both nostrils.

These two twists are closed-body twists in which your belly turns in the opposite direction of the natural flow of your foundation. Your spine and your organs really enjoy this squeeze, but breathing is more difficult. Even when you do these twists with good alignment and a sense of ease, your breath will naturally be quick and short. These twists also have the benefit of opening the outsides of your hips and legs. Those of you who are stiff in the outsides of your hips will find these twists very challenging, yet also extremely beneficial. (For example, many well-toned athletes will feel a strong resistance to moving in this way, and yet these very poses will balance many of their other physical endeavors.) You can use props underneath your hips in these poses so that your spine can maintain its length as you twist. You will go much deeper into the twist when you release the internal struggle and resistance that comes from a full-out push. Marichi's Twist 3 maximizes the twist in your spine as your pelvis is locked into a square position by your legs and your spine is isolated. Therefore constantly observe your alignment and breath as you move in and out of these twists. In Lord of Fishes Pose, there is much more opening in the sides of your hips,

although here, too, your spinal twist is maximized. Feel this twist evenly distributed in your hips and spine, from the sides of your hips all the way up to the crown of your head.

Today's sequence begins with the Sun Salutations and standing poses to create activity and heat in your entire body. Cobbler's Pose and Wide Angle Pose prepare you for twisting as they open your hips and ground your legs. The rest of the practice repeats the twists, interspersing them with Cobbler's Pose to re-center you and create symmetry in your body. The practice ends with Cobra Pose to restabilize your sacrum.

FOCUS FOR THIS PRACTICE:

- In the Sun Salutations, focus on an even depth to your groins through the movements and the poses. Notice that one groin will tend to be deeper than the other.

- In the standing poses, broaden your back muscles away from your spine as you maximize the length of your torso.

- In all the twists, lengthen the sides of your waist.

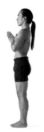 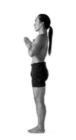 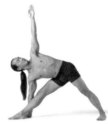 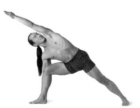

1. Practice two mini **Sun Salutations,** staying in Downward-Facing Dog for 5 breaths.

2. Practice two full **Sun Salutations,** staying in Upward-Facing Dog for 3 breaths and the second Downward-Facing Dog for 5 breaths.

3. Practice **Triangle Pose** for 45 seconds on each side.

4. Practice **Standing Forward Bend** for 30 seconds on each side.

5. Practice **Extended Side Angle Pose** for 30 seconds on each side.

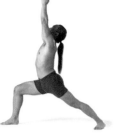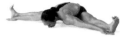

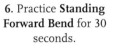

6. Practice **Standing Forward Bend** for 30 seconds.

7. Practice **Warrior 1** for 30 seconds on each side.

8. Practice **Standing Forward Bend** for 30 seconds.

9. Practice **Cobbler's Forward Bend** for 1 minute.

10. Practice **Wide Angle Forward Bend** for 1 minute.

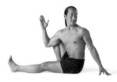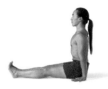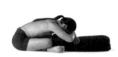

11. Practice **Marichi's Twist 1** for 30 seconds on each side.

12. Practice **Cobbler's Pose** for 30 seconds.

13. Practice **Marichi's Twist 3** for 30 seconds on each side.

14. Practice **Staff Pose** for 15 seconds.

15. Practice **Crossed-Legs Forward Bend** (see page 259) for 30 seconds. Recross your legs the opposite way, and practice again for 30 seconds.

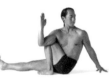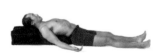

16. Practice **Lord of the Fishes Pose** for 30 seconds.

17. Practice **Cobbler's Pose** with a slight backbend for 30 seconds.

18. Practice **Marichi's Twist 3** for 45 seconds on each side.

19. Practice **Cobbler's Pose** with a slight backbend for 30 seconds.

20. Practice **Lord of the Fishes Pose** for 45 seconds on each side.

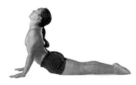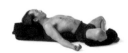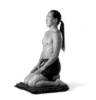

21. Practice **Cobra Pose** for 10 seconds, three times moving slowly.

22. Practice version 3 of **Reclined Cobbler's Pose** for 3 minutes.

23. Meditation. For 5 to 10 minutes, practice **Hero Pose.** Feel the dialogue between the broadness of your back body and length of your front body.

24. Relaxation and Breath Awareness. For 5 minutes, practice version 3 of **Supported Relaxation Pose** (page 268). Feel as though you are smelling the fragrance of the air. Sip the air delicately and consciously.

Both Sideways Wide Angle Pose and Seated Crossed-Legs Twist provide a strong foundation with a clear, elongated waist from which you can turn. Use a lift under your sitting bones to sit your pelvis completely upright, with the top of your sacrum in a natural back-bend. With adequate lift under your sitting bones, you can find quite a bit of movement in your hip sockets to begin the twist. Start your spine spiraling by turning your pelvis and grounding your thighbones. In Wide Angle Twist, the movement of your back thigh toward the ground—even if it slightly lifts from the ground—is the anchor from which the twist begins. From the grounding of your legs, feel the lightness of your pelvis initiate the extension of your lower back. Use this extension to enhance your twist. Likewise, in Crossed-Legs Twist, the thigh that you are turning away from will tend to become ungrounded. Sometimes I even use my hand to press that thigh back down toward the ground as I turn away from it. Both these twists teach you how much space you can find between your pelvis and your thighs; increasing this space brings great relief throughout your body-mind because it deeply enhances your ability to breathe. These two twists also allow you to adjust your pelvis so that you can find the full extension of your spine from the ground with ease.

Today's sequence begins with Downward-Facing Dog, Child's Pose, and standing poses to release your hamstrings as preparation for forward bending. From here, Marichi's Twist 1 awakens your ability to twist. Now that your hips are open and prepared to sit upright, you move on to Seated Crossed-Legs Twist. The Cobbler's Pose that follows is a neutral pose that further opens your hips. The openings created by the previous poses prepare you to practice your first Sideways Wide Angle pose with as much ease as possible. The rest of the poses are variations and repetitions of Seated Crossed-Legs Twist and Sideways Wide Angle Twist, so you can learn the more subtle aspects of these poses and go progressively deeper into them. Remember, repetitions of twists are beneficial, whereas holding them for long periods of time is too harsh on the nervous system. This practice ends with Cobbler's Pose and Reclined Cobbler's Pose to reset the sacrum and equalize the spine.

FOCUS FOR THIS PRACTICE:

- In Downward-Facing Dog and Standing Forward Bend, deepen your groins to fold your pelvis over your thighs and find the maximum opening of your hamstrings. Combine this action with the tuck of your tailbone to protect your hamstrings.

- In the standing poses, deepen your groins, tuck your tailbone, and lengthen the sides of your waist.

- In the twists, ground your legs, broaden your back muscles, and lengthen the front of your spine.

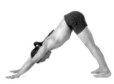   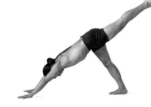 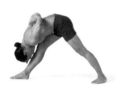

1. Practice **Downward-Facing Dog** for 2 minutes.

2. Practice **Child's Pose** for 30 seconds.

3. Practice **Standing Forward Bend** for 1 minute.

4. Practice version 2 of **One-Legged Downward-Facing Dog** with one leg up behind you for 15 seconds on each side.

5. Practice **Pyramid Pose** for 30 seconds on each side.

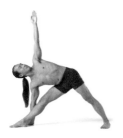 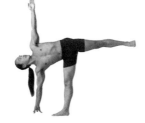 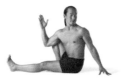

6. Practice **Triangle Pose** for 30 seconds on each side.

7. Practice **Half Moon Pose** for 30 seconds on each side.

8. Practice **Standing Forward Bend** for 30 seconds.

9. Practice **Marichi's Twist 1** for 30 seconds on each side.

  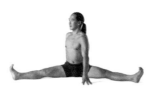

10. Practice **Seated Crossed-Legs Twist** for 30 seconds on each side.

11. Practice **Cobbler's Pose** for 15 seconds.

12. Practice version 1 of **Sideways Wide Angle Pose** for 15 seconds on each side.

13. Practice **Seated Crossed-Legs Twist** for 30 seconds on each side.

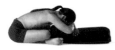 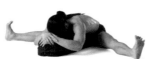 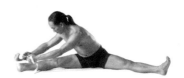

14. Practice **Crossed-Legs Forward Bend** (page 259) for 30 seconds. Re-cross your legs and repeat for 30 seconds.

15. Practice **Wide Angle Forward Bend** (page 264) for 30 seconds.

16. Practice version 3 of **Seated Crossed-Legs Twist** or, if not possible, version 2 of **Seated Crossed-Legs Twist** for 30 seconds on each side.

17. Practice version 2 or 3 of **Sideways Wide Angle Pose** for 30 seconds on each side.

 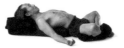 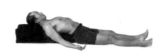

18. Practice **Cobbler's Pose** with a slight backbend for 1 minute.

19. Practice version 3 of **Reclined Cobbler's Pose** for 3 minutes.

20. Relaxation and Breath Awareness. For 5 minutes, practice version 3 of **Supported Relaxation Pose** (page 268). Observe your exhalations and lengthen them, if possible, without straining.

21. Meditation. For 5 to 15 minutes, sit in **Seated Crossed-Legs Pose** in the middle of the room. Meditate on sitting squarely on both your sitting bones, with both groins evenly deep, feeling the even weight of each thigh dropping toward the earth.

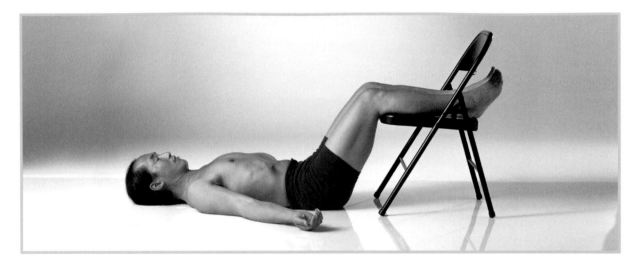

Breath Awareness

For 2 minutes, practice version 2 of Supported Relaxation Pose.

RELAXATION POSE. Version 2 of Relaxation Pose is specified for today because it takes all the weight and tension off your lower back. This pose also makes you aware of how relaxed your calf muscles are (or are not). Consciously soften your calf muscles until they feel like pools of water on the chair. You might have to shift the chair every so often so it carries the weight of your legs more completely. Your legs should not jam down into your hip sockets; they should feel as if they are levitating without creating a pull on your pelvis or spine. With your legs higher than your belly, you will have a better chance at feeling the completions of your exhalations.

BOTTOM OF THE EXHALATION. For 5 minutes, begin to exhale smoothly, without effort. To do this, allow the light touch of your observation to drop into the sensations and sounds of your exhalations.

Now, bring your awareness to the silence at the bottom of your exhalations, feeling them fade into emptiness. There is always a natural pause at the bottom of your exhalations. In this exercise, I want you to look more closely at that pause and become more familiar with that moment. So pause intentionally for 1 or 2 seconds at the bottom of each exhalation. Every so often you will be tempted to pause your exhalation much longer. However, at this point in your practice, try to suspend that tendency or desire and keep pausing the exhalation for only 1 or 2 seconds. If this short pausing or even the observation of the natural moment of emptiness begins to bring more tension or anxiety, stop this technique and go back to scanning your body for relaxation.

If you ever feel so agitated that you feel like you have to get up and move around, this is fine, but when you do so, move slowly, mindfully, and skillfully out of the pose by drawing your knees into your chest and rolling onto your right side.

RETURN TO RELAXATION. For 2 minutes, return to Relaxation Pose and slowly scan your body, from head to toes.

Meditation

For 10 minutes, sit in Hero Pose with a pillow under your hands. Meditate on the very small and gentle rocking of your pelvis from a more round back to a more sway back.

In our culture, there are many stereotypes about meditation that lead many of you to believe that when you meditate, you must sit up straight and stay completely still—as if you were standing at attention in the military—and that internally you must be completely focused, like a warrior with a single task at hand. But in all honesty, meditation postures should be gentle and you should constantly realign your posture from your observation of your breath. Without disturbing your mind, your body can continue its conversation with center and with the way your breath is being absorbed.

ROCKING MOTIONS. Today I am asking you to consciously make small rocking motions with your pelvis, from a more round back on your exhalation to a more sway back on your inhalation. Picture a small lizard on a rock that seems at first glance to be extremely quiet. But as you look more carefully, you detect the movement of the lizard's breath and the beat of its heart undulating and pulsing its body like ripples from a rock thrown into a pond. When you allow your body to pulsate with your breath and your heart, you reduce the tendency for your legs to fall asleep and your body to become stagnant.

YOUR ARMS. The pillow under your hands allows your arms to rest but also reminds you to keep your

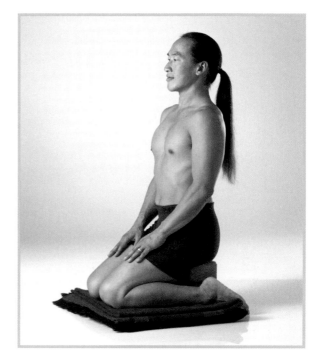

arms from hanging heavily from your chest. Let the pillow teach you how to keep your arms lifted up into their sockets as if they were two poles of a tent lifting the tent upward.

The movement of your pelvis and the lift of your arms keep your body awake and your mind present. To find the best alignment of your arms, hands, and pelvis, observe how your breath flows. Try to maximize the ease and the flow of your breath. As you train yourself in this way, your body will intuitively find a more subtle alignment that allows your mind to go into deeper states of emptiness and receptivity.

WIDE ANGLE POSE

Wide Angle Pose creates a broad foundation from which you lift
and grow your spine.

POINT OF PLAY:
Deepen your sacrum as you
move your thighs back.

Toes and knees straight up

Waist long

Legs extending strongly

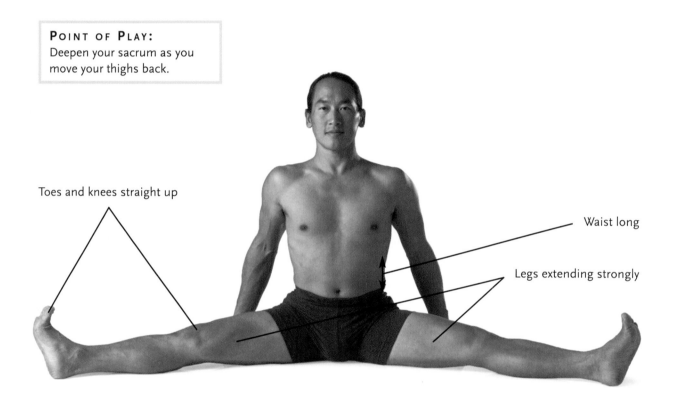

HALF BOAT POSE

Half Boat Pose integrates your torso with your legs
by strengthening your core.

POINT OF PLAY:
Lift yourself higher, and lower
yourself down.

Arms drawn back into sockets

Legs extending strongly

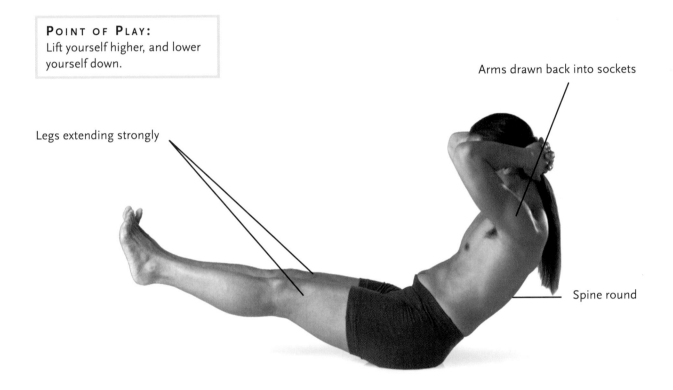

Spine round

ONE-LEGGED DOWNWARD-FACING DOG POSE

One-Legged Downward-Facing Dog Pose allows you to maximize the length
of your spine as you spiral it.

POINT OF PLAY:
On your exhalation, twist
deeper, and on your inhalation, widen your back muscles.

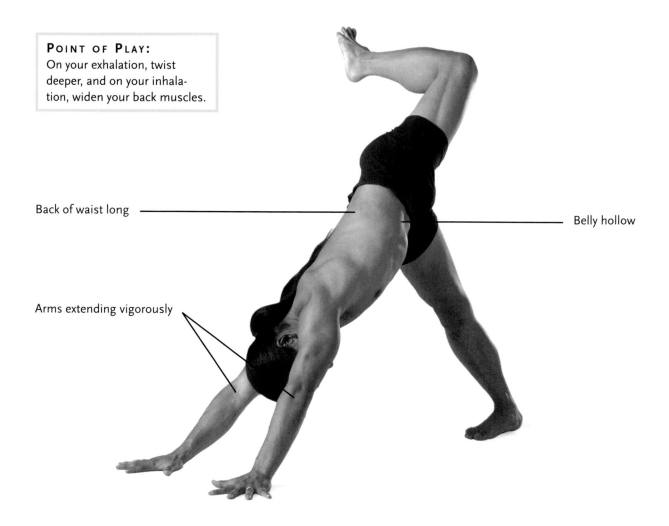

Back of waist long

Belly hollow

Arms extending vigorously

RECLINED LEG STRETCH SERIES, VERSION 3

Reclined Leg Stretch Series, version 3, is an expansive pose that forces you to be attentive to grounding your body and bottom leg while you open your front body.

POINT OF PLAY:
Arch your lower back more and then less.

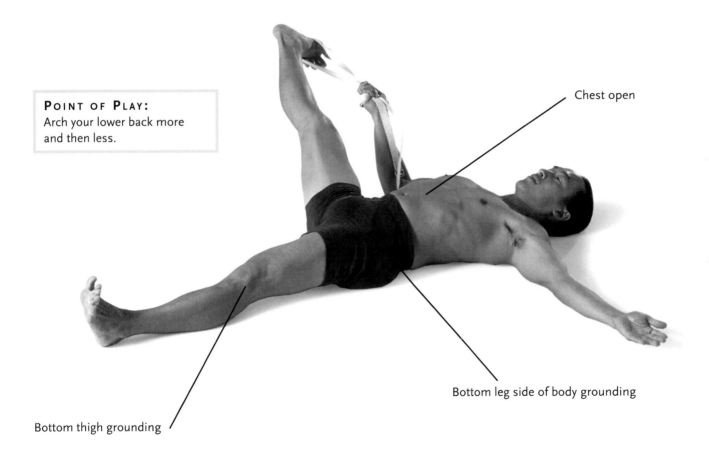

Chest open

Bottom leg side of body grounding

Bottom thigh grounding

RECLINED TWIST

Reclined Twist allows gravity to open your spine
as you focus on surrender.

Natural curve in your lower back

Thighbones moving toward hamstrings

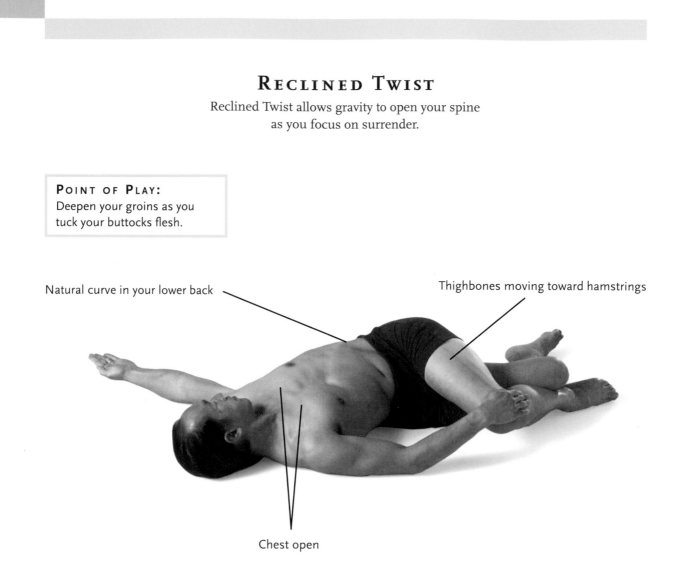

Chest open

RECLINED STRAIGHT-LEG TWIST

Reclined Straight-Leg Twist is a strong twist in which you must utilize your legs and core to maintain integrity in your spine.

POINT OF PLAY:
Play with lengthening your right and then left waist.

Top waist long

Thighbones moving toward hamstrings

Chest open

SIMPLE TWIST

Simple Twist is a graceful twist in which your entire body spirals in the same direction,
allowing ease of breath.

> **POINT OF PLAY:**
> Come in and out of the twist,
> coordinating your movement
> with your inhalation and exhal-
> ation.

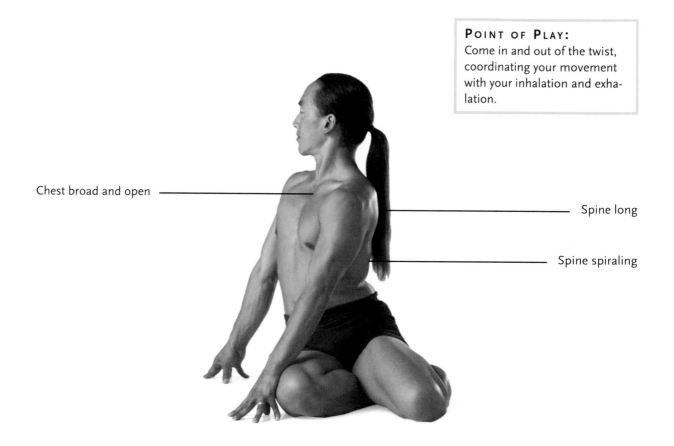

Chest broad and open ——————

Spine long

Spine spiraling

MARICHI'S TWIST 1

Marichi's Twist 1 enables you to use your arms to spiral your torso
and open your heart from the grounding of your legs.

POINT OF PLAY:
Play with lifting your head then
releasing it down.

Shoulder blades moving down back

Shin in armpit

Heel of bent leg just outside sitting bone

Arms in sockets

SEATED CROSSED-LEGS TWIST

Seated Crossed-Legs Twist provides a strong, stable foundation
from which you can ease your spine into a twist.

POINT OF PLAY:
Rock your pelvis from a round
back to a sway back.

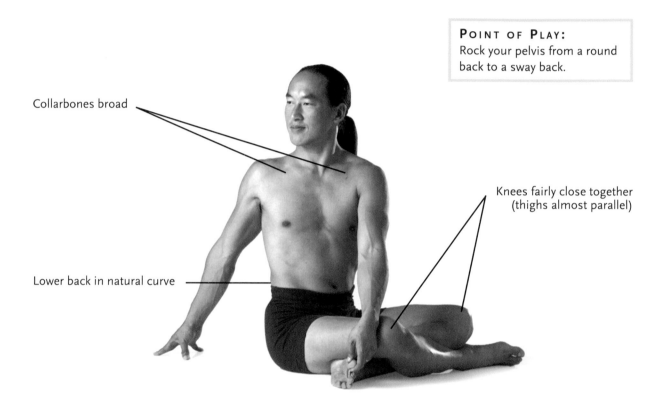

Collarbones broad

Knees fairly close together
(thighs almost parallel)

Lower back in natural curve

SIDEWAYS WIDE ANGLE POSE

Sideways Wide Angle Pose challenges you to ground your legs
and maximize the length of both sides of your waist as you move into the twist.

POINT OF PLAY:
Experiment with turning your torso more or less toward your front leg.

Waist extending

Chest open

Both thighs pressing toward ground

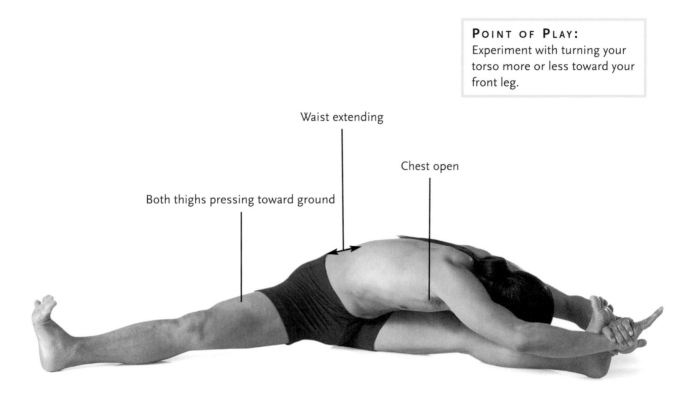

MARICHI'S TWIST 3

Marichi's Twist 3 provides a strong twist as you turn your torso in the opposite direction from the foundation of your legs, massaging your vital organs.

POINT OF PLAY:
Experiment with coming out of the twist and then twisting more deeply.

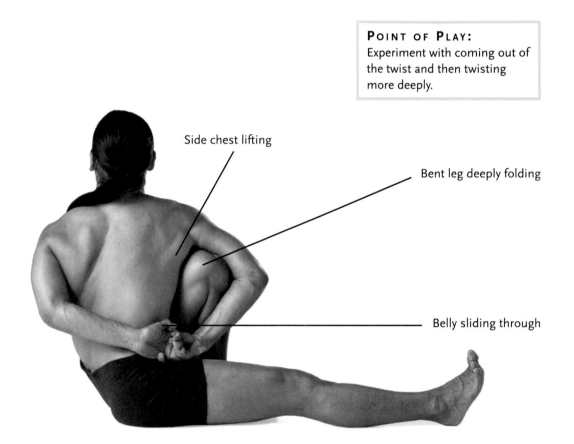

Side chest lifting

Bent leg deeply folding

Belly sliding through

LORD OF THE FISHES POSE

Lord of the Fishes Pose is a liberating twist
that culminates in a broad, open chest.

POINT OF PLAY:
Try sitting on a prop and then
sitting on the ground.

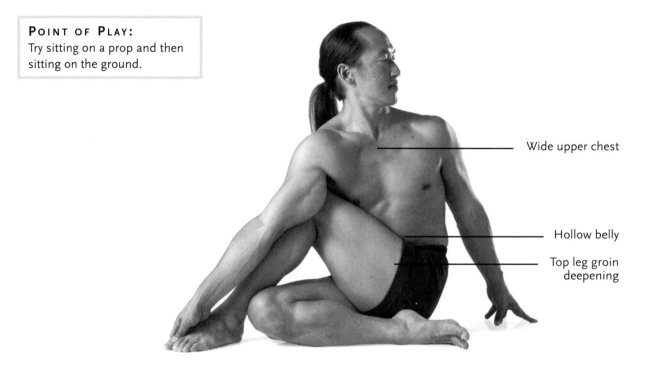

Wide upper chest

Hollow belly

Top leg groin
deepening

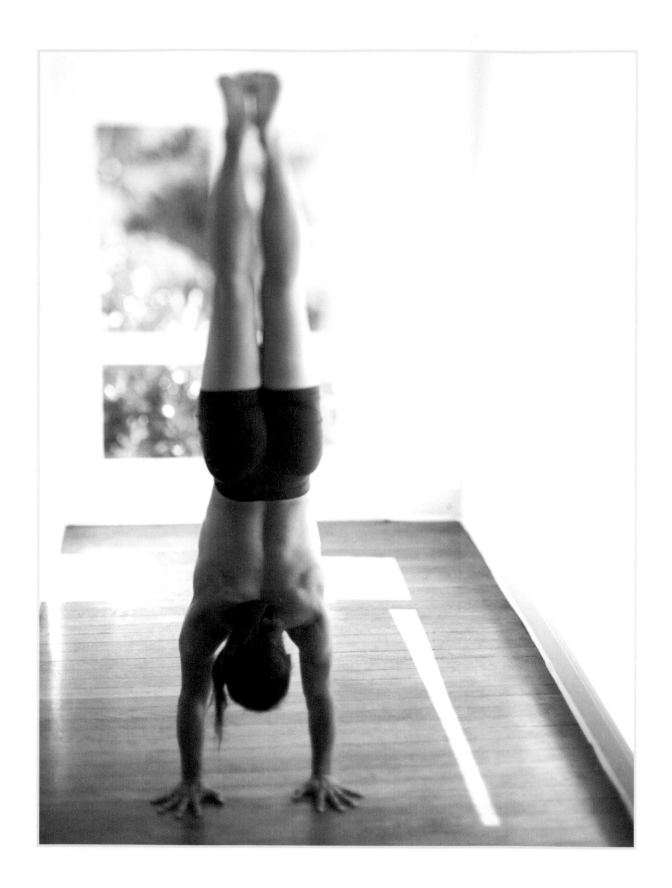

THIS IS TRUE YOGA: THE UNBINDING
OF THE BONDS OF SORROW. PRACTICE
THIS YOGA WITH DETERMINATION
AND WITH A COURAGEOUS HEART.
—*BHAGAVAD GITA*, TRANS. BY STEPHEN MITCHELL

WEEK 5:

Facing the Unknown

WHEN IT COMES RIGHT DOWN TO IT, WE KNOW SO LITTLE ABOUT WHO WE ARE AND THE UNIVERSE around us. As we step into the future, we make calculated guesses about what will happen next and how we will respond, but we are actually clueless for the most part. Therefore, our relationship with the unknown is a very prominent part of our lives. As you move into yoga poses that are not part of your everyday physical and mental vocabularies, you begin to understand your visceral and intellectual ways of dealing with the unknown. By consciously practicing yoga poses that are completely unfamiliar, you conduct an experiment that can teach you how you react in the face of being lost.

Handstand not only turns you upside down but also makes you depend on your arms as your means of solo support. For most of you, this brings a deep fear, not only of the possibility of hurting yourself but also of not knowing what's going to happen. By putting yourself in this situation, you can become acutely aware of how your body reacts and how you can change or relax some of those reactions. So the important thing is not necessarily your ability to do Handstand but rather your discovery of how you can relax in a threatening situation. How can you approach Handstand in a less goal-oriented way? How can you begin to have a childlike playfulness and a sense of fun when you do Handstand, as if the pose were a new Christmas toy that you had no idea how to work?

Shoulderstand is an interesting posture because even though it is an inverted pose, it does not cause a noticeable fear of falling. Nonetheless, the change in orientation and the shift of perspective that it creates are still quite profound. Because of this, Shoulderstand is usually a good pose to start your approach to inversions. Some of you, however, will be afraid that Shoulderstand might cause pain in your neck or upper body. Therefore, taking incremental steps is a good way to move toward Shoulderstand.

About Inverted Poses

If you have experience inverting your body (doing handstands, cartwheels, and headstands), going upside down will not feel foreign. However, many of you have not played with these postures so being upside down will be completely unfamiliar. None of us, however, spend all that much time during a given day upside down, so when you begin to spend 5 to 30 minutes per day in inverted positions, you take on a very different perspective. Being upside down not only changes your view of the world by 180 degrees, but your muscular system also has to respond differently as it supports your body in this orientation. Your organs can find relief as they drop into the upper spaces of the cavity that contains them. It is also very inspiring to learn to do something completely different with your body and to begin to master a pose that is totally out of your daily vocabulary.

When I teach children, the most exciting pose for me to help the kids learn is Handstand. Children learning this pose experience a combination of excitement, silliness, challenge, and general fun. Your fear of the pose may overwhelm your initial childlike responses, but nonetheless, I believe everybody is exhilarated by attempting these poses. It is amazing how empowering it is to feel your full body weight being supported by your arms.

Approach these poses carefully and frequently so your fear and unfamiliarity will slowly be relieved. Spending some time in inverted poses on a daily basis turns your mind inward, relieves stress, and shift your perspective from whatever you are obsessing about.

EMOTIONS. The inverted poses bring your body back to neutral. They place us in a middle ground with our emotional body, where it is not a matter of feeling happy or sad but of being able to feel the clear and neutral space between happiness and sadness. Whatever emotions you experienced before practicing the inverted poses will seem much more diluted so you can observe them without being overwhelmed. In inverted poses, the underlying quality of contentment that is always available to you permeates your consciousness more fully.

FOCUS OF YOUR MIND. Because all of your weight is placed on either your arms, head, or shoulders, the inverted poses focus attention on your upper body, neck, and head. They ask you to be attentive to your alignment, your circulation, and the relationship of your upper spine with your shoulders, arms, and head.

BALANCING. As you practice the inverted poses, you should move toward ease. Not only should you begin to let go of fear and anxiety, you should find your balance in these poses more in the center of your skeleton. For instance, in Handstand—as you line up your forearms right under your upper arms so your elbows are articulating full extension and straightness, and when your upper arms are in line with your torso and your torso is in line with your legs—your skeleton maximizes its ability to support your weight. This refined alignment takes some time to reach, since your joints need to open up and your muscular body needs to support you. But with practice, balancing your body in center—and without effort—becomes a wonderful art of listening and responding. To me this is one of the most important and enjoyable aspects of the yoga poses.

BREATH. Whenever you move into the unknown and respond with fear, you usually grip your breath. However, just being able to observe your breath at all in inverted poses means that you have overcome some of your initial fears. As you observe the way your breath moves, you can adjust the alignment and the action of your muscular skeletal body. As you observe the subtleties of your breath, the quieting of your mind will be profound.

HANDS. As you work your hands in the inverted poses, let them be receptive and responsive. Be sensitive to how your hands are touching either the ground or your body. When your hands overwork, your wrists become tight and more susceptible to injury. From the foundation of your hands, your forearms should have both a sense of grounding through your hands and a rising up from them. In general, your fingers

ANATOMY LESSON

1. Thighbones grounding toward hamstrings

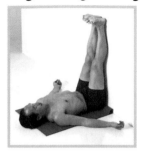 To learn about your thigh-bones, practice version 2 of Legs Up the Wall Pose. Place the heels of your hands on the very tops of your thighs, where they meet your pelvis, and press your thighbones toward your hamstrings, in the direction of the wall. See if you can get this same action in Downward-Facing Dog without the use of your hands.

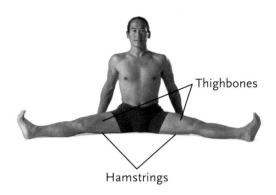

Thighbones

Hamstrings

2. Relaxation of neck

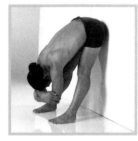 To learn about the relaxation of your neck, practice version 3 of Wall Hang and play with moving your neck around and slowly letting it hang to feel the release and relaxation of your neck muscles.

3. Wakefulness of feet

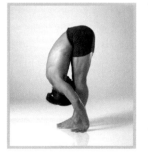 To learn about the wakefulness of your feet, practice Standing Forward Bend and look at your feet as you raise your toes and spread them. As your toes spread, move the balls of your feet away from the heels and lift your arches. Try to maintain as much activity as you can in the arches of your feet as you slowly lengthen your toes back to the ground.

should be lightly spread so you get an even, broad contact with whatever you are touching while the center of your hand feels like it is drawing from its foundation into the lift of your forearms and upper arms. The ease of your breath and the neutral placement of your lower ribs allow your hands to be relaxed and responsive.

SHOULDERS AND ARMS. Let your shoulders and arms feel as if they are both supporting and expressing your heart. Extend your arms from the center of your chest and yet also gather them back into your chest to aid the support of your heart. Let the work of your shoulders and arms feel that the connection with your heart is completely integrated. When you are upside down, any shift in balance is more obvious. The response of your shoulders, arms, and hands to this ever-changing balance becomes an exquisite dance that completely engages your mind.

LEGS AND FEET. Whenever you are upside down, your legs and feet function as a channel for strength and connectivity to your body as well as an important orientation for your mind. When your legs are drawn into center and your legs and feet are active and energized, you get a much better idea of where your body is in space. The more you can orient yourself off the centering action of your legs and feet, the more your mind will let go of its fear.

LOWER BACK. As you turn upside down initially, you tend to collapse into your lower back. Use the reach of your legs upward to support the length and ease of your lower spine. Those of you whose shoulders are tight may not be able to find the proper alignment in your upper body, which will make your lower body compensate for this lack of extension. As you practice these poses, you will increase your ability to open your shoulders, extend your legs, and relieve the jamming in your lower back.

DAY 1: LEARNING THE VARIATIONS

The first practice in this week builds progressively so that you have many preparations for both Handstand and Shoulderstand. For some of you, there will be variations that you may not even be able to attempt. If this is the case, stay with the variations that are possible and continue to develop toward approaching these challenging variations. I believe if you are consistent in approaching these poses over a long period of time—say, six months to a year—the postures will develop organically and substantially. In Handstand, you will gradually gain strength and confidence so that your arms can support your weight. You will also gain sensitivity to the alignment of your arms, which will provide you with more responsiveness to balance. Just through feeling the alignment of Handstand, whether you are standing on your feet, lying on your back, or standing on your hands, you become familiar with the general organization of the posture. In some ways, constantly approaching the pose and understanding its shape is more important than actually doing the posture.

You may have more of an instant rapport with Shoulderstand because it feels more familiar and less scary than Handstand. However, in some ways Shoulderstand is a far more complex posture, mainly because of the unusual shape of your arms and neck. So give Shoulderstand as much time, consistency, and mindfulness as Handstand. Try to understand the sequencing that I have provided below, both in the variations of each pose and in the progression from one pose to the next. This sequencing will give you the proper warm-up both mentally and physically to attempt the postures. Take time in each variation to feel the effects on your body-mind.

MOVING IN AND OUT OF INVERTED POSES

This week it is especially important to set up for the poses—whether physically setting up your props or mentally setting up your body—so that as you move into the postures you are mindful from beginning to

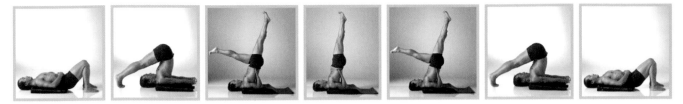

This photo sequence illustrates moving into and out of Shoulderstand.

end. Setting up the foundation for the pose and taking your time to feel your movement toward the pose will help you avoid becoming paralyzed with fear. These poses will also teach you how your intention influences your entire practice. Just as when a runner puts on her shoes, a violinist respectfully takes out his instrument, or a martial artist bows before coming into the practice room, your respect for space, presence of mind, and receptivity set up the necessary foundation for practice. So as you line up your mind and body to move into an inverted pose, approach the pose as single-mindedly as possible. And in any of these postures where we ask you to use props, for example, in Shoulderstand, the folding of the blankets and your mindfulness in setting your foundation are also crucial. Take your time and set your course.

It is just as important to take your time and be mindful as you move out of these postures. People often collapse the pose as they begin to come out, thinking that they have to release to come down. In fact, increase the action of the pose as you lower yourself. For instance, in Handstand, immediately before you begin to bring one leg back to the ground, increase the length of the entire pose up.

PROPS FOR SHOULDERSTAND

To ensure the safety of your neck and to achieve correct alignment, practice Shoulderstand on three folded blankets as shown in the photograph at right.

To set up your props, first stack your three folded blankets so that the neat, folded edges are aligned on top of each other. Then place the blanket stack on the

edge of your yoga mat, so that the neat, folded edges of the blankets extend about 3 inches beyond the mat's edge. Finally, fold the mat over the rough edges of the folded blankets, bringing the edge of the mat about 3 inches short of the neat, folded edge of the blanket stack. You now have a mat/blanket "sandwich," in which the filling (the blankets) extends about 3 inches outside the bread (the mat).

When you go up into Shoulderstand, your shoulders should rest on the neat, folded edge of the blanket stack so your neck easily spills off the edge and your head rests on the floor. Having the blankets only partly covered by the yoga mat means that your upper arms will be on the mat, which will keep them from sliding, but your neck will be on the blanket, which will allow it more freedom of movement.

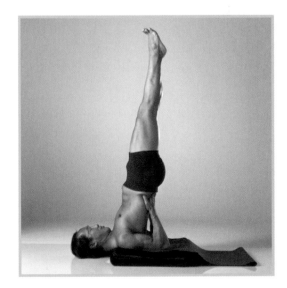

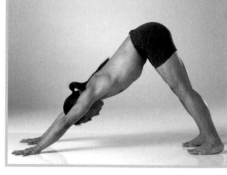

1. Practice **DOWNWARD-FACING DOG POSE** for 1 to 2 minutes. Feel the integration between the length of the sides of your waist, the opening of your chest, and the extension of your arms.

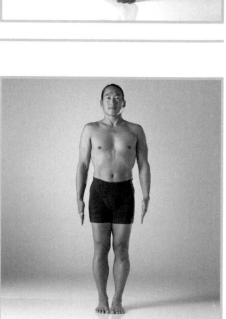

2. Practice **STANDING FORWARD BEND** for 1 minute. Move your shoulder blades toward your pelvis, keeping your arms in their sockets and the sides of your neck relaxed.

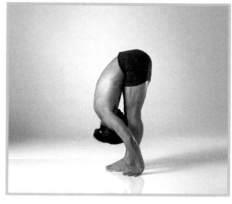

3. Practice **MOUNTAIN POSE** for 1 to 2 minutes. With active, responsive feet, ground your thighbones toward your hamstrings.

4. Try all three versions of **Reclined Mountain Pose,** for 30 seconds in each version.

VERSION 1: On the floor, arms by your sides, soles of your feet pressing into the wall

By using the wall and the floor, you can wake up your legs fully while you have a wonderful awareness of your back body on the ground, eliciting broadness and length. Use the floor to discover which parts of your body can make full contact with the ground as you try to enhance the natural curves of your spine with the grounding of your legs.

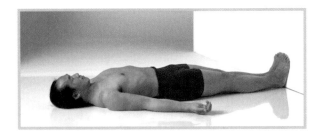

VERSION 2: On the floor, arms stretched out over your head, feet pressing into the wall

This version teaches you how stretching your arms over your head affects your entire spine and rib cage. Attempt to keep your back lower ribs in contact with the floor as your arms reach toward the ground, extending vigorously from your feet. Look for a deeper and deeper relaxation of your neck as you fully wake up your arms and legs.

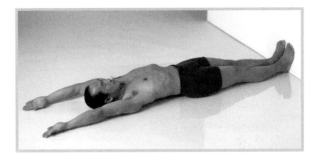

VERSION 3: Blanket roll under your shoulder blades, arms stretched out over your head, feet pressing into the wall

This version emphasizes the opening of your upper chest while giving you extra feedback on the placement of your shoulder blades and upper arms. This helps you understand the difference between opening your upper chest and pushing your lower ribs forward. Challenge your shoulder blades to move up into your rib cage without jamming the spine between them. Search for as much even contact with your feet on the wall as possible, feeling their connectivity to your pelvis, spine, and shoulders.

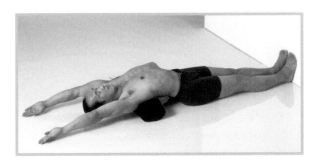

5. Try all three versions of **VOLCANO POSE** *(Urdhva Hastasana)* for 30 seconds in each version.

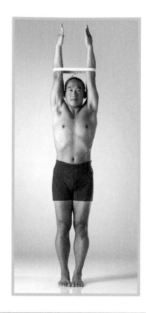

VERSION 1: Strap around your arms, just above your elbows, arms above your head, pressing out against the strap

This version helps you find the full extension of your inner elbows and define the line between your inner shoulder blade, inner arm, and palms. Link the grounding of your thighs toward your hamstrings with the reach of your inner elbows. As you reach your arms, reach your entire rib cage along with them.

VERSION 2: Block between your hands

Having a weight in your hands and something to press into brings you awareness of the alignment of your arms and their extension upward. Support this extension from the length of your waist and the lift of your chest, paying special attention to relaxing your neck. Challenge yourself to find the full integration of your legs, torso, and arms.

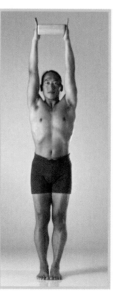

VERSION 3: Facing the wall—toes at the wall—stretch your hands up the wall as you rise up on your toes. Then, lower back down onto your heels, trying to keep your hands at the same height.

By coming up onto your toes, you activate your feet and legs to help you extend your waist, chest, and arms, without pushing your lower ribs forward. As you slowly lower back down to your heels, keeping your feet active, place your forehead on the wall to soothe your neck and facial muscles. Demand as much length as your outer body can muster while at the same time you cool your inner body.

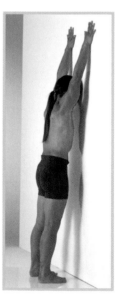

6. Try all three versions of **HANDSTAND PREPARATION** with timing as follows.

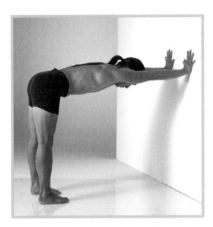

VERSION 1: Right angle against the wall, with hands against the wall, feet on the ground for 30 seconds

Without your arms and torso bearing weight, you can adjust your shoulders to find their optimal alignment and maximum extension. Use the grounding of your thighbones toward your hamstrings as an anchor from which to extend your spine into your hands. Explore different heights of your hands on the wall to maximize the natural curves of your spine.

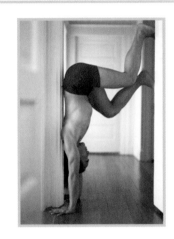

VERSION 2: In a doorway, place your hands on the ground and walk up the doorframe while pressing your spine against the other side of the frame. Repeat several times briefly.

This version is a fabulous way for almost all of you to get on your hands. This pose takes some fear out of Handstand because your entire back is supported and given orientation. You also feel the power of your legs adding to your ability to lift off your arms. Your neck is in line with the rest of your spine—relax it completely. Press your hands strongly into the ground while being sensitive to the alignment of your elbows, shoulders, and wrists (perpendicular to the ground).

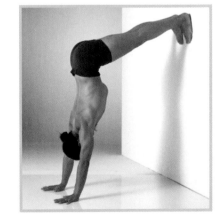

VERSION 3: Hands on the floor legs-distance away from the wall, feet higher than a right angle so your body is closer to a straight line than a right angle. Repeat several times briefly.

This version relies heavily on the muscles of your arms, back, and abdomen and is a little bit more work for your arms than being completely vertical (full Handstand). But because you feel more secure with both the soles of your feet and your hands touching a surface, you can build the strength needed for Handstand without the fear. Leaning the weight of your pelvis toward the wall gives your feet strong, tactile contact with the wall. Challenge yourself to find the full extension of your shoulders by engaging your shoulder blades strongly into your back and lifting your thighs vigorously into your hamstrings.

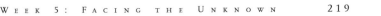

7. Try all three versions of **HANDSTAND** *(Adho Mukha Vrksasana)* with timing as follows.

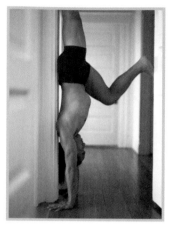

VERSION 1: Doorway handstand, bringing one or both legs vertical into full handstand for about 10 seconds

This version allows you to shift the weight of your legs directly over your hands without feeling completely suspended in midair. It is a great way to let go of your fear and slowly become more secure being on your hands without losing your orientation. Attempt to find as straight a line as possible, from your hands to your top leg.

VERSION 2: Kicking up into handstand, but not getting there. Repeat several times.

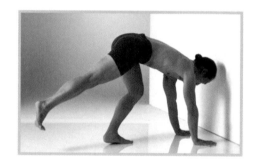

It is more important for you to feel the shift in your weight—the movement of your pelvis from its Downward-Facing Dog position toward a vertical Handstand position—than it is for you to get your legs up to the wall. Rather than being goal oriented, simply enjoy shifting your body weight onto your hands. Keep your neck relaxed and look down at your hands. Take several breaths in between attempts at kicking up to make sure that you are starting from a calm, centered, in-body place.

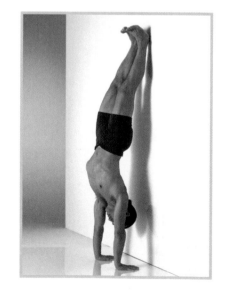

VERSION 3: Full pose, if possible, at the wall for 10 seconds. Repeat once more.

Handstand provides you with the complete exhilaration of being upside down on your own arms. The challenge is to find the full extension of your body by awakening your feet and legs so that they rise away from the ground instead of falling into your arms. Constantly refine your alignment.

8. Try all three versions of **MOUNTAIN POSE** *(Tadasana)* variation for 30 seconds in each version.

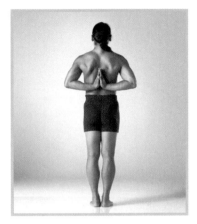

VERSION 1: Hands in *namaste* behind your back

This version of Mountain Pose opens up your shoulders and arms in the opposite direction of Handstand, moving you toward Shoulderstand. Observe how your legs affect the lift of your chest no matter what position your arms are in. Bring your hands closer together and farther up your back while you broaden and lift your collarbones.

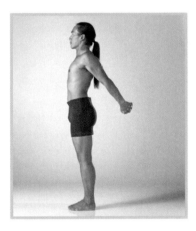

VERSION 2: Hands interlaced behind your back, arms lifting toward shoulder height

This version also reverses the work you did in Handstand, but this time with straight arms. Feel the opening of your upper chest muscles as you try to keep as much broadness in your upper back as possible. As you use your arms, your neck will tend to initiate the action. Instead, relax your neck as you use your arms. Maintain Mountain Pose as vertically as possible as you slowly lift your arms higher.

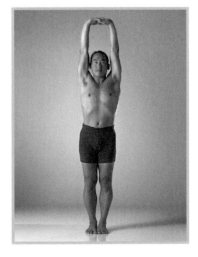

VERSION 3: Hands interlaced, arms raised over your head

This version is a great way to open up your shoulders and wrists because interlacing your hands creates an internal circuit that allows you to feel the alignment of your arms more profoundly. With your feet finding more contact with the earth and your hands in contact with each other, you get a strong sense of your entire skeleton elongating from the earth, skyward into your hands. Imagine yourself with your back on the ground or against the wall, and try to attain as much broadness and length of your entire back body as possible.

9. Try all three versions of **STANDING WIDE ANGLE FORWARD BEND** (*Prasarita Padottanasana*) for 30 seconds in each version.

VERSION 1: Fingertips on the ground, chest lifting, head looking forward

For those of you with tighter hamstrings, being on your fingertips lets you extend your spine fully as you lift your chest and head. With your fingertips and arms directly underneath your shoulders, you can accentuate the lift of your chest and the length of your waist from the anchor of your legs. Because your legs are wide, you can find a deeper folding in your pelvis into the forward bend. Challenge yourself to find strong legs without hyperextending your knees (that is, jamming them into a locked position).

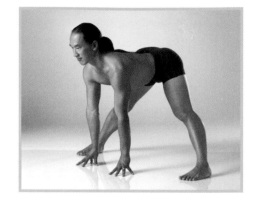

VERSION 2: Head releasing and resting on the ground, a block, or a chair

In this version you find the introspection of a forward bend and an inverted pose plus a full release of all your back muscles. Even with this rounding of your spine, continue to move your shoulder blades into your back and toward your pelvis so that you can truly relax your neck from the foundation of your shoulder blades. As your head is lightly supported, continue to release the tension in your neck.

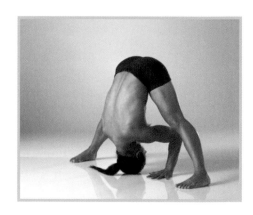

VERSION 3: Hands interlaced behind your back, arms straight, swinging your hands toward the ground

This version prepares you for the movement of your shoulders in Shoulderstand. The weight of your arms opens your shoulder joints with the aid of gravity. Challenge yourself to open your joints and draw your arms into their sockets as you firm your shoulder blades into your back. Be a little careful coming up from this pose because you may feel lightheaded. You can counter this by articulating and grounding your feet. Keep your mind attending to your weight shift and the contact of your feet with the ground.

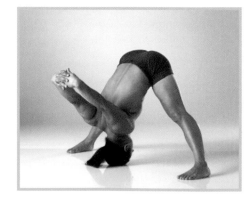

10. Try all three versions of **EAST SIDE OF THE BODY STRETCH** *(Purvottanasana)* for 30 seconds in each version.

VERSION 1: Hips and legs on the ground, elbows bent, chest lifting

This version isolates the opening of your chest and shoulders. Play with the way your shoulders insert into their sockets to feel a wonderful integration between your upper arms, collarbones, and shoulder blades. With your hands and arms in this position, find the backbend in your upper chest. Ground your legs to fully lift your chest and awaken your spine.

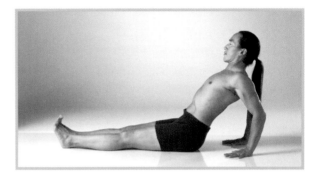

VERSION 2: Table Pose. Straighten your arms and lift your hips, but keep your knees bent.

In this version, your arms are straight, giving you a strong, direct channel between your hands and the lift of your chest. With bent legs, you are able to lift your legs more completely. With your pelvis this high, your chest can find its full opening, allowing you to let your head fall backward with a relaxed neck. Feel the way the strength of your arms and legs open up your front body as you maintain the broadness and length of your back body.

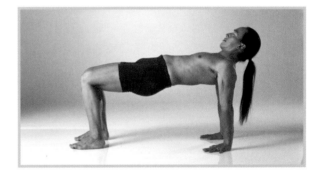

VERSION 3: Full pose, with legs straight

This pose fully awakens your back body to elongate and open your front body. The challenge is to maintain the internal spiral of your legs along with the contact of your inner feet as you slowly lift your pelvis higher and higher. To get the full opening of your chest so that your head can release backward, transfer the strength of your legs into the lift of your chest. If dropping your head back feels like it jams your neck, keep your head up and look down at your legs. Feel your tactile feet coordinating with the suppleness of your belly and the internal rotation of your legs.

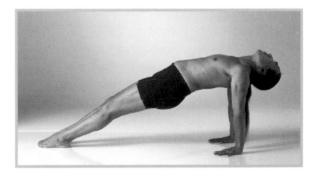

11. Try all three versions of **WALL SHOULDERSTAND** *(Salamba Sarvangasana)* variation for 30 seconds to 1 minute in each version.

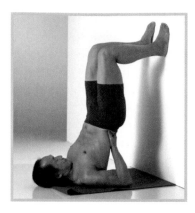

VERSION 1: Soles of your feet on the wall, legs bent

With your legs bent, you can adjust your body to any height, which allows you to find the foundation of your arms and the relaxation of your neck. Even though your legs are bent, keep your thighbones moving toward the backs of your legs. This keeps your groins and belly open as a channel between your legs and torso. Challenge yourself to move toward a vertical position and yet bear more weight on your arms and shoulders without putting any more tension in your throat or neck.

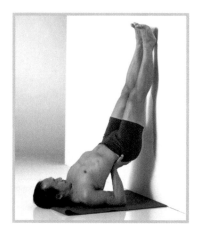

VERSION 2: Legs straight, pelvis supported by palms of your hands

This version provides your pelvis with support so you can begin to understand the restorative quality of Shoulderstand. Because there is no emphasis on being vertical and the weight is off your head, you can get the general position of Shoulderstand without any of its severity. Begin to understand the softness of your brain, the relaxation of your eyes, and the ease of your neck. The challenge is to keep your elbows and arms close enough together so they act as a real support system. Press your arms into the blanket or the mat as your side chest lifts toward the ceiling.

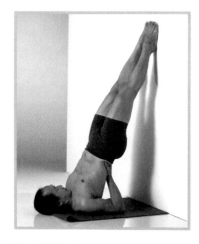

VERSION 3: Full pose, with legs straight and hands supporting midback

This version gives you the full experience of Shoulderstand with the support of the wall. For those of you who are not able to get completely vertical, supporting the pose with your legs against the wall allows you to work on the alignment and action of your arms without straining them or having them bear your full weight. Also, using the wall lets you vary the height of your chest, making sure that you don't overstrain your neck. Use the wall to bring awareness to your feet and activate the backs of your legs.

12. Try all three versions of **PLOW POSE** *(Halasana)* for 30 seconds in each version.

VERSION 1: Feet on a chair, arms extended, fingers interlaced

For those of you who have tight hamstrings, this version allows you to extend your spine completely and to use the grounding of your legs toward your hamstrings as a way to lift out of any tendency to sag onto your neck or arms. With your fingers interlaced, ground your arms and hands on the floor or blankets. Turn your arms fully under your chest so that you are on your arms and not the base of your neck.

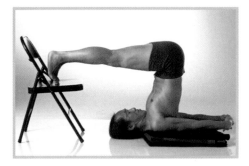

VERSION 2: Feet on a chair, hands supporting your back

This version brings you into the full foundation of Plow Pose and Shoulderstand, challenging you to keep your arms rotated under your chest while you press your hands firmly against your back. Work your arms strongly as you soften any effort in your neck, face, and sense organs. A key to understanding both Plow Pose and Shoulderstand is your investigation into the relaxation of your neck and the strengthening of your upper arms into the ground.

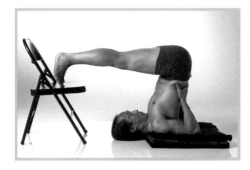

VERSION 3: Full pose, with feet on the floor, arms extended, fingers interlaced

This version opens your back body while slightly rounding your spine, bringing you into the quietness of a forward bend (though some of you may feel somewhat claustrophobic and constrained). Reawaken your feet and legs to keep them from collapsing toward your face. Learn to work your legs and feet vigorously while at the same time softening your eyes, tongue, and throat. Try to find as much traction and elongation of your torso as possible.

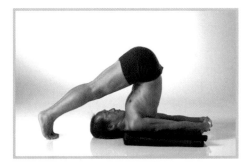

13. Try all three versions of **SHOULDERSTAND** *(Salamba Sarvangasana)* for 30 seconds in each version.

VERSION 1: Legs bent, knees opening away from each other, feet apart, thighs parallel to the ground (like Happy Baby Pose)

In this version your legs help counterbalance any inability to be completely vertical, allowing you to maintain the natural curves of your lower back. Because your muscles do not have to work to keep you upright, you will find this version a very relaxed pose. Your groins and belly stay soft, which allows your breath to flow much more easily. However, with your legs this relaxed, it is important to keep your thighbones grounding toward your hamstrings to maintain the full ease of your breath. Use this balance and ease to focus more on aligning and strengthening the foundation of your arms and shoulders.

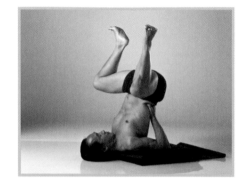

VERSION 2: One leg straight up, one leg parallel to the ground. Do both sides.

Dropping one leg parallel to the ground gives you a counterbalance so you balance more on your shoulders than on your neck or the back of your head. Keep your pelvis square and use your legs to elongate your torso, finding their reach in opposition to your arms. As you balance on your shoulders, continually let go of any tension in your neck.

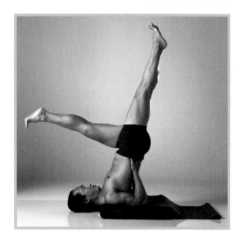

VERSION 3: Full pose, with both legs straight up

The full pose will soothe your nervous system, even if you are struggling with this pose. Your eyes can see your entire body, which lets you refine the alignment and evenness of your legs. For those of you who can get vertical and find true balance in this pose, challenge yourself to get more work from your arms and legs. We all need to let go internally and find as much ease and space inside this pose, no matter what our capability is.

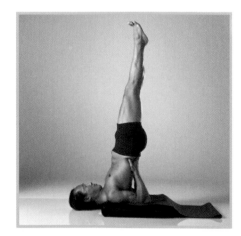

14. Try all three versions of **FISH POSE** *(Uttana Padasana)* for 15 seconds in each version.

VERSION 1: Legs bent, chest lifted, top of the head on the ground

This version allows you to focus on the depth of your groins and the complete backbending of your spine. You can fully utilize your arms and legs to pump the arch of your spine and the lift of your chest. Your head and neck also help complete the bridge of your spine, propelling your chest upward. Though your legs are bent, your thighbones moving away from your pelvis down into your hamstrings aid you in breathing completely. Try to create an arch in your spine that is as even as possible.

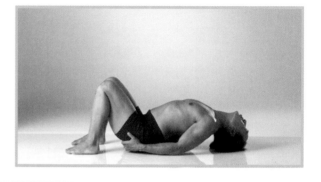

VERSION 2: Legs extended along the ground, top of the head on the ground, elbows pushing into the ground

In this version your legs become a stronger counterbalance to your torso, enabling you to lift your chest farther. Mindfully extend through the backs of your legs, keeping the sharpness of your legs as a main ingredient for this version. The more you can work your legs and arms, the more your chest will be lifted fully so that you can find the relaxation of your neck. Keep pumping the energy of your legs and arms into the circle of your spine.

VERSION 3: Full pose, with legs in the air, arms in the air, hands together

In this version your legs are in the air, which naturally pulls your spine even further into a backbend. Bringing your hands together in *namaste* creates an internal interconnectedness, giving you an awareness of your shoulder blades and upper arms supporting the openness of your heart. The full activity of your feet allows you to find the full strength of your legs—this is the foundation for the extension and arch of your spine. Vigorously work your arms and legs to awaken fully the backbending of your torso, neck, and head.

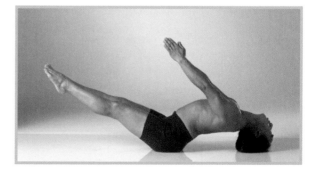

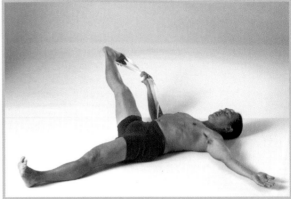

15. Practice the **Reclined Leg Stretch Series** (straight-leg, sit-up, and leg-to-the-side) for 30, 15, and 30 seconds for the versions, on each side. In all three versions, continue to increase the contact of your bottom leg on the ground.

16. Practice version 1 of **Cobbler's Pose** for 3 minutes. As you slowly increase the length of your spine, increase the feeling of space inside your brain, your neck, and your torso.

Relaxation and Breath Awareness

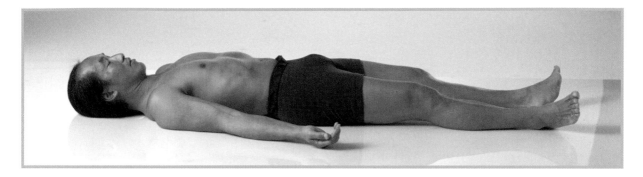

17. For 5 minutes, practice Relaxation Pose, with your arms above your head, loosely holding your elbows. With a smooth, slightly extended inhalation, feel how your breath naturally moves into your upper chest. After 2½ minutes, reverse the cross of your arms so the other forearm is on top. If this position irritates your shoulders, place a blanket or a pillow underneath your arms.

Meditation

18. For 5 to 15 minutes, sit in Seated Crossed-Legs Pose or Half Lotus against the wall, with support under your pelvis. Quickly scan your entire body, repeatedly.

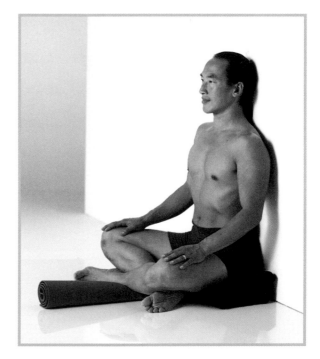

DAY 2: LEARNING RECLINED MOUNTAIN POSE AND HANDSTAND PREPARATION

In Reclined Mountain Pose and Handstand Preparation, you will learn about the relationship between your hands, arms, shoulders, and torso. In Reclined Mountain Pose, having the ground as a reference helps you understand your alignment by bringing your awareness to the muscles you are contracting or releasing. In this pose, the activity of your legs shows their obvious effect on the elongation of your waist and the reach and strength of your arms. Regardless of whether or not you get up into Handstand, you can use Reclined Mountain Pose as a variation that will give you many similar benefits on the musculoskeletal level.

Understanding how to keep your elbows fully extended is an important aspect of learning Handstand. Without the proper elbow alignment, your arm muscles have to work much harder to keep your arms from collapsing. Tightness in your shoulders can cause your lower back and lower ribs to go into an exaggerated sway, stressing your lower back and wrists. In the Handstand preparations you go from mildly pressing into the wall to having your entire body weight on your arms and your hands. Using the wall and the doorway gives your mind substantial orientation and security, which allows release of most of your fear. You can then concentrate on how your arms and

hands and shoulders are working into the extension and lift of your torso. Try not to stay frozen in one position, but be playful on your arms, making small movements with your shoulders, torso, and pelvis over the foundation of your hands. This movement helps make your arms, hands, and shoulders responsive to bearing your body weight.

Today's sequence includes standing poses that all involve the extension of your arms. At the end of the practice you balance the movement of your shoulders with East Side of the Body Stretch and Supported Bridge Pose. Reclined Leg Stretch Series and Reclined Hero Pose release your body and prepare you for relaxation.

FOCUS FOR THIS PRACTICE:

- In the Sun Salutations, awaken your feet by splaying your toes, lifting your arches, and finding a tactile relationship to the ground.

- In Downward-Facing Dog and the standing poses, ground your thighbones toward your hamstrings.

- In Handstand Preparation and Reclined Mountain Pose, find the maximum reach of your arms as you relax your neck.

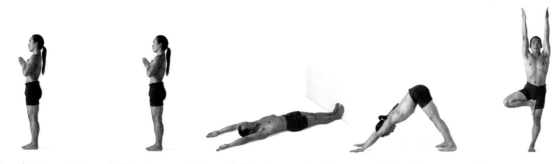

1. Practice two mini **Sun Salutations,** staying in Downward-Facing Dog for 5 breaths.

2. Practice two full **Sun Salutations,** staying in Downward-Facing Dog for 5 breaths.

3. Practice version 2 of **Reclined Mountain Pose** for 30 seconds.

4. Practice **Downward-Facing Dog** for 1 to 2 minutes.

5. Practice **Tree Pose** for 30 seconds on each side.

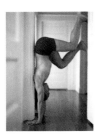

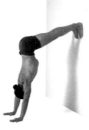

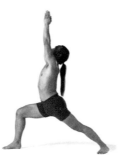

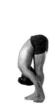

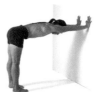

6. Practice **Extended Side Angle Pose** for 45 seconds on each side.

7. Practice **Standing Forward Bend,** holding your elbows, for 30 seconds.

8. Practice **Warrior 1** for 30 seconds.

9. Practice **Standing Forward Bend,** holding your elbows, for 30 seconds.

10. Practice version 1 of **Handstand Preparation** for 30 seconds.

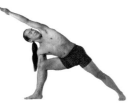

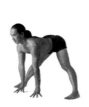

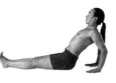

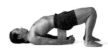

11. Practice version 2 of **Handstand Preparation,** repeating several times without holding.

12. Practice version 1 of **Standing Wide Angle Forward Bend** for 30 seconds.

13. Practice version 3 of **Handstand Preparation** for 10 seconds.

14. Practice version 1 of **East Side of the Body Stretch** for 30 seconds.

15. Practice **Supported Bridge Pose** for 1 minute.

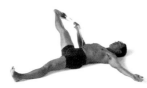

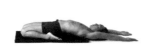

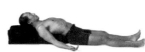

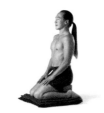

16. Practice the **Reclined Leg Stretch Series** (straight-leg, sit-up, and leg-to-the-side) for 30, 15, and 30 seconds for the versions, on each side.

17. Practice **Reclined Hero Pose** for 1 to 2 minutes.

18. Relaxation and Breath Awareness. For 5 minutes, practice version 3 of **Supported Relaxation Pose** (page 268) with a smooth, slightly extended inhalation. For the first $2^{1}/_{2}$ minutes, place your thumbs in your armpits as in version 2 of Mountain Pose.

19. Meditation. For 10 minutes, sit in **Hero Pose** and meditate on grounding and releasing your thighbones down as you find full length in the sides of your waist and balance your chest over your pelvis.

DAY 3: LEARNING VOLCANO POSE AND WALL SHOULDERSTAND

Because the action and positions of your arms in Volcano Pose and Wall Shoulderstand are virtually opposite, the two poses are often combined within a practice to balance each other. Doing these two poses in combination puts your shoulder joints through their full range of motion, increasing their range and providing muscular strength. These poses balance each other energetically as well. Volcano Pose, which represents Handstand, is very active and energetic, while Wall Shoulderstand cools your body and quiets the mind. Volcano Pose, the logical successor to Reclined Mountain Pose and Handstand Preparation, provides the full alignment of Handstand, letting you play more with the pose because you are not bearing your body weight. In Volcano Pose, you also learn the importance of the strength and extension of your legs to achieving the full extension of your torso and your arms. Try to incorporate the alignment of your back body you learned from Relined Mountain Pose into Volcano Pose, so when you reach your arms over your head, you keep your back body both long and broad. As you activate your legs, arms, and torso, continually relax your neck.

Wall Shoulderstand is the first step in the journey to learning one of yoga's most beneficial poses, Shoulderstand. You use the wall not so you can push into a vertical position but rather so you have the option of moving your torso and pelvis in many different relationships to your shoulders, neck, and head. In these versions, your legs and back muscles will tend to get tired, so do not try to hold this pose for a long time. What you are trying to accomplish with Wall Shoulderstand is finding a deeper understanding of how you can create a foundation with your shoulders and arms. Continue to ask yourself how much contact you can find with your upper arms so that you are more on your shoulders, not on the back of your head or your neck.

Today's sequence begins with three versions of Volcano Pose to prepare you for Handstand and to open your body for the standing poses. From the standing poses, you move into East Side of the Body Stretch as the preparation for Wall Shoulderstand. You finish the practice with Legs Up the Wall and Cobbler's Pose to release any tension in your neck created by Wall Shoulderstand and to transition from the more active practice to relaxation and breath awareness.

FOCUS FOR THIS PRACTICE:

- In the Sun Salutations, ground your thighbones toward your hamstrings.

- In Downward-Facing Dog, Handstand Preparation, and the standing poses, let your feet be alive and supple. Move your feet to discover their relationship with your legs.

- In Volcano Pose and Wall Shoulderstand, relax your neck.

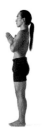 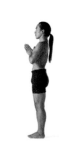 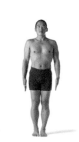 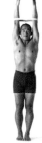 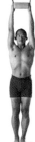

1. Practice two mini **Sun Salutations,** staying in Downward-Facing Dog for 5 breaths.

2. Practice two full **Sun Salutations,** staying in Downward-Facing Dog for 5 breaths.

3. Practice the **Core Strengthening Series** twice, with 1 breath in each pose.

4. Practice **Mountain Pose** for 1 minute.

5. Practice version 1 of **Volcano Pose** for 30 seconds.

6. Practice version 2 of **Volcano Pose** for 30 seconds.

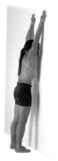
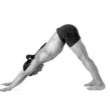
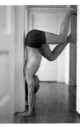
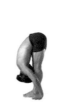
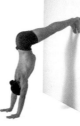
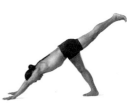

7. Practice version 3 of **Volcano Pose** for 30 seconds.

8. Practice **Downward-Facing Dog** for 1 to 2 minutes.

9. Practice version 2 of **Handstand Preparation** for 15 seconds (if you can hold it).

10. Practice **Standing Forward Bend** for 1 minute.

11. Practice version 3 of **Handstand Preparation** for 5 seconds. Repeat several times.

12. Practice version 2 of **One-Legged Downward-Facing Dog,** with one leg up in the air, for 30 seconds on each side.

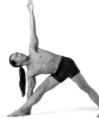
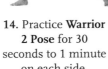
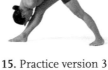

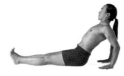

13. Practice **Triangle Pose** for 1 minute on each side.

14. Practice **Warrior 2 Pose** for 30 seconds to 1 minute on each side.

15. Practice version 3 of **Pyramid Pose** for 30 seconds on each side.

16. Practice version 3 of **Standing Wide Angle Forward Bend Pose** for 1 minute.

17. Practice version 1 of **East Side of the Body Stretch** for 30 seconds.

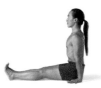
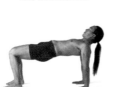
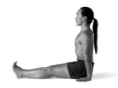

18. Practice **Staff Pose** for 30 seconds.

19. Practice version 2 of **East Side of the Body Stretch** for 15 seconds.

20. Practice **Staff Pose** for 30 seconds.

21. Practice version 3 of **East Side of the Body Stretch** for 15 seconds.

22. Practice **Staff Pose** for 30 seconds.

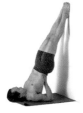
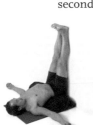
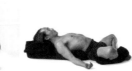
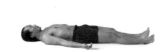

23. Practice all three versions of **Wall Shoulderstand** for 30 seconds in each version.

24. Practice **Legs Up the Wall Pose** for 5 minutes.

25. Practice **Reclined Cobbler's Pose** for 3 minutes.

26. Relaxation and Breath Awareness. For 5 minutes, practice **Relaxation Pose** with the heels of your hands on your side lower ribs

and with your fingers on your front lower ribs. Focus on breathing into your lower ribs with smooth inhalations and exhalations.

27. Meditation. For 5 to 15 minutes, sit in **Seated Crossed-Legs Pose** and meditate on how your breath is moving through your torso.

Day 4: Learning Handstand and Plow Pose

As you approach Handstand, it is critical to take small steps. When you start to practice kicking up, it is not important for you to kick up strongly. Instead, push and kick with your legs in a way that moves your pelvis up and over your hands. Learn to gradually feel the shift of weight from your feet to your hands so that when you eventually do kick up into Handstand, it will come through the coordination of many subtle movements and not just an aggressive, wild throwing of your legs and pelvis. You will learn how to integrate your breath, the push of your legs, and the swing of your pelvis, all in a graceful arc of your lower body moving over your upper body. Relaxing your eyes and gazing toward a specific point on the floor is another way to establish your foundation, both mentally and physically. As you begin to get up into Handstand, your mind can become extremely disoriented. At this point, you can reorient yourself by pressing your hands into the ground and reaching your legs together and up into your feet.

Plow Pose is a preliminary pose for learning Shoulderstand. With your feet either on a chair or on the ground, you can readjust the foundation of your arms, neck, and head as you push your legs up toward the ceiling. Place your arms into a Shoulderstand position and then use your legs to bring your torso and spine more vertical, coming much closer to the actual position of Shoulderstand. Often Plow Pose makes

you feel claustrophobic, so use the downward grounding of your arms and the lifting action of your legs to create more space in your waist and neck.

Today's sequence begins with Sun Salutations and the Core Strengthening Series to awaken your entire body and emphasize your core. The standing poses that follow fully awaken your legs so that as you begin to do Handstand Preparation and Handstand itself, you will be able to orient yourself off your legs and your core. The backbends prepare you to practice Shoulderstand, creating the necessary chest opening and spinal awareness for Wall Shoulderstand and Plow Pose. The sequence ends with Fish Pose to balance your neck both from Shoulderstand and Plow Pose.

Focus for this practice:

- In the Sun Salutations, the Core Strengthening Series, Downward-Facing Dog, and the standing poses, align your neck to optimize the ease in your neck and head.

- In the backbends, ground your feet. Spread your toes, lift your arches, and press down through your heels.

- In Handstand and Plow Pose, ground your thigh-bones strongly into your hamstrings as you press your legs together.

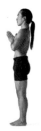 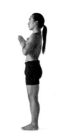 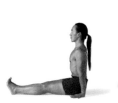

1. Practice two mini **Sun Salutations,** without taking extra breaths in any pose.

2. Practice two full **Sun Salutations,** without taking extra breaths in any pose.

3. Practice the **Core Strengthening Series** twice. On the second round, bend slightly forward in Wide Angle Pose and the last Cobbler's Pose and stay for 1 minute each.

4. Practice the **Reclined Leg Stretch Series** (straight-leg, sit-up, and leg-to-the-side) for 30, 15, and 30 seconds in the versions on each side.

5. Practice version 1 of **One-Legged Downward-Facing Dog** for 30 seconds on each side.

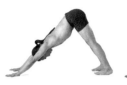

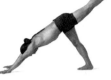

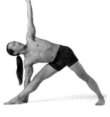

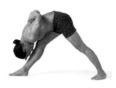

6. Practice **Downward-Facing Dog Pose** for 1 minute.

7. Practice version 2 of **One-Legged Downward-Facing Dog Pose** for 30 seconds on each side.

8. Practice **Standing Forward Bend** for 1 minute.

9. Practice **Triangle Pose** for 30 seconds on each side.

10. Practice **Pyramid Pose** for 30 seconds on each side.

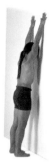

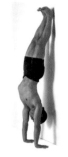

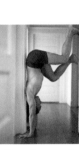

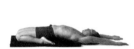

11. Practice **Volcano Pose** for 1 minute.

12. Practice version 2 of **Handstand Preparation** for 5 to 10 seconds. Repeat several times.

13. Practice all three versions of **Handstand.** If you get up, stay for 10 to 20 seconds.

14. Practice **Reclined Hero Pose** for 1 to 2 minutes.

15. Practice **Camel Pose** for 15 to 30 seconds.

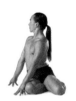

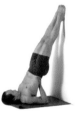

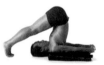

16. Practice version 3 of **Upward Bow Pose** for 5 seconds, if you can do this pose. Repeat several times.

17. Practice version 1 of **Cobbler's Pose** for 3 minutes.

18. Practice **Simple Twist** for 30 seconds to 1 minute on each side.

19. Practice all three versions of **Wall Shoulderstand** for 30 seconds each.

20. Practice all three versions of **Plow Pose** for 30 seconds each.

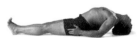

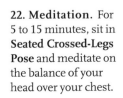

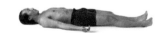

21. Practice **Fish Pose** for 15 to 30 seconds.

22. Meditation. For 5 to 15 minutes, sit in **Seated Crossed-Legs Pose** and meditate on the balance of your head over your chest.

Don't hesitate to make small, subtle movements with your head to inquire more deeply about the nature of true center.

23. Relaxation and Breath Awareness. For 5 minutes, practice **Relaxation Pose,** breathing into your lower, middle, and

upper lungs as evenly as possible. Focus on smooth, extended inhalations and exhalations.

Today's sequence will deepen your relationships with Handstand and Shoulderstand and teach you to connect these poses to the standing poses and a full yoga practice. In the larger scheme of a yoga practice, Handstand and Shoulderstand become the main axis around which the other poses revolve. Attempting Handstand every day will awaken your body-mind like no other pose. Handstand is often used at the very beginning of a practice to quickly engage your mind and body into focusing in the here and now. Practicing Shoulderstand near the end of your practice cools the fire that comes from the previous part of the practice, allowing you to feel the coolness of the evening after a hot afternoon. As you practice both these postures, you must do more than simply go up and stay in the pose; you must continue to refine the balance, action, and surrender of the pose. Which actions enable you to lift and center yourself more deeply? What do you need to let go and release in order to further enhance the way your breath moves through these poses?

For some of you, one or both of these poses might be instantly frustrating or lead to frustration. So set your course, find your relaxation, clear your mind, and once again approach the pose. Learning to relax in the face of difficulty can have profound effects both on your practice and on your life outside the yoga room.

The beginning of today's sequence opens your body in the shape of Handstand in various orientations to gravity. By doing this, you prepare your body to do full Handstand. All these poses, including Handstand, are great poses to start any practice. After Handstand, the standing poses utilize the vigor and alertness created by the previous poses. Your body will be awake, and your focus and observation more keen. You then prepare your arms and chest for Shoulderstand with Standing Wide Angle Forward Bend, East Side of the Body Stretch, and Plow Pose. The sequence ends with Reclined Leg Stretch Series and Fish Pose to balance the Shoulderstand.

FOCUS FOR THIS PRACTICE:

- Throughout the practice, feel the relationship between the grounding of your thighbones into your hamstrings and having alive, articulate, and supple feet.

- In Handstand and Shoulderstand, work your arms strongly as you release your neck.

- During Relaxation and Breath Awareness, let the tension in your legs and feet dissolve.

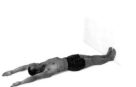

1. Practice version 2 of **Reclined Mountain Pose** for 1 minute.

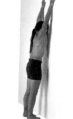

2. Practice **Volcano Pose** for 1 minute.

3. Practice **Downward-Facing Dog** for 1 minute.

4. Practice **Standing Forward Bend** for 1 minute.

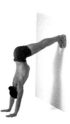

5. Practice any version of **Handstand Preparation** for 15 to 30 seconds.

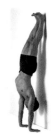

6. Practice version 2 or 3 of **Handstand** several times.

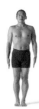 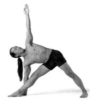

7. Practice **Mountain Pose** for 1 minute.

8. Practice **Standing Forward Bend** for 30 seconds.

9. Practice **Triangle Pose** for 30 seconds on each side.

10. Practice **Standing Forward Bend** for 15 seconds.

11. Practice **Extended Side Angle Pose** for 30 seconds on each side.

 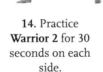 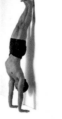

12. Practice **Standing Forward Bend** for 15 seconds.

13. Practice **Warrior 1** for 30 seconds on each side.

14. Practice **Warrior 2** for 30 seconds on each side.

15. Practice **Standing Forward Bend** for 30 seconds.

16. Practice version 2 or 3 of **Handstand** several times. If you get up, stay for 10 to 20 seconds.

17. Practice version 3 of **Standing Wide Angle Forward Bend** for 15 to 30 seconds.

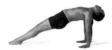 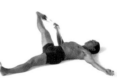 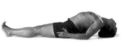

18. Practice **East Side of the Body Stretch** for 30 seconds.

19. Practice all three versions of **Plow Pose** for 30 seconds each.

20. Practice all three versions of **Shoulderstand** for 30 seconds each.

21. Practice the **Reclined Leg Stretch Series** for 30, 15, and 30 seconds for the versions on each side.

22. Practice **Fish Pose** for 15 to 30 seconds, or repeat several times for shorter lengths of time.

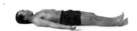

23. Relaxation and Breath Awareness. For 5 to 10 minutes, practice **Relaxation Pose** and breathe evenly and smoothly through both sides of your

lungs. Without creating any tension, focus on the smoothness and evenness of your inhalations and exhalations as you take full breaths.

24. Meditation. For 5 to 10 minutes, sit in **Hero Pose** and meditate on the placement of your shoulders and the relaxation of your neck. Most of us need

to bring our upper arms lightly back and up without using our neck muscles.

DAY 6: BREATH AWARENESS AND MEDITATION

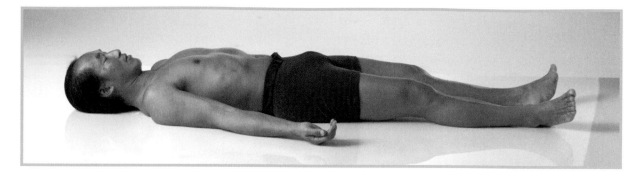

Breath Awareness

For 2 minutes, practice version 3 of Relaxation Pose with extra emphasis on feeling the broadness of your back body and its receptivity both to the ground and to your front body dropping toward it.

RELAXATION POSE. In this version of Relaxation Pose, you are attempting to return to a completely neutral body. If your body does not feel as if it is in a neutral position—especially if your head feels like it is being thrown back—place a small prop, like a folded blanket, underneath your head. If your lower back doesn't feel at ease in this position, use a support (such as a rolled blanket) under your thighs. However, I believe it is important—even after finding the Relaxation Pose that works best for you—to return periodically to the unsupported version of Relaxation Pose to see if you can find ease without any props. Feel the contact of your back body with whatever you are lying on and use this contact to observe how much you are dropping into the ground. For the first 30 seconds, try to create as much symmetry as possible, not just from right to left but from front to back and top to bottom. Then after 30 seconds of making subtle adjustments, put your adjusting to rest. Begin to accept and receive whatever sensations arise.

EQUAL INHALATIONS AND EXHALATIONS. As you inhale and exhale, observe how evenly your breath moves into every part of your being, mindfully letting go of the gripping and tension wherever you find it. The breath awareness technique I am introducing to you today is making your inhalation and exhalation equal in length. To do this, begin to count the length of your natural inhalations and exhalations. Instead of trying to change the ratio, just use counting as a way to observe what the ratio is between your inhalation and your exhalation. Then, keep on asking yourself whether there is any obstruction that you can let go of that might create more equality. For example, if your inhalation is shorter than your exhalation, ask yourself: what is obstructing my inhalation? After a few minutes of observation, begin to shorten whichever is longer, the inhalation or the exhalation. If this feels completely unnatural, you might try lengthening whichever is shorter. Or maybe you can find a happy medium where your inhalation and exhalation can be relatively the same length. Let yourself reside in this rhythm for the next 5 to 10 minutes. Allow this rhythm to relax you more deeply, dropping you toward the ground. Let this deeper relaxation smooth and elongate your breath naturally.

Meditation

For 10 minutes, sit in Seated Crossed-Legs Pose away from the wall. Make sure you sit with the natural curve in your lower back (on a prop high enough so you can have a natural sway in your lower back). Place your hands in *namaste,* allowing receptivity as well as a lift of your sternum.

For the first minute, focus on the balance of your head over your heart. Scan your body from the crown of your head to the soles of your feet, noticing when your mind begins to wander away from observing the sensations of your mind, body, and breath.

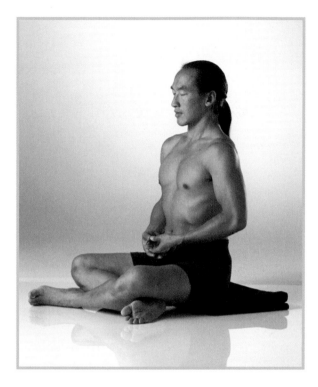

LOWER BACK. One of the most effective meditations that I do is to focus on the feeling of my lower back, keeping my lower back light, moment by moment, to get more space and more breath without too much effort. The natural curve of your lower back is a slight backbend that is not rigid, with a gentle undulation between being straighter and being in a deeper backbend.

As you listen to your breath, you will understand when you are working too hard to lift your spine. Your balancing act between relaxation and effort and between habit and mindfulness will become a subtle interplay. The exquisite nuances revealed from your observation will bring balance and contentment to your inner body. The beauty sometimes becomes so great that it may make you shy away from the practice of meditation. But complementing the large external movements of your everyday life by going inside and sitting with the minute and the subtle will bring balance to your life.

RECLINED MOUNTAIN POSE

Reclined Mountain Pose teaches you to align your posture
by using the floor as a reference.

POINT OF PLAY:
Keep your neck soft and your
arms in their sockets as you
move your shoulder blades
down toward your pelvis.

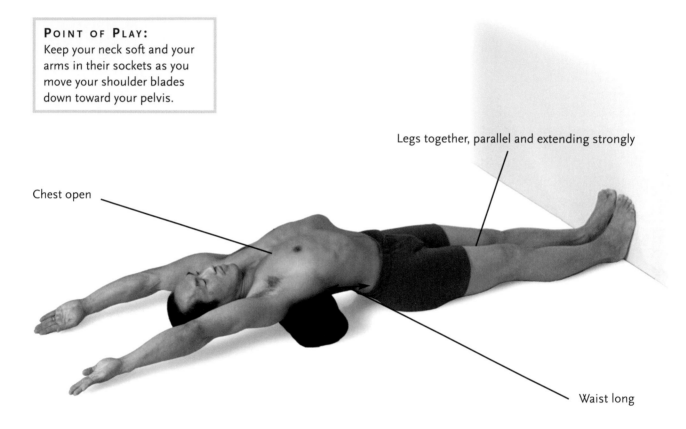

Legs together, parallel and extending strongly

Chest open

Waist long

VOLCANO POSE

Volcano Pose teaches you how the length of your spine depends on the strength and alignment of your legs.

POINT OF PLAY:
First maximize the reach of your entire body and then soften the reach to find relaxation in your neck and sense organs.

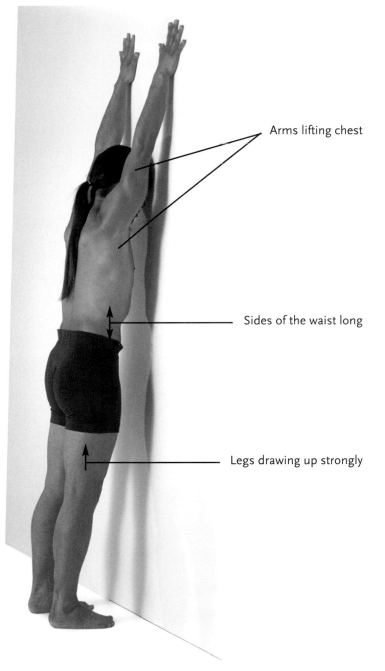

Arms lifting chest

Sides of the waist long

Legs drawing up strongly

HANDSTAND PREPARATION

Handstand Preparation teaches you how to reach
and align your torso and arms.

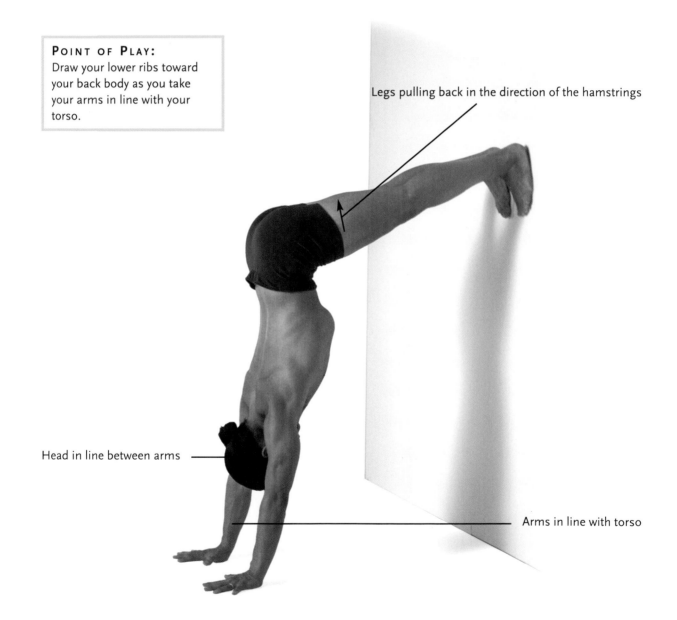

POINT OF PLAY:
Draw your lower ribs toward
your back body as you take
your arms in line with your
torso.

Legs pulling back in the direction of the hamstrings

Head in line between arms

Arms in line with torso

HANDSTAND

Handstand awakens and invigorates your entire body
as it builds your confidence.

POINT OF PLAY:
As you extend your arms
strongly, find an ease of
breath.

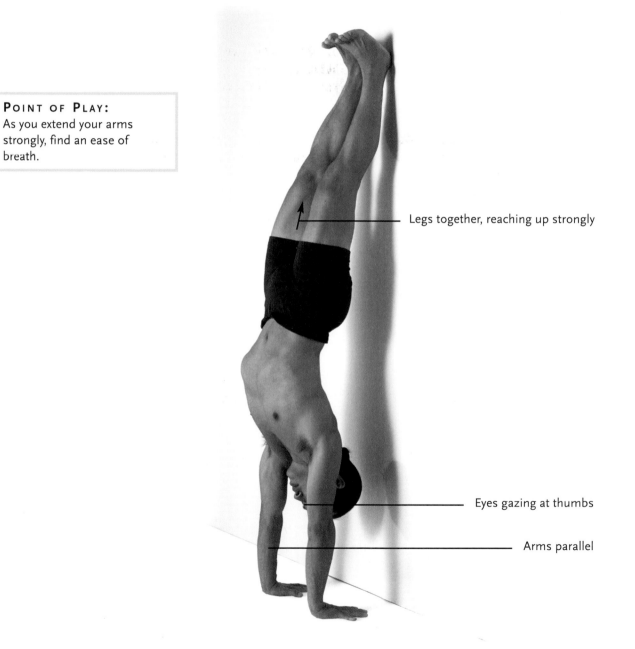

Legs together, reaching up strongly

Eyes gazing at thumbs

Arms parallel

MOUNTAIN POSE VARIATION

This variation of Mountain Pose challenges you to maintain the lift of your chest as you use your arms to loosen the chest muscles that bind your breath.

POINT OF PLAY:
Drop your chest and lift your arms, then lift your chest and lower your arms.

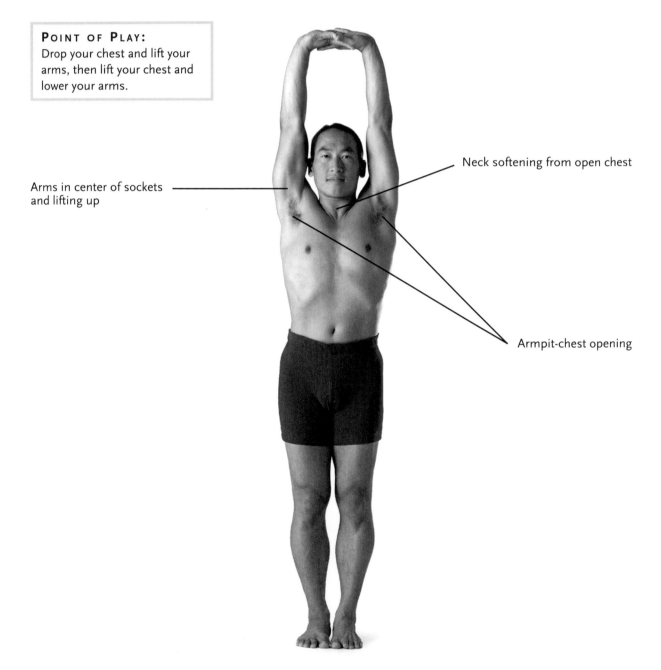

Arms in center of sockets and lifting up

Neck softening from open chest

Armpit-chest opening

STANDING WIDE ANGLE FORWARD BEND

Standing Wide Angle Forward Bend provides the benefits of an inverted pose without putting weight on your neck or creating a sense of fear.

POINT OF PLAY:
Press your inner heel into the ground and lift your arches.

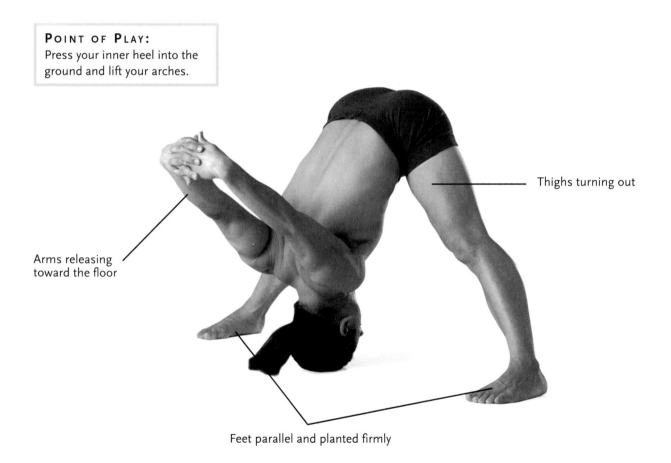

Thighs turning out

Arms releasing toward the floor

Feet parallel and planted firmly

EAST SIDE OF THE BODY STRETCH

East Side of the Body Stretch opens your chest and the front of your pelvis intensely
while invigorating your entire body.

POINT OF PLAY:
Lift your hips higher and drop
your groins more.

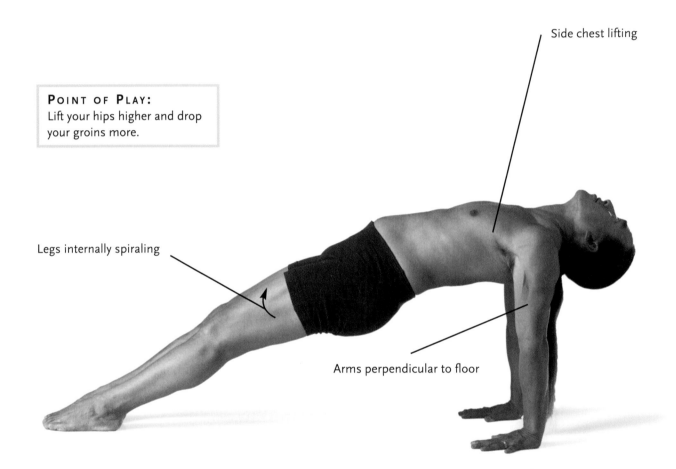

Side chest lifting

Legs internally spiraling

Arms perpendicular to floor

WALL SHOULDERSTAND

Wall Shoulderstand soothes your nerves without overworking your arms or stressing your neck, allowing you to control how high you want to go.

POINT OF PLAY:
Ground your thighbones toward your hamstrings as you deepen your sacrum into your body.

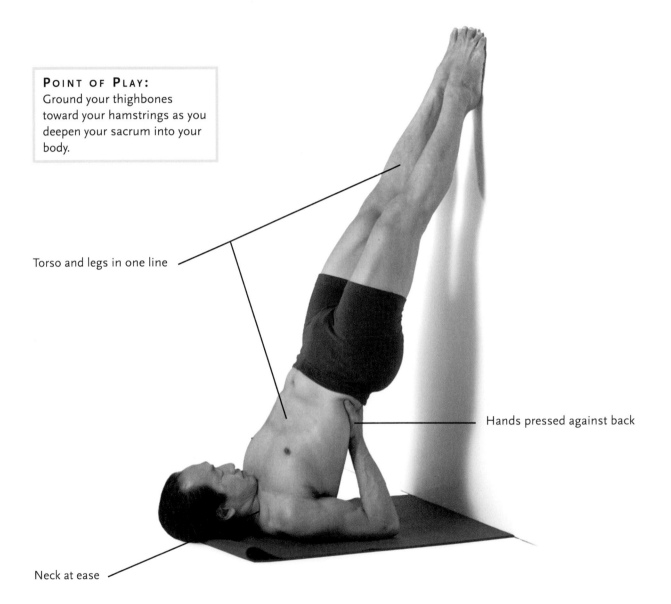

Torso and legs in one line

Hands pressed against back

Neck at ease

PLOW POSE

Plow Pose combines a forward bend with an inverted pose to open your back body and quiet the input to your senses, allowing you to look inward.

POINT OF PLAY:
Relax your eyes and throat as you ground your arms.

Thighbones pressing up toward hamstrings

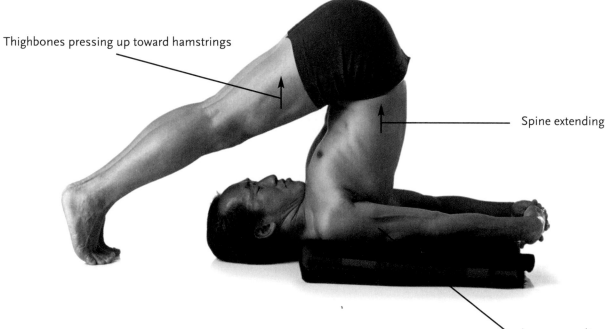

Spine extending

Arms grounding

SHOULDERSTAND

Shoulderstand soothes your nervous system
and balances the effects of Headstand in your practice.

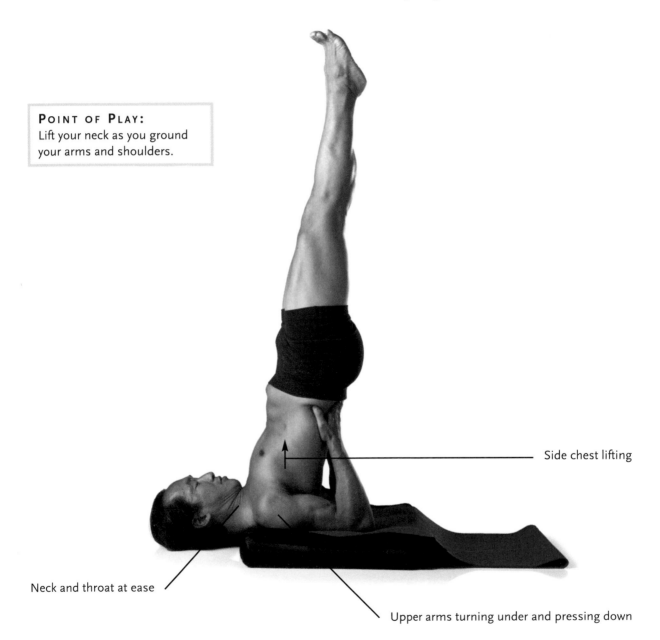

POINT OF PLAY:
Lift your neck as you ground
your arms and shoulders.

Side chest lifting

Neck and throat at ease

Upper arms turning under and pressing down

FISH POSE

Fish Pose integrates your neck with the rest of your spine
and charges your spine with the work of your arms and legs.

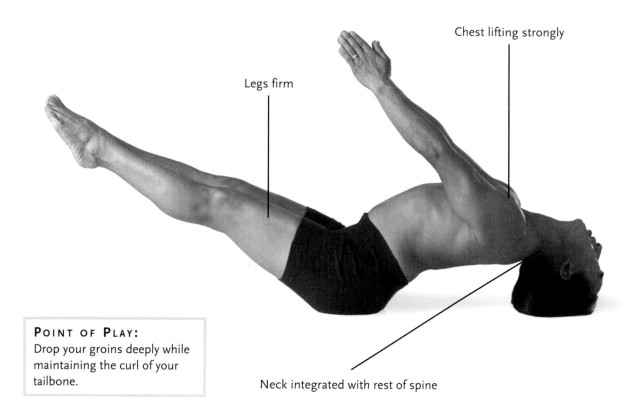

Legs firm

Chest lifting strongly

Neck integrated with rest of spine

POINT OF PLAY:
Drop your groins deeply while
maintaining the curl of your
tailbone.

THE RESOLUTE IN YOGA SURRENDER

RESULTS, AND GAIN PERFECT PEACE;

THE IRRESOLUTE, ATTACHED TO RESULTS,

ARE BOUND BY EVERYTHING THEY DO.

—*BHAGAVAD GITA*, TRANS. BY STEPHEN MITCHELL

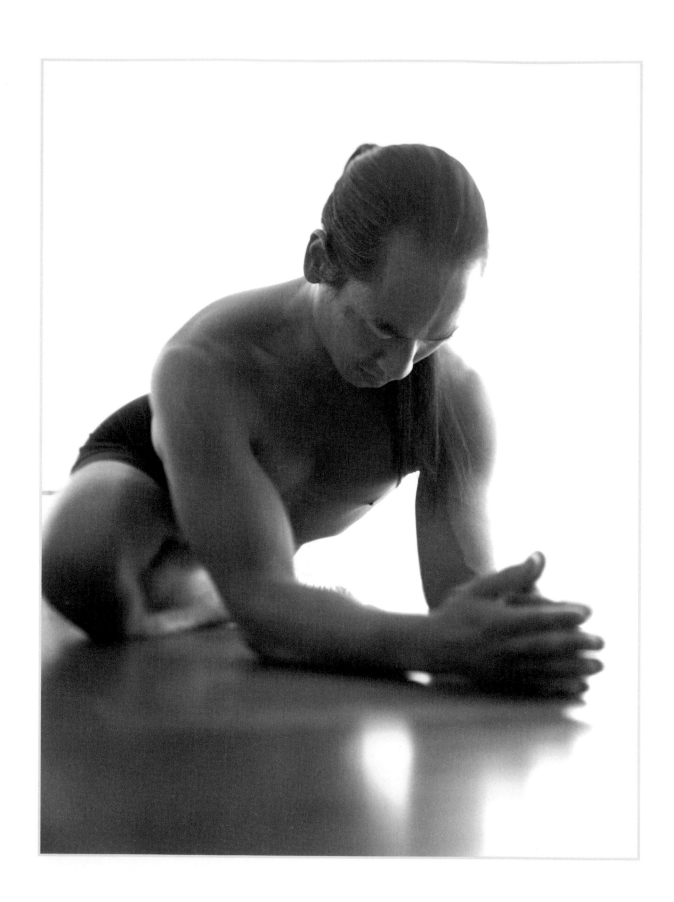

WEEK 6:

Listening Inward

A FREQUENT RESPONSE PEOPLE HAVE WHEN YOU ASK THEM THESE DAYS HOW THEY ARE IS, "I'M SO busy." Many of us have filled up our schedules in the outside world to the point where there is no time or energy for looking inward. When I was in Bhutan recently, I saw young children on the hillsides who gave me the feeling that they were completely integrated with their environment, just as if they were part of the hillside, with their consciousness interwoven both inwardly and outwardly. Can you find a little bit of time to turn inward to the point where you are fully present in the moment and where all internal movement is as fully observed as external movement is?

As you use the forward bends and restorative poses to turn inward, you quiet all input coming into your senses, not by removing yourself from external stimuli, but by not attaching yourself to anything that is moving in and out of your body. The forward bends literally fold you so that your senses (eyes, ears, mouth, and nose) turn toward yourself. Going into a forward bend is like spinning yourself into a cocoon. The forward bends turn your senses inward, allowing you to observe what is taking place within your body.

In the restorative poses, you begin to be able to observe the sensations of your body without identifying with them. You ask your nervous, muscular, circulatory, and digestive systems to minimize their need to work. And you keep exploring "nondoing" as a way to get a clearer and clearer look at the core of your being. As surface noise begins to quiet, the deep inner workings of your mind, body, and breath become more exposed.

When an animal goes to sleep, the movement of its breath becomes its dominant characteristic. Likewise, when you are doing forward bends or restorative poses, the way your body is receiving your breath should be one of your most prominent observations. You also more readily observe the way your mind wanders, moving in and out of different perceptions and thoughts. Both your breath and your mind have habitual patterns. In restorative poses, these patterns become more apparent in your general field of awareness.

By turning inward, you start to realize how much of your life takes place within the boundaries of your mind and body. As you move deeper and deeper inward, you see how many of your external perceptions are biased by your internal emotions and sensations. The way you typically identify yourself only superficially defines you. But what about the part of you that is not superficially defined? You are like the new moon in the shadow of the rest of the moon, with your superficial self-identification only hinting at the circumference of the entire sphere of your being. By going deeply inward, you begin to see the roots of many of your actions and to understand why you are as you are in the world.

ABOUT FORWARD BENDS

Forward bends are some of the most familiar shapes your body will take in yoga. Consider that when you sit, your position is basically a habitual forward bend. And you've probably done some stretching by bending forward over your legs. However, the forward bends in yoga are not about collapsing or lethargy. They are quieting poses, but your internal movement should be clear and strong. It is necessary for the vitality of your forward bends that the action of your legs and arms supports both your spine and upper chest, even as you surrender to the internal quietness of the poses. The release you receive in the muscles of your back, your neck, and the backs of your legs can create an extraordinary letting go of your entire body-mind. Whether you do forward bends actively or as restorative poses, your main emphasis should be on an equal release throughout your entire back body while your front body continues to have space to receive and breathe.

ABOUT RESTORATIVE POSES

Restorative Poses come in all forms, including backbends, forward bends, inversions, and twists. However, their common thread is that these poses are supported so you use very little muscular effort. When doing restorative poses, focus on simply letting go and allowing the circulation of your breath and mind to be more integrated in your body. Restorative poses are advanced postures because they demand that your mind be present when there is no strong physical calling. But just by practicing yoga you are continually trying to integrate your mind, body, breath, and spirit. Letting your mind stay involved in the subtle movements of your body eventually becomes an exquisite joy. Lie back and listen. Our society is one that defines itself as "busy" and doesn't innately understand the place and need for such poses. However, your ability to use this book wisely will partly depend on your finding a way to integrate restorative poses into your regular practice.

EMOTIONS. Often your emotions become more apparent as you move into forward bends and restorative poses because external input is reduced. Even though some of you may find forward bends physically excruciating while others may find them quite pleasurable, the actual position of turning inward highlights the emotions in all of us. In the restorative poses, because there is little feedback from physical stimulus, your emotions surface. Because of this, you might have a difficult time staying with these poses. Ground yourself by focusing on your breath and gradually building the length of time you stay in postures.

FOCUS OF YOUR MIND. In restorative poses, focus your mind on watching the even release of your body as reflected in the evenness with which your entire body absorbs your breath. If you scan your body in these postures, starting from the crown of your head and going to the soles of your feet, you begin an

ANATOMY LESSON

1. Wide sitting bones and tailbone drawing under

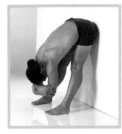

To learn about your sitting bones and tail-bone, practice version 3 of Wall Hang, lifting and widening your sitting bones as high up the wall as possible. Now draw your tailbone between your sitting bones and toward your pubis. Feel the interplay between these two actions.

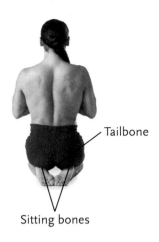

Tailbone

Sitting bones

2. Evenly active and elongated spine

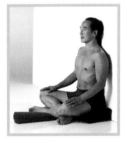

To learn to evenly activate and elongate your spine, sit in version 1 of Seated Crossed-Legs Pose. Now, very slowly elongate your spine as evenly as possible from the base to the crown of your head. Feel how your back muscles can stay broad and evenly supportive.

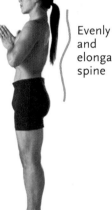

Evenly active and elongated spine

3. Sacrum and shoulder blades deep into body and communicating with each other

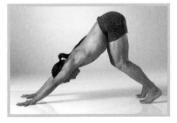

To learn about the relationship between your sacrum and shoulder blades, practice version 1 of Downward-Facing Dog, maintaining the natural curves of your spine as much as possible. Firm both your sacrum and your shoulder blades deep into your body so your front body receives them. As your sacrum and shoulder blades press into your body, observe the communication between them.

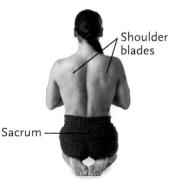

Shoulder blades

Sacrum

internal, subtle adjustment that allows for mindfulness throughout your entire body. The movement of your breath and your ability to be mindful leads to optimum balance.

CHEST. No matter which restorative pose you are in or how deeply you move into your forward bends, your chest should move easily with the rise and fall of your breath. The energy of your arms and legs should still support your chest, even if your back is rounded.

ARMS. Use or place your arms to encourage the release of your entire body. In the forward bends, if you pull too much with your arms, your body will react with a natural fear response that will begin to shut down its receptivity. Pulling with your arms in the right amount creates a deeper absorption and flow of breath and a sense of integration and evenness throughout your body. In restorative poses, the proper support of your arms creates an evenness of

your breath throughout your head, neck, and upper chest.

LOWER BACK. In all these postures, adjust your lower back so it feels integrated with your entire body. If you are experiencing any extra stress in your lower back, change your setup or your action inside the pose. Practice the forward bends in a way that creates a feeling of traction and release in your lower back instead of stress or strain.

NECK AND HEAD. The placement of your neck and head should flow with your torso. Periodically play with their position to find clarity and ease. In all these postures, soften your sense organs and create more receptivity. For instance, let your eyes feel as if they are falling deeply into their sockets as they turn downward to look at your heart. Allow your sense organs to feel as if they are turning inward to witness the movements and feelings of your inner body.

DAY 1: LEARNING THE VARIATIONS

When you practice forward bends, learning variations is more important than ever. You will probably tend to force and pull deeply into forward bends. However, if you do this in the hip-opening poses (such as all versions of Crossed-Legs Forward Bend), forcing will put excess strain on your knees. In addition, in the straight-leg forward bends (one or two legs straight), aggressiveness can lead to a strained lower back. While you play with these variations, learn to observe how your entire body is opening.

For people who find forward bends very difficult, these poses will take persistence. To move toward openness in these poses, it is better to do version 1 or 2 of a pose daily rather than occasionally trying to force yourself into version 3.

For the restorative poses, versions 1, 2, and 3 are not necessarily progressive; instead, they are each full poses that are useful at different times.

Both the forward bends and restorative poses require a very minute, subtle listening. Continually scan your entire body from head to toe. As you ob-

serve your body, you will find unconscious areas of tension and holding that you can release. Many of the setups for these poses are fairly elaborate, but setting up the foundations for these poses is crucial for receiving their benefits. If you take your time in the beginning, you will be able to stay in the poses much longer and the depth of your release and integration will increase.

MOVING IN AND OUT OF FORWARD BENDS AND RESTORATIVE POSES

As you move into forward bends, set up a strong foundation. The major hinging of your forward bend takes place in your hip sockets, so use your legs to create a strong grounding that allows your pelvis to move more freely. Before you move into the forward bend, check to see whether your pelvis comes to a vertical position (it is practical to use your hands at this point to observe accurately). If it does not, prop your pelvis up until it comes to vertical, so when you come forward there will not be excessive pulling or strain in your lower back. Please move slowly into the forward bends so that you can find an even rounding in your spine connected with a constant elongation. As you slowly move forward, observe a letting go.

Before you move into the restorative poses, set up your props as meticulously as possible because when your body begins to rest deeply. any asymmetry will be exaggerated.

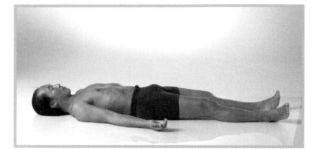

Then, adjust your body so that the props open and support your body and your body feels even, balanced, and content. Often when you lie down on props, your skin slightly catches in a certain direction. If possible, adjust your body so that the movement of your skin catches in a direction that enhances the opening of your posture and allows your skin to feel broad, receptive, and moveable. For example, when the bolster is under your back in Supported Relaxation Pose, the skin of your shoulder blades should be drawn down away from your neck, but you don't want that skin to feel pinched.

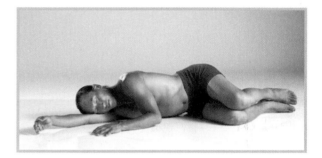

When you come out of the forward bends or restorative poses, move slowly while making the transitions. To come out of a forward bend, reground your foundation and slowly bring your spine back to vertical, vertebrae by vertebrae, with as much elongation

as possible. To come out of a restorative pose, if possible, draw your knees into your chest and turn to your side, as shown above; sitting up abruptly destroys the calming effect.

After coming out of all these poses, sit with a neutral spine for a few moments to let your spine and all the spinal muscles regroup in their natural positions.

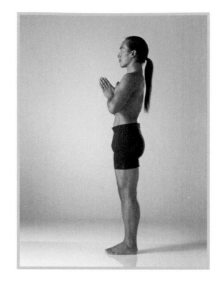

1. Practice two mini **SUN SALUTATIONS,** staying for 5 breaths in Downward-Facing Dog. Emphasize the broadness and openness of the muscles and skin of the backs of your legs.

2. Practice two full **SUN SALUTATIONS,** staying for 5 breaths in Downward-Facing Dog. Allow your spine to move fluidly and evenly.

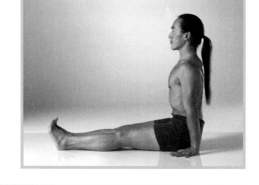

3. Practice the **CORE STRENGTHENING SERIES** twice. Focus on grounding your legs. The second time around, stay in your final Cobbler's and Wide Angle Poses (bending forward) for 1 minute.

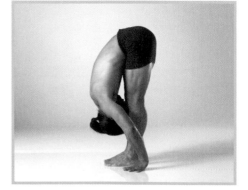

4. Practice **STANDING FORWARD BEND** for 1 minute. Focus on grounding your legs.

5. Try all three versions of **Crossed-Legs Forward Bend** *(Sukhasana)* for 30 seconds in each version on both the left and right sides.

VERSION 1: Feet in crossed-legs position; head resting on your hands, a bolster, or the seat of a chair

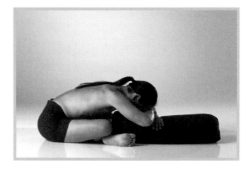

When you support the weight of your head and body on a prop, your back muscles and hips feel like they can let go. This version acquaints you with the quiet, inward-turning nature of forward bends, where there is more a sense of letting go than of stretching. Widen and draw your sitting bones backward away from your knees as you feel your tailbone moving toward your pubis. Search for the completion of your exhalation.

VERSION 2: Legs in ankle over knee (shin over shin) position; head on your hands, a bolster, or the seat of a chair

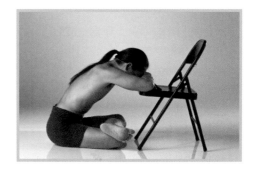

The position of your legs in this version intensifies the opening in your hips, especially combined with the forward bend. Support yourself high enough so that your body has some release instead of clenching in pain. Let yourself enjoy the shape of the pose without feeling you have to get a deep stretch or heavy sensation. While doing this pose, you confront some of your body's deepest physical and emotional bindings. Support your head and chest at a level that keeps your spine evenly active and elongated, from your tailbone to the crown of your head.

VERSION 3: Legs in Half Lotus; head resting on your hands, a bolster, or the seat of a chair

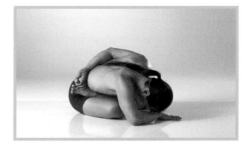

When your legs are able to take this shape, you will find that having your foot buried in your belly with your legs deeply folded is soothing. You feel the support for your lower back and sacrum from your front body and the placement of your legs. With your legs in Half Lotus you begin to understand the circuitry of Full Lotus, which provides a feeling of completion and wholeness. Observe the position of your sacrum and shoulder blades. Deepen them into your body and feel their relationship to each other.

6. Try all three versions of **COBBLER'S FORWARD BEND** (*Baddha Konasana*) for 30 seconds in each version.

VERSION 1: Against the wall, bolster behind your lower back

With your legs in this position, it is very difficult to maintain the natural curve of your lower back. Sitting at the wall against a bolster provides support so that the muscles of your back will not be solely responsible for lifting your chest. If you cannot get your sitting bones close to the wall or if knees are extremely high, sit on a prop. This version lets you stay much longer in the posture, slowly easing your legs open with their own weight and through conscious release. Try to widen and bring your sitting bones back toward the wall as you bring your tailbone under toward your pubis to gain support and elongation from the depth of your abdominal muscles.

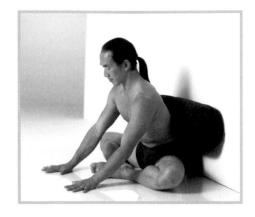

VERSION 2: Head on a bolster that is placed (perpendicular) between your legs

This foundation of your legs in Cobbler's Pose naturally rounds your back and tucks your tailbone. Evenly round your entire spine and drop your head on the bolster to create a congruous feeling throughout your body. The goal is not to bring your head to the bolster, but to have the support high enough so your head soothes itself by resting on the bolster. Search for evenness in the activity and elongation of your spine. Look for the completion of your exhalations and the evenness of your breath.

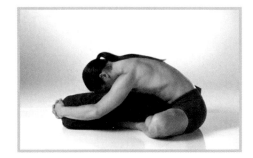

VERSION 3: Full pose, without props

Being in full contact with the floor with the outsides of your legs, the floor of your pelvis, and your forehead provides a deep internal release that may surprise you. As you draw yourself down to the floor, it is tempting to overuse the pull of your arms, but continue to stay focused on releasing inside your hip sockets, especially in the depths of your groins and pubis. The challenge is to be patient and let the pose fold naturally, with your sacrum and shoulder blades deepening into your body. Observe any restrictions.

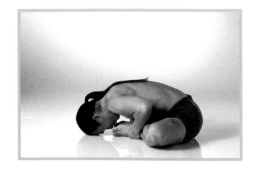

7. Practice the **RECLINED LEG STRETCH SERIES** for 30 seconds in the straight-leg version, 15 seconds in the sit-up version, and 30 seconds in the leg-to-the-side version, on each side. In all versions notice the broadness at the back of your top leg, your lower back, and your sacrum that allows the breath to move easily into these areas.

8. Try all three versions of **ONE-LEGGED FORWARD BEND** (*Janu Sirsasana*) for 30 seconds in each version, on each side.

VERSION 1: Sitting against the wall, hips on a blanket, bolster behind your lower back

Many of us have a tendency to pull into the forward bends. However, you will benefit greatly from just sitting upright with your legs in this position. The wall and the bolster let you do this without straining or overusing the muscles of your back body. When you stay in this pose for longer periods of time, the opening in back of your straight leg and in the hip of your bent leg will begin to occur naturally. To create a good foundation and a deep internal lift, widen your sitting bones, move them toward the wall, and draw your tailbone under toward your pubis.

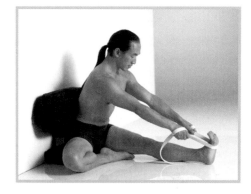

VERSION 2: Head resting on a bolster or chair so spine is evenly elongated

When you rest your body forward on a surface, all your back muscles begin to unwind, releasing tension from your legs, pelvis, and back body and from the back of your neck. Often in forward bends, less is more, and patience and breath become two main ingredients to letting go the tension and tightness of your calves, hamstrings, hips, and back muscles.

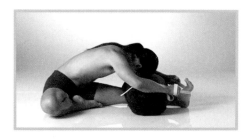

VERSION 3: Full pose, with head resting on shin

In this version you learn how active arms can further the release of your back body. Keep your shoulder blades moving away from your neck as the pull of your arms encourages your chest to move forward. The challenge is not to become overly aggressive but instead to listen to how much pull is beneficial. As you fold deeply upon yourself, let there remain a feeling of spaciousness and harmony.

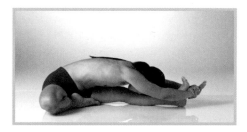

9. Try all three versions of **SUPPORTED DOWNWARD-FACING DOG** *(Adho Mukha Svanasana)* variation for 30 seconds in each version.

VERSION 1: Hanging Dog, with a strap around a doorknob or hook on the wall

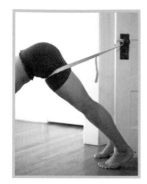

This version allows you to get the proper direction of the movement of your thighs, along with full traction on your lower back. By hanging on the strap, you take all the weight off your arms so you can continue to walk your hands forward to find the maximum elongation of your lower back and waist. The pull on your thighs that moves them into your hamstrings provides an ease of breath all the way down into the base of your pelvis.

VERSION 2: With a block at its highest height, your legs bent, a strap just below your elbows

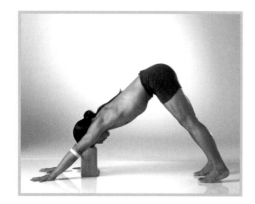

The strap helps support the full extension of your arms so the alignment of your arm bones can easily support some of the weight of your body. Placing your head on the block allows you to rest the weight of your head so your neck can let go completely, and resting your forehead on a surface helps cool your nervous system. Bending your legs allows those of you who are very tight to move the weight of your pelvis and torso in the direction of your legs. To find the natural curves of your lower back, widen and lift your sitting bones as you draw your tailbone under.

VERSION 3: With the block at its lowest height, with straight legs (if your head is not touching the block, this is not for you)

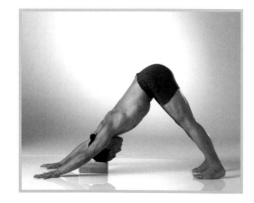

This version maximizes the opening of your shoulders and upper chest while you release the back of your neck. As you move more deeply into this restorative Downward-Facing Dog, press your shoulder blades and sacrum into your body and feel the muscular connection between the two. Your upper chest and shoulder joints have to open to a much greater extent. Be careful that you don't compensate for the lack of opening in your shoulders by pushing your lower ribs forward. Don't hesitate to go back to version 2 any time this version feels like a strain or inhibits your breath.

10. Try all three versions of **SEATED FORWARD BEND** *(Paschimottanasana)* for 30 seconds in each version.

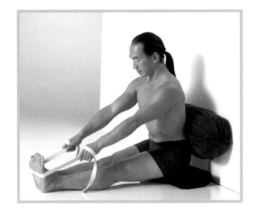

VERSION 1: Sitting against the wall, on a prop if necessary, a bolster behind your lower back

If many of us would spend time sitting against the wall with straight legs—even without the intention of bending forward—we would achieve both flexibility and release of tension in the backs of our legs. Focus at the root of your pelvis (widen your sitting bones as your tailbone naturally draws under) to keep yourself folding in the proper place with adequate support.

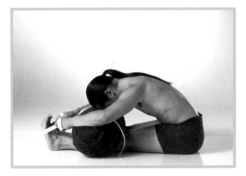

VERSION 2: Head resting on a chair or on a bolster placed on your legs

This version completes the forward bend in the sense that your entire back body is allowed to release. Prop yourself up high enough so that while you are surrendering, your spine is evenly rounded, from your tailbone to the back of your skull. This ensures that your whole back opens without one area being overstressed.

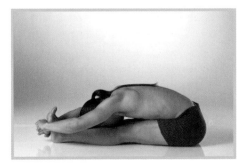

VERSION 3: Full pose, head resting on shins

This version is much more active than versions 1 and 2, both in your legs and in your arms. As your arms begin to pull, your legs have to ground proportionately and extend more strongly. Continue to deepen your sacrum toward your front body as your shoulder blades drop down your back and find their muscular connection with your sacrum. This action continues to support and elongate your front body, so as you turn inward and fold deeply, your front body is not compressed.

11. Try all three versions of **WIDE ANGLE FORWARD BEND** (*Upavista Konasana*) for 30 seconds in each version.

VERSION 1: Against the wall, bolster behind your lower back

For some of you, having your legs spread and straight will make it easier to sit upright, while others will find this leg position creating even more resistance to keeping your body upright. The wall in this version brings you awareness of the position of your spine and supports your back muscles so they do not have to overwork. The resistance in your legs will slowly release. Do not rely completely on the wall, but begin to create internal support, starting from the wideness of your sitting bones and the grounding of your legs.

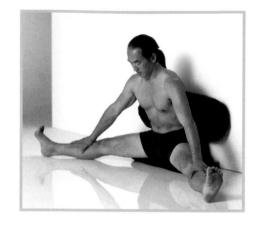

VERSION 2: Head on a bolster placed (perpendicular) between your legs

Once your body becomes capable of a forward bend in this wide-leg position, this version is a deeply restorative pose. Your body feels like it can rest on the bolster or chair with great ease, naturally spilling forward between your legs. The challenge is to keep your legs and feet active to promote as deep a grounding as a coming forward.

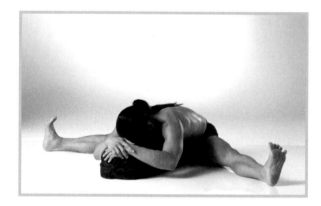

VERSION 3: Full pose, head touching the ground

For most of you the full pose is not as comforting as the supported version, so your ability to dig deep into the fear and tension of your back body becomes heightened. Don't let the weight of your body coming forward pull you from your anchor; keep your knees and toes pointing straight upward so that you don't roll onto or strain your inner legs. Rather than focusing on bringing your head to the ground, focus on creating the depth of your sacrum and the support of your shoulder blades.

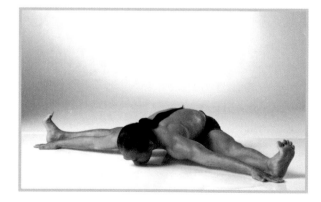

12. Try all three versions of **RESTORATIVE CHILD'S POSE** *(Balasana)* variation for 30 seconds in each version.

VERSION 1: A bolster (perpendicular) under your chest

Supporting your chest with the bolster so that the middle of your back is higher than your sacrum encourages the fold of your legs and gives your front body tactile contact, which enables your body-mind to relax deeply. It is not necessary to activate the wideness of your sitting bones or the drawing under of your tailbone, but be mindful of how the base of your spine feels and how your breath is flowing in this area. Challenge yourself to stay awake, observing the layers of tension that you shed and the new depths of relaxation that you reach.

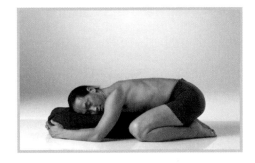

VERSION 2: Bolster (perpendicular) under your chest, folded blanket under your shins (your feet hanging off the back)

For many of you, one of the tightest parts of your body is the front of your shins and feet. When you decrease the opening and stretch in this area—by letting the angle be less acute—your body will be less confronted or challenged. This sends a message to your nervous system that it can let down its guard and be completely supported. Focus on observing the naturalness and depth of your exhalation. Without any effort, this action allows your spine to be even and elongated.

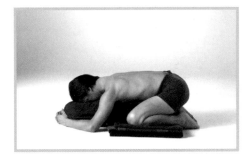

VERSION 3: Folded blanket under your shins (feet hanging off the back), a bolster under your buttocks, and two bolsters (perpendicular) under your chest

This version creates even less bending in your hip joints and provides more support for your torso. Having your chest higher than your pelvis without forcing your pelvis to fold deeply provides extreme comfort, alleviating any downward pressure on your neck and head. Imagine your sacrum and shoulder blades falling deeply into your body.

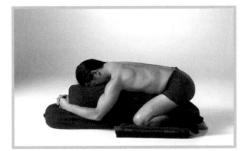

13. Try all three versions of **Restorative Backbend** *(Viparita Dandasana)* variation for 30 seconds in each version.

VERSION 1: Cross bolsters backbend

This version creates a very even, subtle backbend that will elicit a good feeling as well as a profound opening. Opening your upper chest is one of the most important movements that we can do in yoga because most of us habitually protect and close our heart chakra. To reverse that tendency brings you closer to balance around true center. Keep your legs strong and maintain your awareness of your pelvis while you open your chest, and explore the connection between legs, pelvis, and chest.

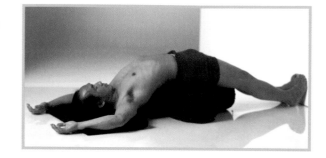

VERSION 2: Rectangular blanket or block under sacrum (low version of Supported Bridge Pose)

When your sacrum is slightly lifted, you get the benefit of an inversion without overly challenging the opening of your hip flexors or lower back. The evenness that comes to your spine allows a profound evenness of your breath. Your pelvic organs recede deeply into a sacrum that is rising to meet them, relaxing your internal organs. Follow the completion of your exhalation, consciously relaxing your vital organs more and more.

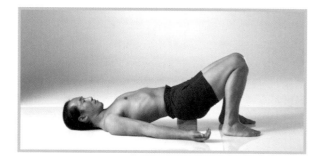

VERSION 3: Over the seat of a chair (with legs through the chair back), head supported

This version allows you to find a complete opening without having to overwork. In this full backbend, you can move and make adjustments as you feel the subtle alignment of your legs and arms supporting the arch of the spine. Learn how to catch the bottom tip of your shoulder blades with one edge of the chair while your buttocks flesh is dragged by the chair's other edge. Find the full elongation of your spine while your shoulder blades and sacrum deepen. Remain active in the pose, ensuring length and broadness of your entire spine.

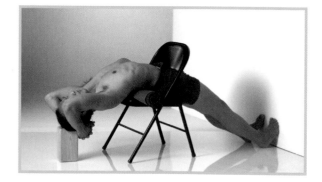

14. Try all three versions of **RESTORATIVE PLOW POSE** *(Halasana)* for 30 seconds in each version.

VERSION 1: Legs bent, thighs and knees on the chair seat, ankles on the backrest, back rounded, arms over your head

In this version, you evenly round and fold your body, much like Child's Pose with a different orientation. The emphasis is not on lifting but on using the weight of your legs and the rounding of your back to open the muscles of your back body and neck. Continue to adjust your weight and the position of the chair so that the posture is completely comfortable. Feel your inhalation moving between your sitting bones and tailbone.

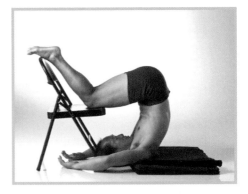

VERSION 2: Knees and shins resting on a chair seat, a blanket under your shoulders (like Shoulderstand), hands in Shoulderstand position

In this version you actively create a foundation with your arms to allow more lift in your entire torso. Your legs—even though they are extended—should provide traction for your spine. Some of you (depending on your height) may need to put blankets on the chair seat so that as your legs are resting they are pushed upward by the support. This not only grounds your legs but also suspends your spine. As your spine relaxes, adjust the position of your legs and arms for evenness and elongation of your spine.

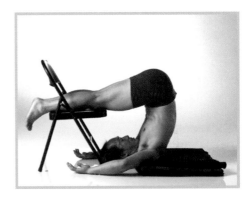

VERSION 3: Arms clasped behind your back (knees bent or straight as in version 1 or version 2)

By clasping your hands behind your back, you turn your arms under your chest, taking any weight off the base of your neck. As you create this strong foundation, learn how to relax the muscles of your back. Position the chair and your legs so that your back muscles can be suspended and not responsible for the ease of your neck. Although your emphasis in this pose should be on surrender, focus as well on your sacrum and shoulder blades as they deepen and press into your body.

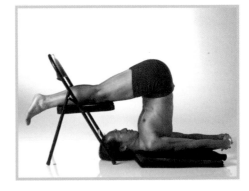

15. Try all three versions of **SUPPORTED RELAXATION POSE** *(Savasana)* variation for 1 minute in each version.

VERSION 1: Mountain Brook Pose, with support under your legs, chest, and head

This pose supports and creates contact under three important parts of your body: your thighs, kidneys, and neck. This support allows the vulnerable posture of Relaxation Pose to be more accepted by your body's survival mechanisms. The support also creates a graceful undulation through your body, allowing for deeper relaxation. To anchor this fluid pose, stay focused on the base of your pelvis. Observe your natural breath within this Relaxation Pose. Ask yourself: How smooth is my breath? Is my inhalation or my exhalation longer? Is my inhalation easy? Is my exhalation easy?

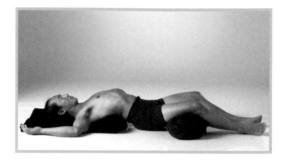

VERSION 2: Calves resting on the seat of a chair

Resting your calves on the seat of a chair removes the possibility that the pull of your legs will strain your lower back. It also reminds your calf muscles to surrender their holding and their responsibility for balancing your body, enhancing the internal evenness and suppleness of your spine. Adjust the chair so that the weight of your legs feels mainly supported by the chair, creating a sense of floating in your abdominal cavity, sacrum, and lower back. Observe your natural breath within this Relaxation Pose, asking yourself the same questions as in version 1.

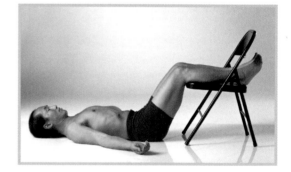

VERSION 3: Bolster (lengthwise) supporting your chest and head

This version opens your chest and creates traction in your lower back. Even though your chest is more open, psychologically the pose feels less vulnerable than unsupported Relaxation Pose. Having your head higher than your chest and your chest higher than your pelvis—without the responsibility of your back muscles holding them up—brings more alertness to your mind, more opening to your heart, and more grounding to your legs. Let the bolster support the depth of your sacrum and shoulder blades and encourage a deep absorption of your breath. Observe your natural breath within this Relaxation Pose, asking yourself the same questions as in version 1.

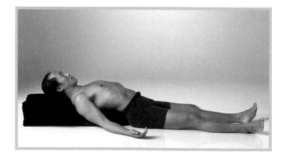

MEDITATION

16. For 5 to 10 minutes, sit in Seated Crossed-Legs Pose, and meditate on the extension and smoothness of your exhalation.

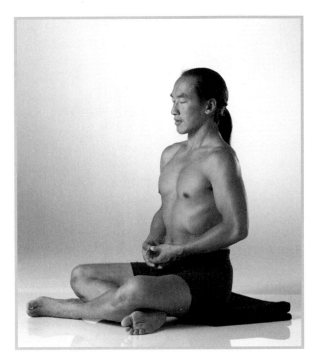

Cobbler's Forward Bend and Wide Angle Forward Bend are both symmetrical forward bends with wide-open thighs. However, Cobbler's Forward Bend is a hip opener, while Wide Angle Forward Bend opens your hamstrings and the insides of your legs. Many times Cobbler's Pose precedes Wide Angle Forward Bend because it opens your hips and when you do Wide Angle Forward Bend afterward some of the difficult resistance has already been addressed. In both poses, grounding your thighbones creates the anchor from which you can begin to release forward. Coming forward slowly and being mindful of exactly where the resistance lies informs you exactly where you have to let go. Because these poses are symmetrical forward bends, they are good poses with which to start and end a forward bend practice.

Today's sequence begins with Supported Downward-Facing Dog Pose and Wall Hang to open up the backs of your legs and extend your spine. From this opening, you move into the Core Strengthening Series, which incorporates both Cobbler's Pose and Wide Angle Pose. These poses build the foundation needed for Cobbler's Forward Bend and Wide Angle Forward Bend. Cobbler's Pose with a slight backbend and Seated Crossed-Legs Twist ease your spine before you begin your forward bending. You then move into the forward bend section of the practice. Cobbler's Forward Bend and Wide Angle Forward Bend are repeated several times to let you slowly work through the resistance in your hamstrings and inner legs. The sequence ends with Restorative Child's Pose to rest your back. Please finish this practice with relaxation and breath awareness in Supported Relaxation Pose to counter all the forward bends.

FOCUS FOR THIS PRACTICE:

- In Downward-Facing Dog and Wall Hang, widen your sitting bones and draw your tailbone between them.

- In Cobbler's Forward Bend and Wide Angle Forward Bend, evenly elongate your spine.

- During Relaxation and Meditation, deepen your sacrum and shoulder blades into your body.

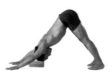

1. Practice **Supported Downward-Facing Dog Pose** for 2 minutes.

2. Practice **Wall Hang** for 1 minute.

3. Practice the **Core Strengthening Series** three times, with a single breath in each pose.

4. Practice **Cobbler's Forward Bend** for 1 minute.

5. Practice **Cobbler's Pose** with a slight backbend for 15 seconds.

6. Practice **Seated Crossed-Legs Twist** for 30 seconds on each side. Repeat with the opposite cross of your legs.

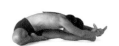

7. Practice **One-Legged Forward Bend** for 1 minute on each side.

8. Practice **Cobbler's Forward Bend** for 30 seconds.

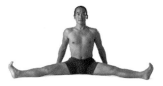

9. Practice **Wide Angle Pose** for 1 minute.

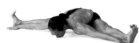

10. Practice **Wide Angle Forward Bend** for 1 minute.

11. Practice **Cobbler's Pose** with a slight backbend for 15 seconds.

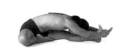

12. Practice **One-Legged Forward Bend** for 1 minute on each side.

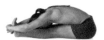

13. Practice **Seated Forward Bend** for 1 minute.

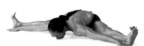

14. Practice **Wide Angle Forward Bend** for 1 minute.

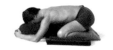

15. Practice **Restorative Child's Pose** for 3 minutes.

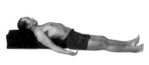

16. Relaxation and Breath Awareness. For 5 minutes, practice version 3 of **Supported Relaxation Pose.** Practice slightly elongated, smooth inhalations moving into your belly and inner thighs.

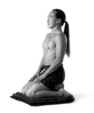

17. Meditation. For 5 to 10 minutes, sit in **Hero Pose** against the wall. Meditate on the relaxation of your inner thighs.

DAY 3: LEARNING ONE-LEGGED FORWARD BEND AND SEATED FORWARD BEND

Both One-Legged Forward Bend and Seated Forward Bend quiet your mind and soothe the agitation of your nervous system and body. One-Legged Forward Bend is an asymmetrical pose, which creates less resistance to your being able to bend forward than when you bend with two straight legs. It also has the element of a twist, which releases the sides of your lower back. Because of this twist, you have to be careful not to torque your sacrum by pulling too strongly over your straight leg. For those of you who are tight, Seated Forward Bend may be frustrating because of the amount of resistance it creates, but the symmetry of the pose makes it much easier to find evenness between the two sides of your body and in the rounding of your spine. If you respect the resistance that comes from attempting to bend forward, you will gradually find a great release of all the muscles of the backs of your legs and torso.

Today's sequence begins with poses that awaken your body and generate energy. You then move on to standing poses interspersed with Standing Forward Bend to open up your hips and hamstrings. These poses work your legs at the same time as they release

your legs, the action you need to take in forward bends. The transition from the standing poses to the forward bends begins with Crossed-Legs Forward Bend. You then move on to One-Legged Forward Bend and Seated Forward Bend. Cobbler's Pose is used in the forward bend section as a neutral pose to release any tension or overbending in your spine. The sequence ends with Cobbler's Forward Bend and Wide Angle Forward Bend to release your hips and back. Practice the relaxation and breath awareness postures, Supported Relaxation Pose and Reclined Cobbler's Pose, to return your spine to neutral.

FOCUS FOR THIS PRACTICE:

- In the standing poses, press your sacrum and shoulder blades toward your front body. Feel the relationship between the two.

- In One-Legged Forward Bend, play with your spine to create length and evenness.

- In Seated Forward Bend, widen your sitting bones and tuck your tailbone.

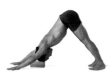 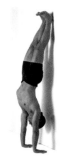 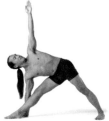

1. Practice **Supported Downward-Facing Dog** for 2 minutes.

2. Practice **Standing Forward Bend** for 1 minute.

3. Practice **Handstand** for 30 seconds.

4. Practice **Triangle Pose** for 1 minute on each side.

5. Practice **Standing Forward Bend** for 1 minute.

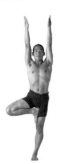

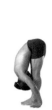

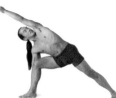

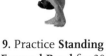

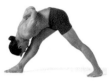

6. Practice **Tree Pose** for 30 seconds on each side.

7. Practice **Standing Forward Bend** for 30 seconds.

8. Practice **Extended Side Angle Pose** for 45 seconds on each side.

9. Practice **Standing Forward Bend** for 30 seconds.

10. Practice **Pyramid Pose** for 1 minute on each side.

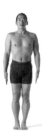

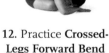

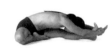

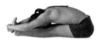

11. Practice **Mountain Pose** for 30 seconds.

12. Practice **Crossed-Legs Forward Bend** for 1 minute on each side.

13. Practice **One-Legged Forward Bend** for 1 minute on each side. Repeat again on both sides. Keep the first round easy, and allow yourself to go deeper on the second round.

14. Practice **Cobbler's Pose** with a slight backbend for 30 seconds.

15. Practice **Seated Forward Bend** for 1 minute. Sit briefly in Staff Pose, and then repeat. Keep the first forward bend easy, and allow yourself to go deeper with the second one.

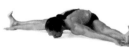

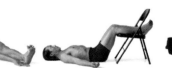

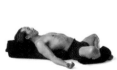

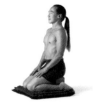

16. Practice **Cobbler's Forward Bend** for 1 minute.

17. Practice **Wide Angle Forward Bend** for 1 minute.

18. Relaxation and Breath Awareness. For 5 minutes, practice version 2 of **Supported Relaxation Pose.** With your hands on your belly, observe the

pause at the end of your exhalation and slightly lengthen it.

For 5 minutes, practice version 3 of **Reclined Cobbler's Pose.**

19. Meditation. For 5 minutes, sit in **Hero Pose.** Meditate on the natural curves of your lower back.

Day 4: Learning Restorative Backbend and Restorative Plow Pose

Restorative Backbend and Restorative Plow Pose are natural counterposes but because both are very gentle, incorporating them within the same practice can be very quieting for the mind. Eventually the amount of time that you can spend in these poses can be increased to 5 minutes or longer, allowing your body to fall deeply into opening. In the Restorative Backbend your body has time to digest how it feels to have an open front body. Restorative Plow Pose suspends your body while the back of your torso feels like it is draped from your legs, convincing the muscles of your back to let go. Restorative Backbend is a pose with which you might end or begin an energetic practice, while Restorative Plow Pose is usually reserved for the end of a practice because it takes you inward so deeply. When you are fatigued, either or both of these poses can be very beneficial for restoring your energy.

Focus for this practice:

- As you set up for your restorative poses, maximize the length and evenness of your spine. Position your sacrum and shoulder blades mindfully.

- In seated meditation, set up by widening your sitting bones and tucking your tailbone.

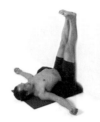

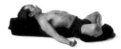

1. Practice version 3 of **Legs Up the Wall Pose** for 5 minutes.

2. Practice version 3 of **Reclined Cobbler's Pose** for 5 minutes.

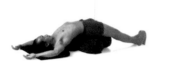

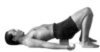

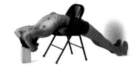

3. Practice all three versions of **Restorative Backbend** for 1 minute in each version, in this order.

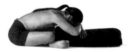

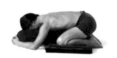

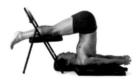

4. Practice version 1 of **Crossed-Legs Forward Bend**, with your head resting on a bolster or the seat of a chair, for 1 minute on each side.

5. Practice **Supported Child's Pose** for 5 minutes.

6. Practice all three versions of **Restorative Plow Pose** for 1 minute in each version.

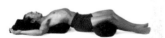

7. Relaxation and Breath Awareness. For 5 to 10 minutes, practice version 1 of **Supported Relaxation Pose.** Elongate your inhalations and exhalations slightly as you relax your sense organs.

8. Meditation. For 5 to 10 minutes, sit in **Seated Crossed-Legs Pose** at the wall. Meditate on maintaining the lift of your torso with as little effort as possible.

DAY 5: LEARNING SUPPORTED RELAXATION POSE

You usually stay in Relaxation Pose for 5 to 10 minutes and sometimes even longer. At first you might think that it would be wonderful to lie down for this long, but as you lie down without moving for an extended period of time, you may find that your body can become quite irritated. Any small asymmetry or tweak becomes exaggerated by the relative quietness of the rest of your body. Those of you who have problem lower backs might even find that lying flat on the ground is impossible for longer than a minute or so. Therefore these three variations of Relaxation Pose make it possible to hold the pose much longer. The version where you place your legs on the seat of a chair takes the weight of your legs off your lower back and eliminates any torque. The version where your torso is supported by a bolster creates a suspension and traction for your lower back at the same time it opens your chest. You will notice quite a difference between having your legs higher than your chest and your chest higher than your legs. In Mountain Brook Pose, your body is supported in critical areas so that it will be fully convinced it can safely let go. To fully support the back of your torso provides a tremendous sensation of relief, as your back body lets go of its habitual tensions and can be much more supportive and responsive. These quiet openings sometimes create the deepest shifts in your posture and in your psyche.

Today's sequence begins with Supported Child's Pose and Crossed-Legs Forward Bend to release your back muscle so that when you lie down for the Relaxation Pose these muscles will release deeply into the earth. You then move on to Restorative Backbend versions 1 and 2, which open your front body so that in the Relaxation Pose your front body will be just as open as your back body. The Supported Relaxation Poses are sequenced so you begin with a forward bend, follow the forward bend with a backbend, and end with Mountain Brook Pose, which is a combination of both a forward bend and a backbend.

FOCUS FOR THIS PRACTICE:

- Throughout the practice, spread the skin of your back evenly. When you set up, find the ease and evenness of your spine and continually readjust as necessary.

- In Supported Relaxation Pose, turn your shoulder blades under toward your pelvis and widen them away from your spine. Make sure your sacrum feels balanced and comfortable.

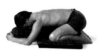 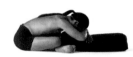 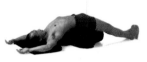 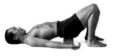

1. Practice **Supported Child's Pose** for 5 minutes.

2. Practice version 1 of **Seated Crossed-Legs Forward Bend**, with your head on a bolster or chair, for 2 minutes on each side.

3. Practice version 1 of **Restorative Backbend** for 2 minutes.

4. Practice version 2 of **Restorative Backbend** for 2 minutes.

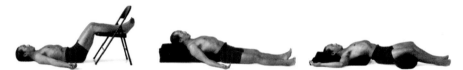

5. Practice all three versions of **Supported Relaxation Pose** as follows: version 2 for 3 minutes, version 3 for 3 minutes, version 1 for 5 minutes.

6. Meditation. For 10 minutes, practice **Seated Crossed-Legs Pose**. Meditate on releasing your legs into the earth as you gradually elongate your spine into its natural curves. Feel the lift of your chest from wide, relaxed back muscles created by the practice. Meditate on expanding your awareness from the center of your body outward.

7. Breath Awareness. For 5 minutes, practice **Seated Crossed-Legs Pose** with your legs crossed in the opposite way from your meditation pose. On your inhalations, feel the broadness of your back body. On your exhalations, feel the length of the front of your spine.

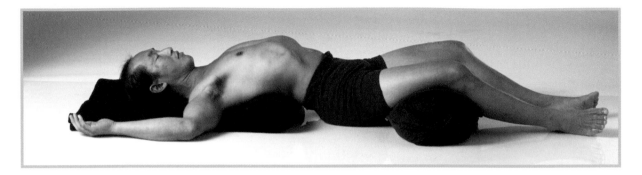

Breath Awareness

For 3 minutes, lie in version 1 of Supported Relaxation Pose.

MOUNTAIN BROOK POSE. This version of Relaxation Pose creates a feeling of movement as you are relaxing. For many of you, this pose will coax your breath naturally into your body. When your body is supported and freed up in just the right places, your nervous system is convinced that it is safe to let go of all protections and restrictions. Your body feels much more calm and steady, as when a friend touches you on the back when you need support. Sometimes too much contact creates a pulling away or a lethargic sleepiness. But Mountain Brook Pose tends to awaken your body without disturbing its ability to soften and relax completely. For some of us this support may seem a bit jarring or mildly uncomfortable at first, but if you consistently practice this pose, you will find a great companion.

ALTERNATE NOSTRIL BREATHING. As you find your mental seat, play with alternate nostril breathing, more as a visualization than a physical manipulation. The technique is this: Imagine you are inhaling up the entire right side of your body, from the sole of your right foot all the way up through your right leg and the right side of your torso and in through your right nostril. As you exhale, imagine that you are exhaling from the top of the left side of your skull, down through your left nostril, and all the way through the left side of your torso, left leg, and out through your left foot. From here, you inhale up the left side of your body, starting from the sole of your left foot, continuing up your left leg and through the left side of your torso, inhaling through your left nostril and the left side of your neck and head. Then exhale through the right side of your body, starting from the right side of the crown of your head, then continuing through your right nostril and through the right side of your torso and arm, down through your right leg and out the sole of your right foot.

This represents one full cycle of alternate nostril breathing. It doesn't really matter if you are actually alternating nostrils. Simply imagine a circulation of breath from the right to the left and then from the left to the right. Feel like a river that makes a U-turn from the right to the left side and then changes directions from the left to the right side. After doing this for 10 to 20 cycles, return to smooth, slightly elongated inhalations and exhalations for about 3 minutes, feeling your breath moving through both left and right nostrils and sides of your body as evenly as possible. Remind yourself that every inhalation can create deeper relaxation, especially for your neck, head, and sense organs. The exhalation will allow you to feel like your entire being fades into emptiness.

Meditation

For 5 to 15 minutes, sit in Seated Crossed-Legs Pose (or Half Lotus, if possible). Make sure your knees and ankles are not jammed or aggravated. Feel the activity of your feet and legs giving rise to your spine. Meditate on your mind becoming more quiet as you continue to focus on your legs and arms supporting your posture.

From this week of forward bends, you might feel that your body and mind have a chance to become more quiet and turn more inward the way the night becomes darker and quieter until 3 or 4 A.M. There is a natural curve to meditations. Initially you focus on your posture and your breath just like when you first get in bed. You squirm and move until you find a position that you can settle in. As you find your body beginning to quiet, you can meditate on your breath and let your breath adjust your posture more minutely. From here, you can let that go and feel everything— your mind, your body, and your breath—fade into emptiness.

QUIET MIND. It is sometimes difficult to distinguish between a mind that is wandering, a mind that is falling asleep, and a mind that is becoming very quiet. Usually when your mind is very quiet, you still maintain mindfulness of your posture and breath, no matter how far in the background. When you catch yourself wandering or falling asleep, you will probably notice that your habitual posture has begun to reassert itself and your breath has become more erratic.

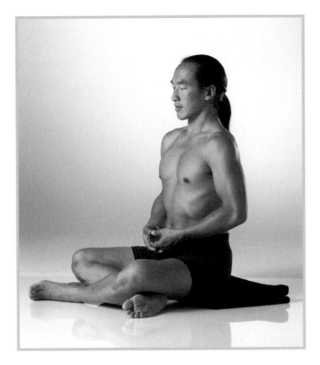

These states of mind are difficult to navigate, and as you go into deep states of awareness and meditation, they become more indescribable. As I look back on my meditation experiences, I am filled with feelings of balance, contentment, peace, and exquisite beauty. These feelings are often strongly juxtaposed by pain in the body, disturbance in the heart, and uncontrollable flights of the mind. Not knowing what is going to arise day by day, you learn how to surrender more completely to what happens without expectation and without purpose.

CROSSED-LEGS FORWARD BEND

Crossed-Legs Forward Bend opens your hips and allows you to bend deeply forward,
rounding your spine to turn completely inside.

POINT OF PLAY:
Rock your pelvis back and
forth with the rise and fall of
your breath.

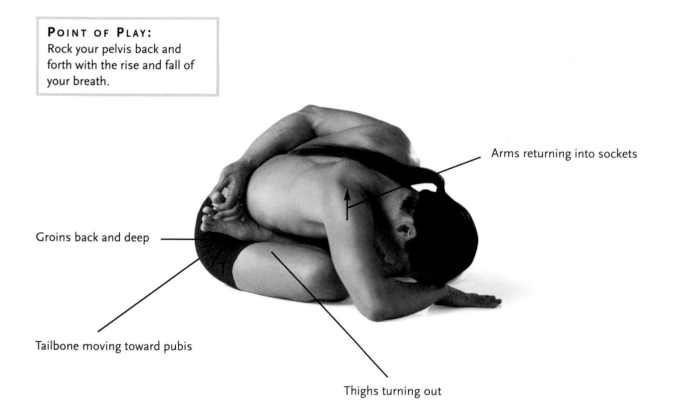

Arms returning into sockets

Groins back and deep

Tailbone moving toward pubis

Thighs turning out

COBBLER'S FORWARD BEND

Cobbler's Forward Bend opens your legs to ground you with the earth.

POINT OF PLAY:
Move your groins back as you
turn your thighs out.

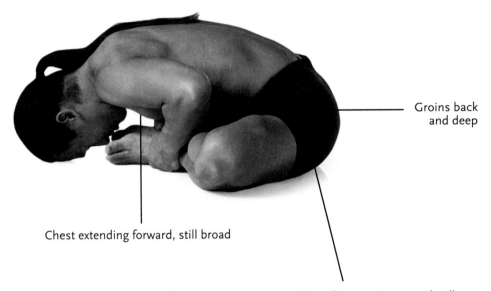

Groins back
and deep

Chest extending forward, still broad

Tailbone moving toward pubis, pubis moving toward tailbone

ONE-LEGGED FORWARD BEND

One-Legged Forward Bend opens your hips and hamstrings and releases your back
as it gradually soothes the irritation from your body.

Spine rounding evenly

POINT OF PLAY:
POINT OF PLAY:
Let the sitting bone on your
bent leg side lift off the
ground, but move your tailbone more toward your pubis.

Groins moving back equally

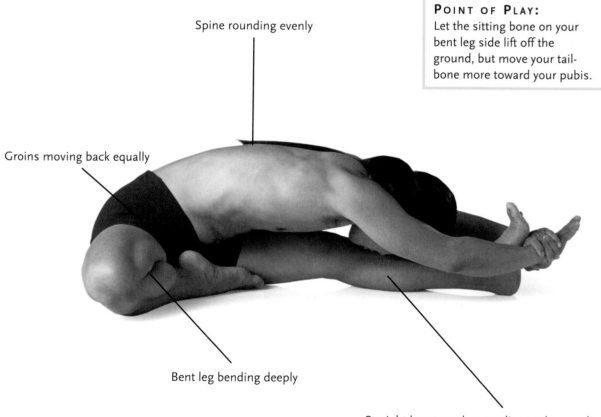

Bent leg bending deeply

Straight leg strongly extending and grounding

SUPPORTED DOWNWARD-FACING DOG

Supported Downward-Facing Dog soothes your nervous sytem
as you fully extend your body.

POINT OF PLAY:
Bend and straighten your legs
to maximize the traction of
your spine.

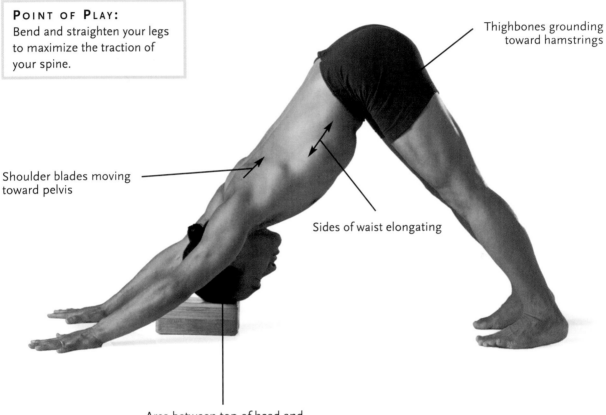

Thighbones grounding
toward hamstrings

Shoulder blades moving
toward pelvis

Sides of waist elongating

Area between top of head and
forehead resting on block

SEATED FORWARD BEND

Seated Forward Bend turns you deeply inward,
allowing you to learn to let go of the resistance in your back body and in your mind.

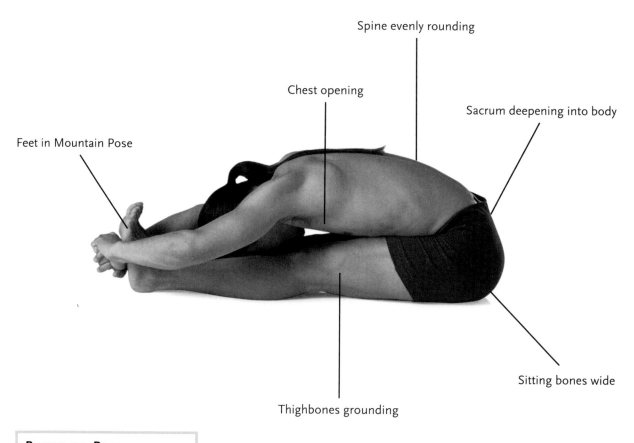

Spine evenly rounding

Chest opening

Sacrum deepening into body

Feet in Mountain Pose

Sitting bones wide

Thighbones grounding

> **POINT OF PLAY:**
> Deepen the top of your
> sacrum into your body as you
> tuck your tailbone toward your
> pubis.

WIDE ANGLE FORWARD BEND

Wide Angle Forward Bend opens your leg muscles
as it grounds you with its wide foundation.

Knees and toes pointing straight up

Thighbones grounding down and back

Sacrum deepening into body

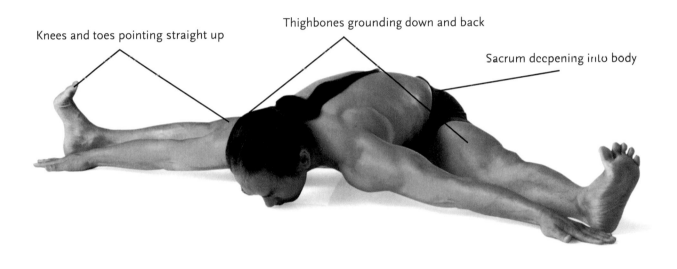

POINT OF PLAY:
Move your tailbone toward
your pubis as you extend your
chest forward.

RESTORATIVE CHILD'S POSE

Restorative Child's Pose opens the back of your torso while soothing your nervous system and releasing the back of your neck.

POINT OF PLAY:
Allow your legs to fold deeply as your back gently rounds, then periodically elongate your spine and drape your body farther forward on your legs.

Spine gradually and evenly rounding

Neck relaxing

Weight of body dropping toward heels

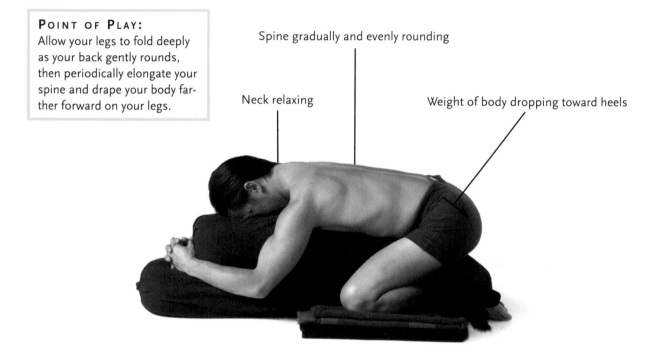

RESTORATIVE BACKBEND

Restorative Backbend passively but profoundly opens your front body,
especially your heart center.

POINT OF PLAY:
Tuck your buttocks flesh away
from your waist as you extend
and ground your thighs.

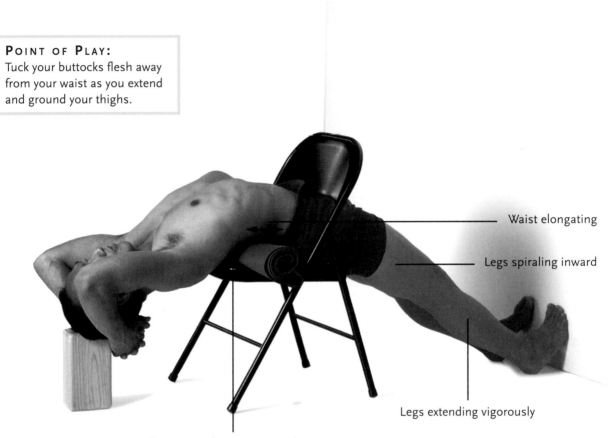

Waist elongating

Legs spiraling inward

Legs extending vigorously

Support under your upper chest

RESTORATIVE PLOW POSE

Restorative Plow Pose brings you into both a forward bend and an inverted position,
which quiets your nervous system and allows you to focus on your emotional body.

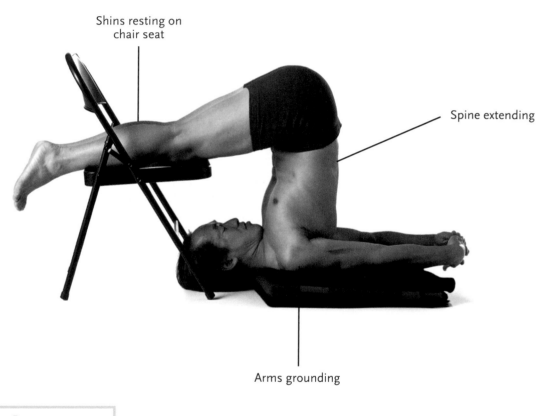

Shins resting on
chair seat

Spine extending

Arms grounding

POINT OF PLAY:
Move your legs more toward
the direction of your feet and
then toward the direction of
your hips.

SUPPORTED RELAXATION POSE

Supported Relaxation Pose grounds your legs
and opens your heart as it restores you deeply.

> **POINT OF PLAY:**
> Increase the broad attentive-
> ness of your mind while deep-
> ening the relaxation of your
> body.

Head slightly higher than chest

Legs dropping completely

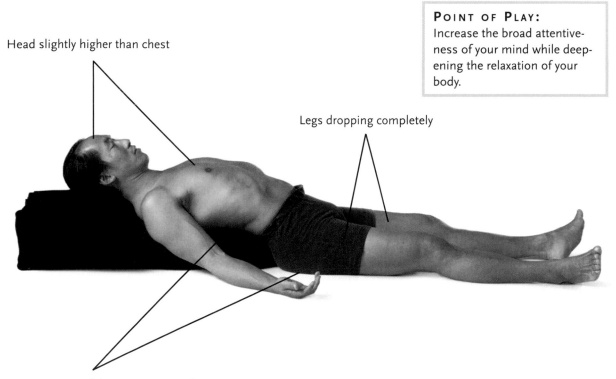

Spine supported, hips unsupported

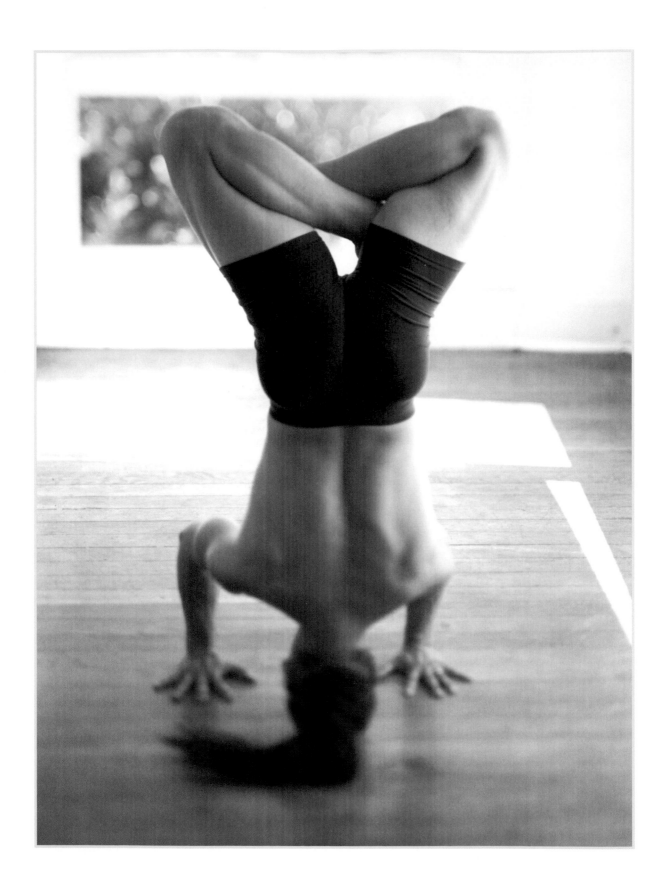

THE SECRET IS JUST TO SAY "YES!" AND JUMP OFF FROM HERE. THEN THERE IS NO PROBLEM. IT MEANS TO BE YOURSELF, ALWAYS YOURSELF, WITHOUT STICKING TO AN OLD SELF.

—SHUNRYU SUZUKI, *Not Always So*

WEEK 7:

Changing Orientation

IS THERE A CHANCE FOR YOU TO CHANGE THE ORIENTATION FROM WHICH YOU SEE THINGS? IS THERE any way to shift the axis from which you spin your reality? Can you be an actor for the day? Can you walk behind someone and imitate his movements and posture? Can you pick a remote thought deep inside your mind to focus on? Is your normal orientation the "real you"?

By putting yourself in Headstand, you turn your world upside down. Your chemistry and your sensory perceptions change radically. At first, it may be completely disconcerting, disorienting, and nerve-racking. But as your fear diminishes, a deep solace arises. Headstand can be a very simple way to see your life from a very different point of view. It can help you question how you normally see life and help you take it less seriously. Eventually it is a relief to take other points of view and move away from thinking that your perspective, thoughts, and emotions comprise the greater truth. Letting go of your "concrete" orientation allows more space in your life for humor and relaxation.

Often our emotions are embedded in our physical habits and when you begin to change your physical posture, emotions that are locked in that physical structure can arise. Headstand forces you to address your habitual posture in your neck, shoulders, and upper torso. The emotions in your neck and shoulders are often in the form of tension and as you balance your upper body, this tension is released, as well as any emotional content that created that tension.

But more than anything, doing Headstand feels like *relief*. It's a relief for your legs, your internal organs, your spine and back muscles, and even your head. And the relief that comes from Headstand may make you realize that you can have this same relaxation in your normal physical orientation. Once you realize you can let go of the tension of your body and still be in the world effectively, you may learn how to discard the tension much more quickly.

ABOUT HEADSTAND

Headstand has been the keystone of my practice. I practice this pose, along with Shoulderstand, almost every day. If I'm traveling and can't practice any other poses, I try to practice Headstand and Shoulderstand. After I took the time to understand Headstand and become fluent in it, it became a pose of ease, meditation, and solace.

For some people, learning Headstand can be a great challenge. The fundamental requirements for creating a beneficial posture include finding the proper alignment of your neck and upper body and the strength of your arms. For many of you, it will be a great achievement just to get up into Headstand, but this is only the beginning. We all need to continually hone our awareness of our alignment and balance in this pose.

Even though I've been doing Headstand for more than 22 years, finding the sweet spot where my entire body is light and floating is still not an everyday occurrence. But I find that regardless of whether or not my Headstand drops me into that blissful center, the general benefits and effects of the pose are still profound. Headstand quiets my mind more than any other posture. The constant dialogue of my entire body with my movement in and out of center keeps my mind present. The light pressure on the top of my head that comes from centering my entire body on it has a deep comforting effect throughout my nervous system. I have done many different sequences and practices throughout the years, but the practices that include both Headstand and Shoulderstand always feel very fulfilling and complete.

All my own teachers taught me—and my own experience confirms this—that Shoulderstand should follow Headstand somewhere in the practice. Most often Headstand comes in the beginning or middle of the practice, with Shoulderstand done at the end.

EMOTIONS. Even though Headstand is a very centering pose, emotionally it is a fiery pose that heats up the body and can elicit strong emotions. The act of doing Headstand centers your mind and heart. So as your emotional body is awakened by the energy moving from your legs and arms toward your heart

center, your mind has a chance to really observe it. When you come down from Headstand, you may feel as though you have cleared some of the bindings that come from holding on to your feelings.

FOCUS OF YOUR MIND. In Headstand, focus your mind on gathering your legs together into a strong, central channel and balancing them over your head. You must continually refine this balance, using keen observation and intuitive response. As you stay in Headstand for longer periods of time, the quietness becomes more profound and therefore your observation of even more subtle movements around center becomes possible.

BALANCING. Balancing in Headstand for the most part is a matter of becoming more and more familiar with being upside down. Your forearms and the crown of your head create a very sensitive and responsive platform on which to balance. To balance on your head, use your arms, head, and spine to do much of the adjusting. These small movements are very healthy for your spine, and can be integrated in your everyday life and posture. Though these areas are very sensitive, they are weaker than your legs and pelvis, so take your time building both your strength and your subtle alignment.

BREATH. When there is fear, your breath will usually be gripped. Being able to observe how your breath moves in Headstand allows you to adjust your alignment much more minutely. Eventually your observation of your breath also allows you to let go of your fear.

SHOULDER BLADES. One of the most important actions in Headstand is to keep your shoulder blades firm against your back and lifting away from your neck. These actions set the foundation for your neck, providing the key to the elongation and ease of your neck in Headstand.

LEGS. Although it may not seem immediately obvious, the way you work your legs is a very important aspect of Headstand. Driving your legs strongly

ANATOMY LESSON

1. The position of your head

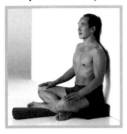

To learn about the position of your head, practice version 1 of Seated Crossed-Legs Pose. With your sacrum and upper back touching the wall, try to bring the back of your head to the wall as you slide your sacrum, upper back, and head farther up the wall. Feel how your head is directly over your chest and your chest is directly over your pelvis.

2. The natural curve of your neck and upper back, and your thoracic spine

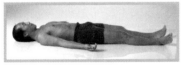

To learn about the natural curve of your neck and upper back, practice in Relaxation Pose with a rolled towel under your neck. Feel how your upper spine between your shoulder blades drops into the ground as your neck rises up away from the ground and moves to the back of your skull. Breathe into both these areas and mentally scan them.

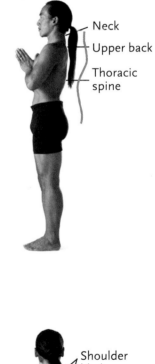

Neck
Upper back
Thoracic spine

3. Hands in relationship to shoulder blades

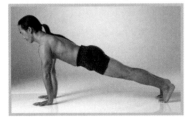

To learn about the relationship between your hands and shoulder blades, practice version 3 of Plank Pose. Feel the firm, even contact of your hands, lengthening and spreading on the ground, as you draw your shoulder blades down toward your pelvis and into your back, broadening them away from your spine. Observe how the action of your shoulder blades affects how the weight of your body is carried on your hands. Respond by pressing your hands even more firmly into the ground.

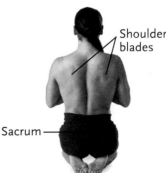

Shoulder blades

Sacrum

together and upward lifts much of the pressure out of your lower back and neck. Your legs also provide your main source of orientation when you are upside down. If your legs are aimlessly flopping around, it is very hard to tell where you are in space.

ARMS. To provide a sound foundation for your Headstand, search for a strong, even grounding of your wrists, elbows, and forearms, while still leaving room for articulation and responsiveness.

HANDS. When you set up your hands for Headstand, interlace your fingers completely but keep your fingers relaxed. For some of you, Headstand will feel better if you keep the palms of your hands together and butt your head against the insides of your wrist. For others, Headstand will feel better if you keep your palms open and place your head inside your hands. Experiment with these two positions and with all the variations in between to see which feels better to your neck and head.

DAY 1: LEARNING THE VARIATIONS

In today's sequence, the Headstand variations and the preparations for Headstand are often more difficult than full Headstand itself. However, this sequence of Headstand preparation poses will help you build the strength and proper alignment for a beneficial Headstand. Therefore, whether or not you can do full Headstand already, you should practice all the variations in this week carefully to learn the many actions that will protect you from possible injury. In today's practice, take a little time between each version to observe how your neck, shoulders, and head feel.

MOVING IN AND OUT OF HEADSTAND

Moving in and out of Headstand is probably the most difficult part of doing the posture. Making the transition from having your legs on the ground to having your legs over your head is not an easy one. You must learn how to maintain the stability of your arms and the length of your neck while you bring your legs and pelvis up above your head. When beginners try to go up into Headstand, they often lose their focus on their foundation and are instead completely absorbed in trying to get their legs up to the wall. You will be much better off keeping your mind primarily focused

on your neck, head, and arms and have your second concern be bringing your legs and pelvis up into Headstand. As long as your foundation stays strong, you can go up into Headstand by hopping with both legs, lifting your legs, or kicking up. Keep observing how the foundation is compromised as you move into the pose.

Many times practitioners will stay too long in Headstand so when they lower their legs to come down, they have no strength left to maintain the foundation. Therefore when you first learn Headstand, I recommend that you make going up and coming down your main focus (rather than staying up). Before going up, ensure that your elbows are directly underneath your shoulders, that the pinkie finger sides of your forearms are firmly planted, and that you have a strong, firm foundation from which to lift. Also, be sure to take your time to place your head properly between your hands.

When you go in and out of Headstand, the gradual shift of your pelvis becomes the crucial factor. When you move into Headstand, propelling your pelvis up over your head is your most important action. When you come down from Headstand, keeping your pelvis in Headstand for as long as possible as you move your legs down toward the ground allows your descent to be soft and graceful.

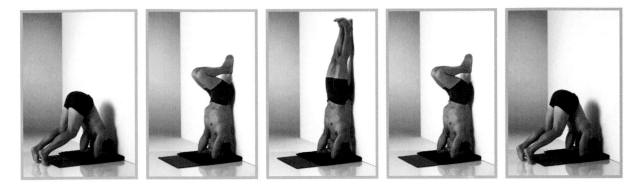

This photo sequence illustrates moving in and out of Headstand at the wall.

DAY 1 PRACTICE

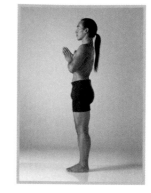

1. Practice two mini **SUN SALUTATIONS,** staying in Down-ward-Facing Dog for 5 breaths. Practice these Sun Saluta-tions leading from your lower body, not from your head and neck.

2. Practice two full **SUN SALUTATIONS,** staying in Down-ward-Facing Dog for 5 breaths. Practice integrating your chest, neck, and head.

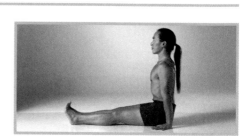

3. Practice **STAFF POSE** for 30 seconds. Focus on keeping your legs together and grounded, and on spreading your toes and expanding the soles of your feet (Headstand legs).

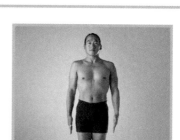

4. Practice **MOUNTAIN POSE** for 1 minute. Focus on posi-tioning your head over your chest, your chest over your pelvis, and your pelvis over your feet.

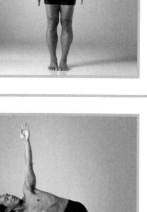

5. Practice **TRIANGLE POSE** for 30 seconds on each side. Position your head slightly in back of your chest, feeling the natural curve of your neck.

6. Try all three versions of **SUPPORTED STANDING FORWARD BEND** *(Uttanasana)* for 30 seconds.

VERSION 1: Bending over back of chair, with support under belly

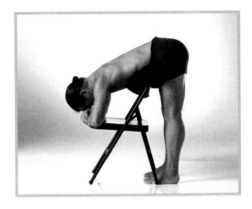

This version provides complete support for your front body while you bend forward. This support allows you to release your back muscles completely without the fear of injuring yourself. For people who are tight, this version allows you to be in the forward bend without straining your lower back. Play with moving your head into slightly different positions in relation to your chest. Feel the effects of moving from a neutral neck to a slightly backbending neck.

VERSION 2: Head resting on the seat of a chair

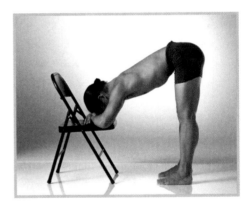

In this version, your forehead rests on the seat of the chair. Your body comes into a forward bend at this point, with a slight inversion as your head is lower than your pelvis. Your main purpose is to find the extension of your spine. Keep your chest from dropping too far down toward the ground and adjust your rib cage to stay in line with the direction of your pelvis and the placement of your head. Feel the natural curve of your neck and upper spine.

VERSION 3: Head on a block (if possible)

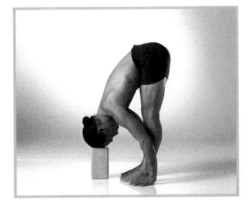

In this version, the top of your head rests on the block, which begins to train you for Headstand. In this pose, you receive many similar benefits as you do from Headstand, as you become aware of your spine with a slight pressure on your head. This is very calming for your nervous system. Touching your hands lightly on the ground, feel their aliveness and their relationship to your shoulder blades as you firm your shoulder blades into your back and up toward your pelvis. Adjust your weight so it is carried by the strength of your legs while at the same time allowing the block to support the weight of your head so your neck is encouraged to soften.

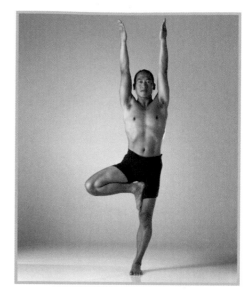

7. Practice **TREE POSE** for 30 seconds on each side. Feel the back of your skull rising upward from the softness of your throat.

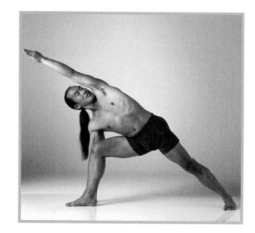

8. Practice **EXTENDED SIDE ANGLE POSE** for 45 seconds on each side. Play with the position of your head, moving more toward a slight backbend with a turn.

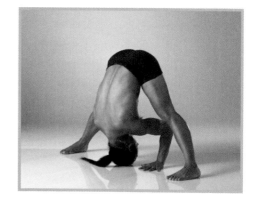

9. Practice version 2 of **STANDING WIDE ANGLE FOR-WARD BEND** for 45 seconds. With your hands planted firmly on the ground, move your shoulder blades into your back and up toward your pelvis.

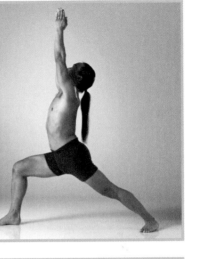

10. Practice **WARRIOR 1** for 30 seconds on each side. Feel the relationship between your fully extended hands and your shoulder blades releasing down your back into your body, lifting the broadness of your collarbones.

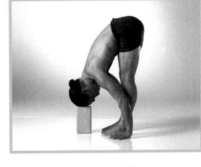

11. Practice any version of **SUPPORTED STANDING FORWARD BEND** for 1 minute. Focus on making your neck as comfortable as possible.

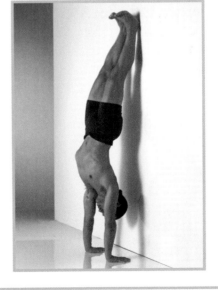

12. Practice **HANDSTAND** for 15 to 30 seconds. Feel the relationship between your broad, firm hands on the ground and your broad, firm, supportive shoulder blades against your back.

13. Try all three versions of **HEADSTAND PREPARATION** for 15 seconds in each version.

VERSION 1: Shins and forearms on the ground, hands interlaced, elbows shoulders-width apart, moving your torso forward and backward

This version builds strength in your arms and helps you learn which position of your arms creates power. It also helps you learn to bring the outsides of your hands and wrists and your entire forearm into good contact with the ground. Move your torso forward and backward at any speed that creates maximum awareness of grounding with the earth and lifting up from there. Keep your neck and head in line with the rest of your spine.

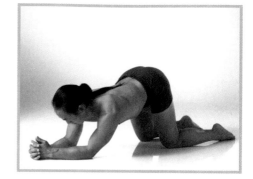

VERSION 2: Circular movements with your shoulders

In this version make circular movements with your shoulders at any speed that creates maximum awareness of the centering of your shoulder socket and the ease of your neck. This variation lets you find the articulation of your shoulder joints and become aware of the constant dialogue between the press of your arms and the ground. Feel the relationship between your upper back and your neck.

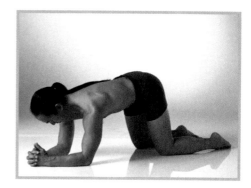

VERSION 3: Repeatedly placing your head on the ground and then lifting it off

This version allows you to experience the physical alignment and some sensations of being in Headstand, without worrying about balance. Feel the relationship between your supple, strong hands and your shoulder blades firming against your back and moving up toward your pelvis. With your head down, continue to lift your shoulder blades as you press your wrists strongly into the ground. Increase this relationship as you lift your head off the ground. Then as you place your head on the ground, feel how the top of your head fits within the triangular shape of your forearms. Make any adjustments to find a strong, tension-free, and responsive foundation of your head and forearms.

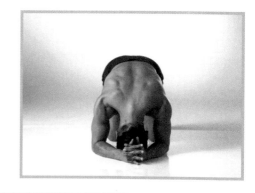

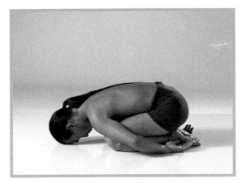

14. Practice version 3 of **CHILD'S POSE** for 1 minute. Rest your forehead on the ground and relax the back of your neck.

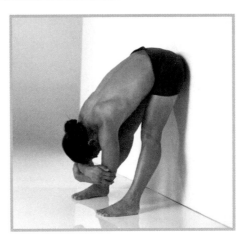

15. Practice **WALL HANG** for 1 minute. Feel the harmonious shape of your entire spine and the weight of your head.

16. Try all three versions of **ELBOW BALANCE** for 15 seconds in each version.

VERSION 1: Downward-Facing Dog with hands in Headstand preparation position, fingers against the wall

This version begins to put a lot of your weight on your arms without requiring you to be completely upside down. It is a good intermediate step if you feel disoriented when you are upside down. The challenge is to keep focusing on the foundation of your arms by lifting your shoulder blades strongly up toward your pelvis. Play around with your head position and challenge yourself to walk your feet closer toward your elbows, raising your pelvis higher and higher.

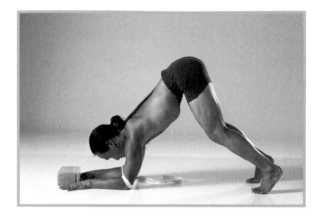

VERSION 2: Arms in Headstand position, legs up the wall (head off the ground)

This version, one of the easiest inverted poses, is a good preparation for Headstand and Forearm Balance (version 3). Some people find this pose easier to learn than Handstand, so you may find it is a good pose in which to become familiar with being upside down. Because your arms are bent and you have a larger foundation on the ground, it is easier for you to get your pelvis above your head, and this is less frightening. Play with arching your neck and looking at the ground and letting your head hang and looking out toward the center of the room, observing how this affects your shoulders, your balance, and your mental orientation.

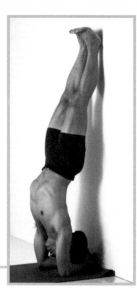

VERSION 3: Forearm Balance (*Pinca-mayurasana*)

This version opens your shoulders more dramatically than the other versions of Elbow Balance. Those of you who have tighter shoulders will tend to compensate by arching your lower back; therefore, you should focus on extending your legs strongly to take the weight of your legs off your lower back. The aliveness of your hands pressing into the ground helps you move your shoulder blades firmly into your back. They also give you strong tactile contact with the ground, helping you articulate your balance. (If you have never tried this pose before, try the foundation without kicking up.)

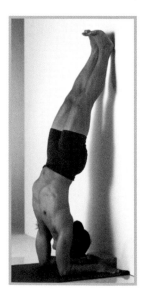

17. Try all three versions of **COW-FACE POSE** *(Gomukhasana)* for 15 seconds in each version on each side.

VERSION 1: Holding your elbow with your opposite hand

This version builds the opening and alignment necessary for Handstand, Forearm Balance, and Headstand. Without this shoulder opening, these inverted poses are much more difficult. Coordinate your movement with your breath, not forcing but feeling the gradual opening of your shoulder joint. The position of your arm behind your head will tend to push your head forward—use the opposite hand to pull your arm farther back, allowing your head to rest against your arm like a pillow.

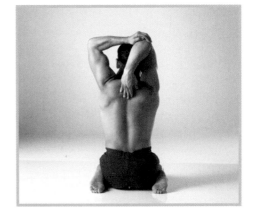

VERSION 2: Using a strap behind your back

This version teaches you about the relationship between your two arms, which are virtually in opposite positions. Your bottom arm is opening for twists and Shoulderstand; your top arm is opening for Headstand, Handstand, and Forearm Balance. As you hold the strap with both hands, reorganize your rib cage, shoulder blades, and upper arms to move toward the alignment of Mountain Pose. Feel the relationship between your neck and your upper back.

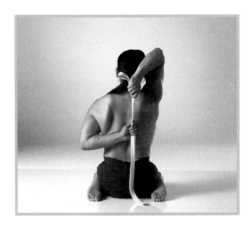

VERSION 3: Clasping your hands behind your back

When you clasp your fingers, it is surprising to find how deeply your internal body releases. The actual touch of fingers to fingers creates an interconnectedness that produces relief. Try to keep your hands supple but not clenched so that you can feel the relationship between your hands and your shoulder blades moving back into their Mountain Pose alignment. Challenge yourself to bring your lower ribs back to center with your head positioned directly over your chest and your collarbones open.

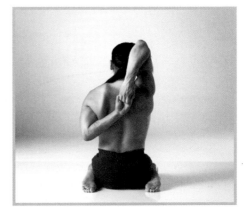

18. Try whichever version of **HEADSTAND** *(Sirsanasa)* you can do presently for 1 minute.

VERSION 1: Back on the floor, with your head against the wall, hands in Headstand position

This version gives you a feeling for the alignment of Headstand. The strength of your legs, the length of your waist, and the light press of your head and arms into the wall lets you feel the internal relationships and orientation of Headstand. Make a mental note of the relationships and architecture of the different parts of your body in this position. Bring special attention to your head position, feeling like the very top of your head is touching the wall.

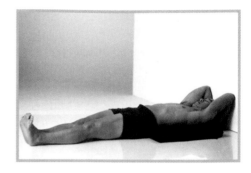

VERSION 2: Headstand against the wall

This version allows you to do Headstand without the fear of falling over. As you become less fearful of being upside down, Headstand becomes one of the most calming poses in yoga. Having the wall behind you when you balance enables your nervous system to release even further. Remember to press your forearms firmly into the ground, lift your shoulder blades toward your pelvis and into your back, and strongly join and extend your legs. With the strong press of your forearms, play with subtle changes to the position of your head until you feel the natural curve of your neck moving into a broad, strong back. This is a version many people return to—even after they can balance in the center of the room—when they are making shifts in their Headstand or trying something new, like Headstand variations.

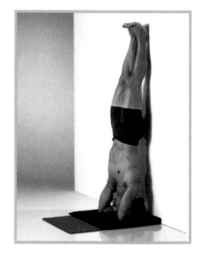

VERSION 3: Headstand in the center of the room

Balancing in the center of the room brings your body to its true center, quieting all that's coming into the core of your body. The more you find the pose's center, the more quiet your Headstand will become, although you gradually have to lose your fear of being in a completely different orientation with less and less feedback. Keep your hands awake, neither hard nor collapsed. This makes your arms—including your shoulder blades—responsive to your ever-shifting balance.

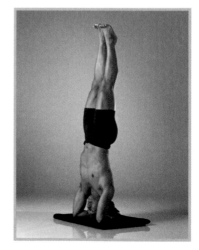

19. Practice version 3 of **CHILD'S POSE** for 1 minute. Resting your forehead on the ground, allow all your neck and back muscles to let go. Feel any compression in your spine be undulated and massaged by your breath.

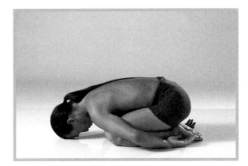

20. Practice **DOWNWARD-FACING DOG** for 1 minute. Find the full reach of your inner arms and the full press of your legs back into your hamstrings so that your head and neck feel suspended and surrendered.

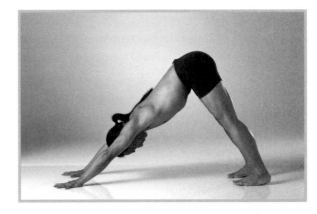

21. Practice version 3 of **RESTORATIVE BACKBEND** for 1 to 2 minutes. Allow the opening of your chest and the gradual backbending of your neck and head to release any compression in your upper spine.

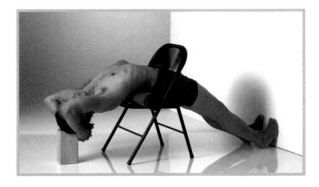

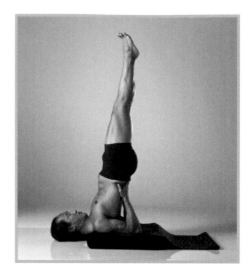

22. Practice **SHOULDERSTAND** for 2 to 3 minutes. As you look toward your chest, feel the quietness and inward turning of all your sense organs.

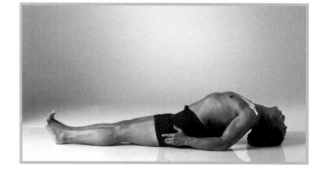

23. Practice **FISH POSE** for 30 seconds. Reintegrate your entire spine by feeling an even, natural arch, moving from the base of your spine to the crown of your head.

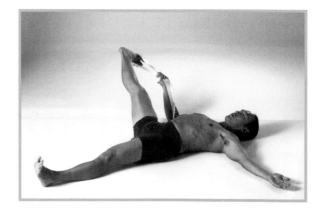

24. Practice the **RECLINED LEG STRETCH SERIES** for 30 seconds in the straight-leg version, 15 seconds in the sit-up version, and 30 seconds in the leg-to-the-side version, on each side. Rest your back body, feeling its broadness and surrender into the earth.

RELAXATION AND BREATH AWARENESS

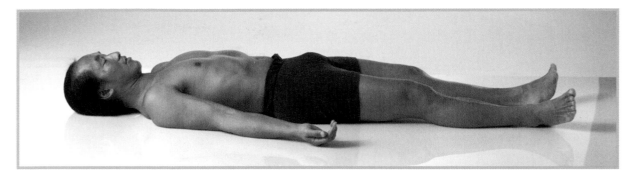

For 3 minutes, practice Relaxation Pose with the top of your head touching the wall. If needed for comfort, place a folded blanket under your head. Observe your natural breath, while consciously relaxing your neck.

For 5 minutes, bring your attention to the entrance of your nostrils and upper lip, and begin to see if you can sensitize yourself to how your breath flows in your nostrils. Using your right thumb, press the soft part of the right nostril to the midline, closing off the flow of air, breathing only through your left nostril. Breathe if possible for about 15 to 30 seconds on that side. Now with the fourth and fifth fingers of your right hand, press the left nostril into the midline

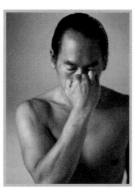

and breathe only through the right nostril. After this, come back to Relaxation Pose, with your hands resting, palms up. Notice again the flow or breathe through your nostrils.

We commonly breathe more dominantly out of one nostril or the other. This usually shifts every 4 hours. In yoga we often try to equalize the way the nostrils are breathing to create a soothing balance in the body.

MEDITATION

For 5 to 10 minutes, practice version 1 of Seated Crossed-Legs Pose, with something light balanced on your head (a paperback book, a one-pound bag of beans or rice, or an eye pillow). Meditate on the gentle length of your spine.

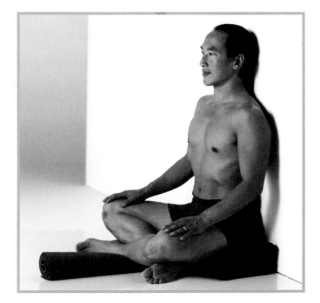

DAY 2: LEARNING HEADSTAND

Today's sequence is a general practice that will prepare you to try Headstand and properly cool down from those efforts. You begin by practicing Downward Facing Dog and Handstand to open up your shoulders and engage your arms. Standing Forward Bend then teaches you to orient your head below your pelvis, while the other standing poses wake up your legs into the reach of your arms and into the length of your neck. You practice Elbow Balance before Headstand to wake up your shoulders and feel the foundation of your forearms. You cool down from Headstand with Child's Pose and Reclined Hero Pose to release any tension from your neck and shoulders. The rest of the sequence balances your entire body from the first part of the practice.

FOCUS FOR THIS PRACTICE:

- In the Sun Salutations, focus on the relationship between your hands and your shoulder blades.

- In the standing poses, play with the position of your head.

- In Headstand Preparation, notice the natural curve of your neck.

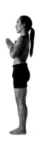

1. Practice two full **Sun Salutations,** holding the second Upward-Facing Dog for 3 breaths and the second Downward-Facing Dog for 5 breaths.

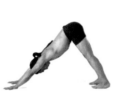

2. Practice **Downward-Facing Dog** for 2 minutes.

3. Practice **Standing Forward Bend** for 1 minute.

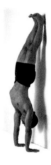

4. Practice **Handstand** for 15 to 30 seconds.

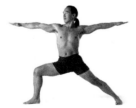

5. Practice **Warrior 2 Pose** for 45 seconds on each side.

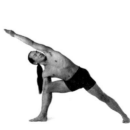

6. Practice **Extended Side Angle Pose** for 45 seconds on each side.

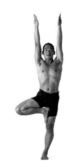

7. Practice **Tree Pose** for 30 seconds on each side.

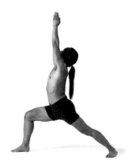

8. Practice **Warrior 1 Pose** for 30 seconds on each side.

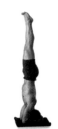 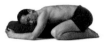 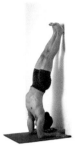

9. Practice **Standing Forward Bend** for 1 minute.

10. Practice all three versions of **Headstand Preparation** for 30 seconds each.

11. Practice any version of **Elbow Balance** for 15 to 30 seconds.

12. Practice any version of **Headstand** that you can do (see if you can get up) for 1 minute.

13. Practice **Child's Pose** for 1 minute.

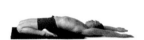 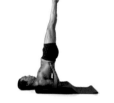 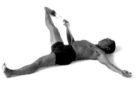

14. Practice **Reclined Hero Pose** for 2 minutes.

15. Practice **Camel Pose** for 30 seconds.

16. Practice **Shoulderstand** for 2 minutes.

17. Practice the **Reclined Leg Stretch Series** for 1 minute in the straight-leg version, 15 seconds in the sit-up version, and 30 seconds in the leg-to-the-side version on each side.

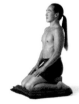

18. Relaxation and Breath Awareness. For 5 minutes, practice version 3 of **Supported Relaxation Pose,** with a weight on the top of your thighs (either folded blankets or sandbags, if you have them). Feel your legs weighted and dropping, as they pull your breath in, in smooth, easy, elongated inhalations.

Imagine that your right leg drops deeper with the weight, and that this encourages you to breathe more into your right nostril. Next, imagine your left thigh is weighted and that you exhale out and then inhale into your left nostril.

Then imagine the right side is more weighted and that you exhale out the right side. As you repeat this pattern, continue to connect the relaxation of your leg with creating deeper breathing in that same-side nostril. Always change the nostril that you use on your exhalation.

19. Meditation. For 5 to 10 minutes, sit in **Hero Pose.** Meditate on grounding your legs with a feeling of activity and circulation moving through them.

DAY 3: PRACTICING HEADSTAND

This practice places Headstand in a very traditional part of the sequence. By warming up with Sun Salutations, by focusing on your center with the Core Strengthening Series, and by waking up the legs in the standing poses, your whole body is in tune to begin Headstand. Doing backbends after Headstand helps restore the natural curve in your neck and reintegrates your neck with the rest of your spine. Shoulderstand allows you to cool down from this fairly strong practice, and Reclined Leg Stretch Series brings you back to a quiet grounding.

FOCUS FOR THIS PRACTICE:

- In the Sun Salutations, focus on the relationship between your neck and upper back.

- In the standing poses, firm your shoulder blades into your back and extend your hands and fingers.

- In Headstand and the backbends, feel and play with minute changes in the position of your head.

1. Practice two mini **Sun Salutations.**

2. Practice two full **Sun Salutations.**

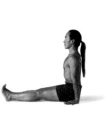

3. Practice the **Core Strengthening Series** twice. On the second round, do a forward bend in the Wide Angle Pose and last Cobbler's Pose and hold each for 1 minute.

4. Practice **Triangle Pose** for 1 minute on each side.

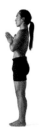

5. Practice **Standing Forward Bend** for 1 minute.

6. Practice version 2 of **Standing Wide Angle Forward Bend** for 1 to 2 minutes.

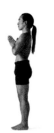

7. Practice any version of **Supported Standing Forward Bend** for 1 minute.

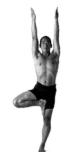

8. Practice **Tree Pose** for 30 seconds on each side.

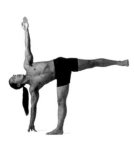

9. Practice **Half Moon Pose** for 30 seconds on each side.

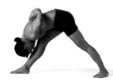

10. Practice **Pyramid Pose** for 1 minute on each side.

11. Practice any version of **Headstand Preparation** for 30 seconds.

12. Practice **Cow-Face Pose** for 30 seconds on each side.

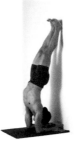

13. Practice **Elbow Balance**, version 3 if possible, lifting your head up and down three times.

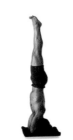

14. Practice **Headstand** for 1 minute, doing whichever version is appropriate for you at this time.

15. Practice **Child's Pose** for 1 minute.

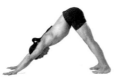

16. Practice **Downward-Facing Dog** for 1 minute.

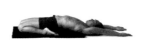

17. Practice **Reclined Hero Pose** for 1 to 2 minutes.

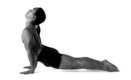

18. Practice **Upward-Facing Dog** for 30 seconds.

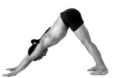

19. Practice **Downward-Facing Dog** for 30 seconds.

20. Practice **Camel Pose** for 30 seconds.

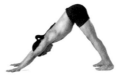

21. Practice **Downward-Facing Dog** for 30 seconds.

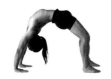

22. Practice **Upward Bow Pose** for 5 seconds. Repeat two more times.

23. Practice version 1 of **Happy Baby Pose** for 1 minute on each side.

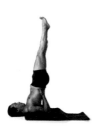

24. Practice **Shoulderstand** for 1 to 3 minutes.

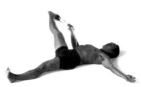

25. Practice the **Reclined Leg Stretch Series** for 1 minute in the straight-leg version, 15 seconds in the sit-up version, and 1 minute in the leg-to-the-side version, on each side.

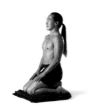

26. Meditation. For 5 minutes, sit in **Hero Pose** against the wall. Meditate on the broadness and extension of your back.

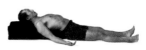

27. Relaxation and Breath Awareness. For 3 minutes, practice version 3 of **Supported Relaxation Pose** and simply observe your breath.

Now use your right hand to block your left nostril and inhale through your right nostril. Then block your right nostril and exhale through your left. Inhale through your left

nostril. Then block your left nostril and exhale through your right. This is a full cycle of *nadi sodhana* breath. Repeat 5 to 10 cycles.

Releasing your hand, scan your body and release any tension. Feel the ease of your breath take you deeper into relaxation.

DAY 4: RESTORATIVE INVERSION PRACTICE

Today's practice is a fairly demanding sequence that I have found to be one of the most restorative practices I have ever done. For almost the entire practice, you will be in an inverted position with your head supported. Spending this amount of time like that creates a radical shift in your body and you will probably come out of this practice feeling extremely different—I myself come out of this practice feeling amazingly light and spacious. For some of you, maintaining certain poses for the suggested timings back to back with the other poses in the sequence may be very difficult. However, if you can persevere and literally go from one pose to the next, you will probably feel an amazing overall effect. This practice more than the other practices in the whole book is highly dependent on its sequence and timing. I find a magical restorative quality to it.

FOCUS FOR THIS PRACTICE:

- In the poses where your head is resting on a block or chair, periodically shift your head position.

- In Headstand and Shoulderstand, focus on the relationship between your hands and your shoulder blades.

- In the restorative poses, breathe into your neck and upper back.

1. Practice version 2 of **Standing Wide Angle Forward Bend** for 2 to 4 minutes.

2. Practice version 2 of **Supported Standing Forward Bend** for 2 to 4 minutes.

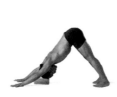

3. Practice version 3 of **Supported Downward-Facing Dog** for 2 minutes.

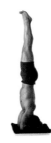

4. Practice **Headstand** for 2 to 4 minutes.

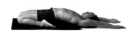

5. Practice **Reclined Hero Pose** for 2 minutes.

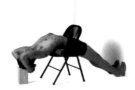

6. Practice version 3 of **Restorative Backbend** for 2 minutes.

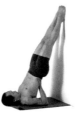

7. Practice **Wall Shoulderstand** for 2 to 4 minutes.

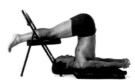

8. Practice **Restorative Plow Pose** for 2 minutes.

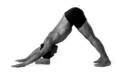

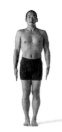

9. Practice **Supported Downward-Facing Dog** for 2 minutes.

10. Practice version 2 of **Standing Wide Angle Forward Bend** for 2 minutes.

11. Practice version 2 of **Supported Standing Forward Bend** for 2 minutes.

12. Practice **Mountain Pose** for 2 minutes.

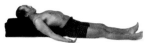

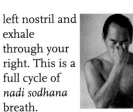

13. Relaxation and Breath Awareness. For 3 minutes, practice version 3 of **Supported Relaxation Pose.**

Now use your right hand to block your left nostril and inhale through your right nostril. Then block your right nostril and exhale through your left. Inhale through your left nostril. Then block your

left nostril and exhale through your right. This is a full cycle of *nadi sodhana* breath.

Repeat 5 to 10 cycles.

Releasing your hand, scan your body and release any tension. Feel the ease of your breath take you deeper into relaxation.

14. Meditation. For 5 to 10 minutes, sit in **Seated Crossed-Legs Pose** on a prop high enough to allow you to maintain the natural curves of your spine. Listen to your breath. Enjoy its ease.

DAY 5: FOCUS ON INVERSIONS

Today's sequence focuses on the traditional inverted poses: Headstand, Shoulderstand, and Plow Pose. The poses in the beginning lead up to Headstand, which is followed by cooling poses. The middle of the practice leads you up to Shoulderstand and Plow Pose, followed by Standing Forward Bend and Seated Forward Bend. These poses allow you to release your neck and neutralize any tension that may have accumulated from doing Shoulderstand and Plow Pose. I believe that after this practice, you will feel an amazing balance in your entire body. You will also begin to realize the profound effects of Headstand and Shoulderstand within any practice. If you spend a small amount of time doing these inverted poses every day and do a practice once a week that has a strong focus on inversions, you will build the necessary sensitivity, alignment, and strength to enjoy these poses for the rest of your life.

FOCUS FOR THIS PRACTICE:

- In all the poses up to and including Headstand, relax your upper back and neck as you refine their alignment.

- In the backbends, observe the relationship between your hands and your shoulder blades.

- In Shoulderstand, Plow Pose, and the forward bends, focus on the placement of your head.

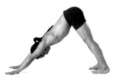 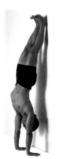 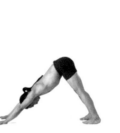 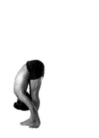

1. Practice **Downward-Facing Dog** for 1 to 2 minutes.

2. Practice **Standing Forward Bend** for 1 minute.

3. Practice **Handstand** for up to 30 seconds.

4. Repeat Steps 1 through 3.

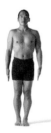 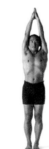 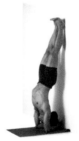 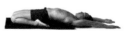

5. Practice **Mountain Pose** for 1 minute.

6. Practice **Volcano Pose** for 1 minute.

7. Practice **Cow-Face** arms while standing in Mountain Pose, two times on each side, for 15 seconds each.

8. Practice version 2 or 3 of **Elbow Balance** for 15 to 30 seconds.

9. Practice **Reclined Hero Pose** for 1 to 2 minutes.

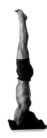

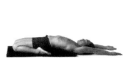
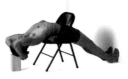

10. Practice **Headstand** for 1 to 4 minutes.

11. Practice **Child's Pose** for 1 minute.

12. Practice **Downward-Facing Dog** for 1 minute.

13. Practice **Reclined Hero Pose** for 1 minute.

14. Practice version 3 of **Restorative Backbend** for 1 to 2 minutes.

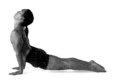
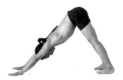

15. Practice **Upward-Facing Dog** for 30 seconds.

16. Practice **Downward-Facing Dog** for 30 seconds.

17. Practice **Camel Pose** for 30 seconds.

18. Practice **Upward Bow Pose** one to three times for 5 seconds each.

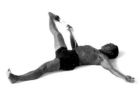
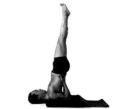
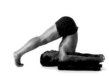

19. Practice the **Reclined Leg Stretch Series** for 1 minute in the straight-leg version, 15 seconds in the sit-up version, and 1 minute in the leg-to-the-side version, on each side.

20. Practice **Shoulderstand** for 1 to 4 minutes, as long as or longer than your Headstand.

21. Practice any version of **Plow Pose** for 1 to 3 minutes.

22. Practice **Wall Hang** for 1 to 2 minutes.

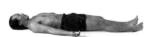

23. Practice version 2 of **Seated Forward Bend** for 1 to 2 minutes.

24. Meditation. For 5 to 10 minutes, sit in **Seated Crossed-Legs Pose**. Meditate on the suppleness and movement of your spine with your breath.

25. Relaxation and Breath Awareness. Sit in **Seated Crossed-Legs Pose** and do 10 to 20 cycles of alternate nostril breathing as described for Days 3 and 4.

For 3 minutes, lie down in **Relaxation Pose** (unsupported, if possible) and focus on relaxing your body completely.

DAY 6: BREATH AWARENESS AND MEDITATION

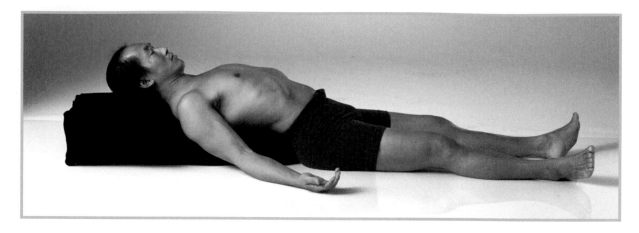

Breath Awareness

For 3 minutes, practice version 3 of Supported Relaxation Pose.

SUPPORTED RELAXATION POSE. In this pose, having your head higher than your chest and your chest higher than your legs creates a position in between sitting up and lying down. The shape of your body supports and opens your heart and lungs and grounds your legs. If your shoulders are tight, you can place a small prop under your arms and hands (folded blankets or towels), but this is not necessary if you are comfortable without them. This version of Supported Relaxation Pose is the preferred reclined position for breath awareness because it supports and opens your chest. The chest opening usually makes it easy for your lungs to take smooth, deep inhalations. Your head position—slightly higher than your chest, in the slightest of forward bends—quiets your mind and allows your sense organs and your attention to move downward toward your heart and lungs. Letting go of the tension of your legs encourages deep relaxation, and this position greatly enhances your ability to do so. This position also prepares you for seated breath awareness and seated meditation because your body becomes used to being more upright. After you have

scanned your body and observed a deep relaxation, you are ready to begin the breath awareness practice.

UJJAYI BREATH. Today's breath practice is the first practice considered a *pranayama* practice rather than simple breath awareness. In *pranayama* the main rule to observe is: Never force your breath. Begin by focusing on slightly closing your throat so that you can hear your inhalations and exhalations. Allow your inhalations and exhalations to be smooth and equal in length, and then gradually elongate both your inhalations and exhalations. If you do this with ease and steadiness for a period of 3 to 5 minutes, you will be practicing *ujjayi* breath—long, deep, smooth absorbed inhalations and long, deep, smooth complete exhalations. It takes years to begin to master this practice. As you progress, your relaxation will become deeper as your inhalations become longer and smoother. Eventually you can reduce the sound of your breath and feel for the quality of absorption. Again, relaxation and observation should always be the main ingredients to any *pranayama* work. When any breath work becomes agitating, return to focusing on relaxation. If you ever feel nerve twitches, your eyes tearing, or ringing in your ears, return to simple relaxation, observing the release of the tension of your body, maybe even without observing your breath.

Meditation

For 10 minutes, sit in Seated Crossed-Legs Pose (or Half Lotus) from Week 6 with the opposite leg on top or in front. Try to balance out the feelings in your hips as much as possible, noticing the weight of your sitting bones on the ground. Meditate on relaxing your sense organs: the backs of your eyes, your inner ears, the bridge of your nose, the root of your tongue, and the receptivity of your skin.

The fifth branch of yoga is *pratayahara,* which means turning your senses inward or withdrawing your senses. In today's meditation I'm asking you to soften all of your sense organs. This creates a much deeper quietness because it shuts down the major stimuli coming into your body. Softening your sense organs doesn't mean that they become unaware of what is taking place outside and inside the body, but rather that they become less affected and stimulated by sensory input. Consider what happens to your body when the phone rings: Your ears perk up and your body prepares to move. But as you learn how to soften your sense organs, you can let this sound enter and dissipate almost as quickly as it registers. Sometimes when you have looked at a bright light and you then close your eyes, you can still see the light because it has left an imprint in your body. As you meditate on relaxing your sense organs, practice

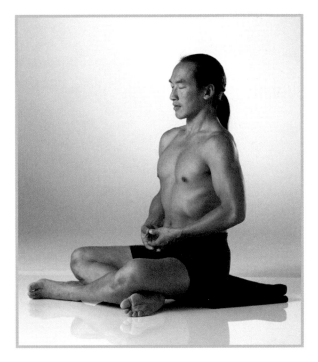

letting go as quickly as possible the effects that the stimulus has inside your body. Continually observing the relaxation of your sense organs can create an immediate balance. This turning inward allows you to respect what is arising from inside your body just as much as you notice what is coming into your body.

POSES OF THE WEEK

SUPPORTED STANDING FORWARD BEND

Supported Standing Forward Bend provides deep rest and relief
as you release your back body and neck.

POINT OF PLAY:
Play with bearing your weight
on the front of your heels
more and more evenly and
completely as you release the
tension from your abdomen.

Shoulder blades moving
down the back

Neck supple

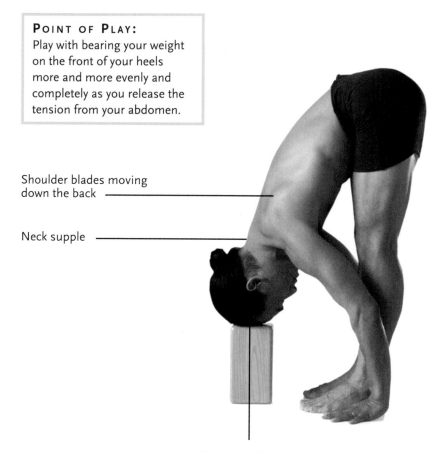

Between top of head and forehead touching prop

HEADSTAND PREPARATION

Headstand Preparation teaches you the actions of your arms and shoulders
that are necessary to support and release your neck.

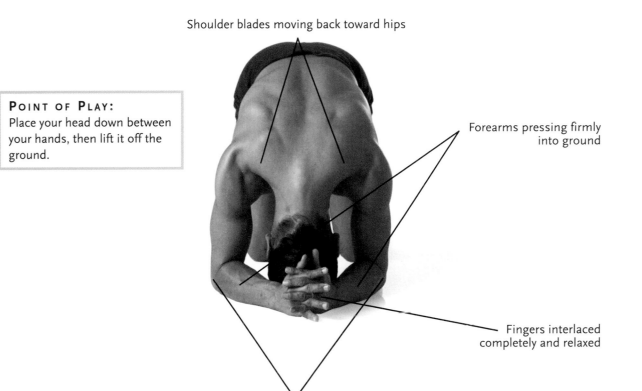

Shoulder blades moving back toward hips

Forearms pressing firmly
into ground

Fingers interlaced
completely and relaxed

Elbows shoulders-width apart

POINT OF PLAY:
Place your head down between
your hands, then lift it off the
ground.

ELBOW BALANCE

Elbow Balance invigorates your entire being
while deeply opening your shoulders.

POINT OF PLAY:
Shift your weight around on
your shoulders and arms as
you relax your neck.

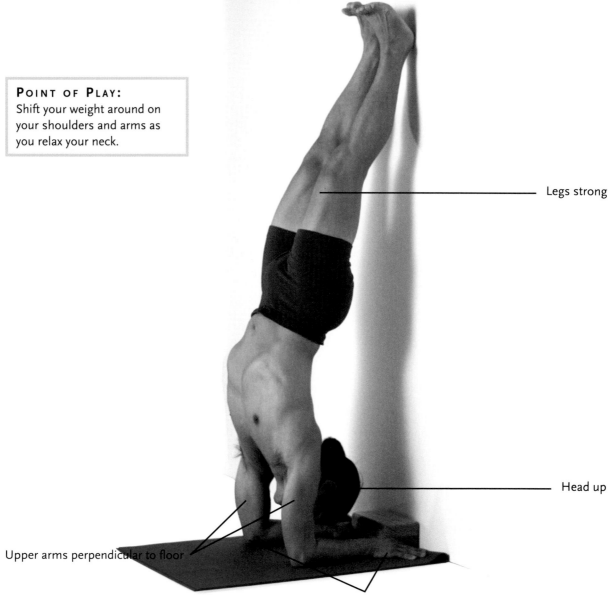

Legs strong

Head up

Upper arms perpendicular to floor

Hands and elbows shoulders-width apart

COW-FACE POSE

Cow-Face Pose releases tension at the base of your neck
while opening your shoulders.

Neck softening

Arms reaching back

Rib cage centered

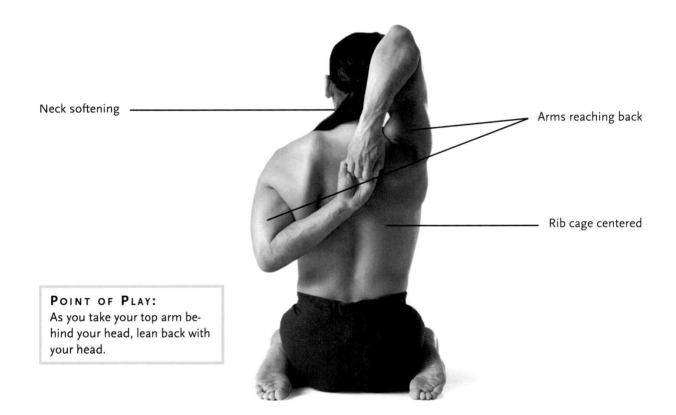

POINT OF PLAY:
As you take your top arm behind your head, lean back with
your head.

HEADSTAND

Headstand calms your nervous system
while teaching you to focus on balance and center.

POINT OF PLAY:
Extend one leg and then the
other. Reach your legs again
and again.

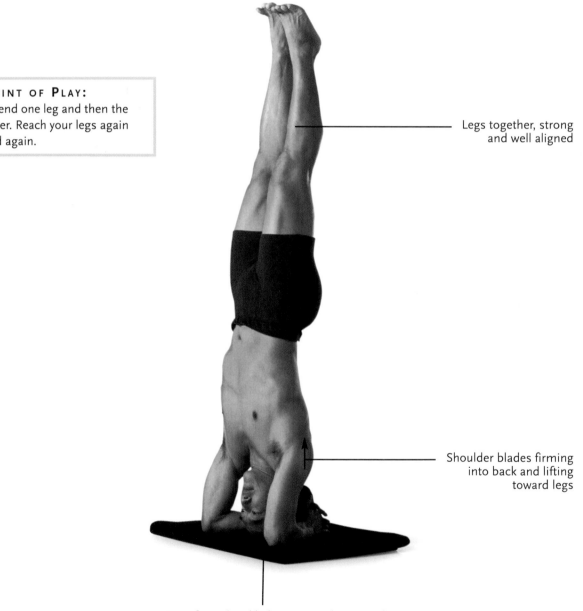

Legs together, strong
and well aligned

Shoulder blades firming
into back and lifting
toward legs

Top of your head balancing on the ground

YOGA, OF COURSE, IS SO MUCH MORE

THAN POSTURES, AND ITS REAL POWER

LIES IN THE DOMAIN OF MIND TRAINING

AND SELF TRANSFORMATION.

—GEORG FEUERSTEIN, *The Deeper Dimension of Yoga*

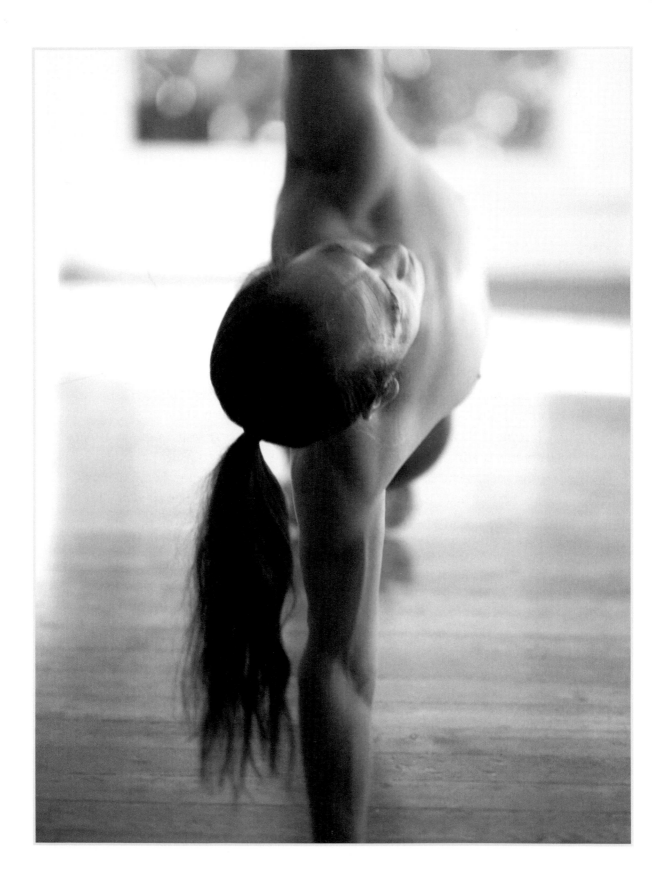

WEEK 8:

Moving toward Balance

THE ELEMENTS OF BALANCE THAT YOU INVESTIGATED IN THE PREVIOUS WEEKS, SUCH AS CONNECTION, vulnerability, receptivity, and being present, are all important aspects of what it means to be balanced in the present moment. Being balanced does not mean that you will never be thrown off balance but rather that you have the means with which to respond as effectively as possible to whatever arises. You will also be able to recover your center and your sense of contentment, again and again. Most events that occur in our lives are either unforeseen or much different than we expected. How can you reorganize, regroup, and find relaxation again deep inside your body in the present set of circumstances? Moment by moment, this is truly a balancing act of an infinite number of factors that we cannot always intellectually organize but have to feel our way through as if we were in complete darkness.

PRACTICING SEQUENCES

During this final week of practice, instead of emphasizing individual postures, I want you to feel the overall choreography of the practices. Try to experience the relationships between the poses. And both during and after a practice, ask how your body, mind, and breath are feeling. When we refer to balance within a yoga practice, we cannot simply address the individual poses. Instead, we look at sequences of poses. In any practice, even if you are going to emphasize a class of poses or a single pose, it is the relationship between a given pose or class of poses and your body and the other poses that creates a feeling of balance.

BALANCED PRACTICES

This chapter presents five balanced practices. Every practice is complete, though each emphasizes a different class of poses. Because your body has its own tendencies, you will find that some of the practices will seem to balance you more. The final practice incorporates all the different kinds of poses in a single overall balanced practice. You will probably find your body humming evenly by the time you get to Relaxation Pose. However, having a practice that emphasizes a particular class of poses, such as the Focus on Backbends, enables you to balance your day. The more you get to know your body and understand the effects of the practices, the more you will be able to decide intuitively which practice will move you toward balance. You might choose a practice to bring balance to your physical body. For instance, if you have worked at your computer all day, you might practice the backbend practice because it is vigorous and the backbends will balance out your posture. You can also choose a practice to bring balance to your emotional body. For instance, if you've had an upsetting day, you might practice the forward bend practice to soothe your nervous system on a vigorous movement practice, like Focus on Standing Poses, to ground yourself. There are no set formulas for emotional, mental, and physical balance. But experiencing the effects of the different practices in this chapter is a good beginning to learning how to move toward balance on a daily basis.

BALANCING YOUR BODY

Students often observe that one side of their body is really different than the other side of their body and they ask me: Should I do my difficult side more often than my easy side so that I can balance myself out? I wish it were this simple. Balancing the body is far more complicated than just trying to create muscular symmetry. Doing poses that are easy and that you enjoy along with those that are more challenging does begin to create more balance in your body. There is no need to do only your difficult side, nor is it good to do only the poses that are easy for you. In moving toward balance, it is often a sequence of many different poses that begin to create an internal balance in your body. A practice that incorporates breath, movement, and mental awareness leads to both physical and mental contentment.

ABOUT BALANCED PRACTICES

Through your previous seven weeks of practice, I provided you with a variety of balanced practices, which followed this general structure.

OPENING AND CENTERING. The practices almost always start with Downward-Facing Dog, Sun Salutations, or the Core Strengthening Series. These poses awaken your body, giving you space to observe your breath, thoughts, and physical sensations, without being dangerous or extreme in the openings they create. They are accessible postures that you can do immediately without overwhelming feelings of resistance.

If you have been very active before a practice or you are physically or emotionally fatigued, you may wish to start your practice by doing a restorative pose, such as Legs Up the Wall or version 3 of Reclined Cobbler's Pose.

HEART OF THE PRACTICE. After you have awakened and centered yourself, you are ready to move into the heart of the practice. This part of the practice is an inquiry in which you delve deeply into a pose (and the relationship among poses), such as standing poses, backbends, twists, or forward bends.

The heart of the practice can include Handstand or Headstand, along with the poses you are emphasizing. These poses keep your mind fully awake and light a fire inside the investigation and inside your body. The standing poses are often the prelude to both Headstand and the postures you are investigating because they give you a substantial foundation from which to research the unknown.

REFLECTIVE SECTION. The reflective section of the practice includes Shoulderstand, a seated pose, and possibly a restorative pose, such as Legs Up the Wall. These poses help you turn inward and reflect on the effects of the prior poses, allowing you to digest that information and absorb it deeply.

MEDITATIVE SECTION. Relaxation Pose or Reclined Cobbler's Pose begin your transition into the meditative part of the practice. These poses quiet your body and allow your mind to be aware of subtle movements and feelings. In this part of the practice you turn your awareness to your breath. You then move on to seated meditation. As you steady your breath and quiet your body movements, the patterns of your mind can be revealed.

DOING THE BALANCED PRACTICES

You can practice the sequences presented in this chapter in innumerable ways. By changing what you focus on, you keep the sequences fresh and find many insights, both about the topic you are investigating and about how your body and mind work. Here are some suggestions:

ANATOMY. Use your yoga practice to explore different parts of your anatomy, changing your specific focus from day to day or week to week. For example, practice all five balanced practices in this chapter focusing on your feet. The next week, focus on your neck. As you focus on different parts of your anatomy, you will learn about that part of your body and its relationship to the poses and your entire being. Often I will focus on an area of my body that is not feeling in balance or that I hardly ever feel. You can also focus on the relationship between two different parts of your body. Some interesting relationships to explore are:

- Lower back and neck
- Legs to arms
- Soles of the feet and floor of the pelvis
- Floor of the pelvis with crown of head
- Legs to spine
- Arms to heart
- Head to heart
- Belly to hands
- Belly to feet
- Tailbone to head

PHILOSOPHICAL CONCEPTS. Use your yoga practice to explore philosophical concepts. For example, explore the concept of "nonviolence" in your practice by asking yourself what it means to be nonviolent in the poses. You could focus on any of the *yamas* or *niyamas* of yoga, such as *santosa* (contentment), *tapas* (self-discipline), or other yoga concepts you learn about in class or through your readings.

EMOTIONS. Use your yoga practice to explore your emotions. Ask yourself how you feel in the individual poses and how the practice as a whole affects your emotional state. For example, you might start your practice angry and then observe what effect the poses have on that anger.

SENSES. Use your yoga practice to explore your senses. For example, focus on your eyes and ask yourself: What do I see during my practice? Where do my eyes move in the poses? When am I actually seeing with my eyes and being conscious of what I see? Or you could pick a specific point to look at in every specific pose—a certain point on the wall in Mountain Pose or the index finger of your top hand in Triangle Pose. To explore your sense of touch, try practicing in the dark and navigating your way through the poses using only the physical sensations of your body.

DAY 1: FOCUS ON STANDING POSES

The standing poses in this sequence balance your body in and of themselves, as they include forward bends (Standing Forward Bend, Pyramid Pose, and Wide Angle Standing Forward Bend), backbends (Warrior 1 and to some degree Extended Side Angle), and mild twists (Triangle Pose and Half Moon). Doing Standing Forward Bend between each of the standing poses lets you observe the effects of the previous pose on your body, to re-center your mind and body, and to restore your legs from the demands of the previous pose.

The standing poses are a great workout for your legs so this sequence counterbalances the standing poses with poses that turn your body upside down, including Handstand, Headstand, and Shoulderstand.

These poses help restore your legs, recirculating and returning the blood in your legs back to your heart. Child's Pose and Reclined Hero Pose also rest and restore your legs. These poses along with the inverted poses quiet your mind and transform the vigorous energy created by the standing poses into a more quiet meditative state. Camel Pose further opens up the fronts of your legs and body to prepare you for Shoulderstand and releases any holding in your front body, preparing you—along with Shoulderstand—for Relaxation Pose. The Reclined Leg Stretch Series not only encourages the muscles of your back body to rest, but also actively opens up the backs of your legs so that when you lie down for Relaxation Pose, your back body can melt into the ground.

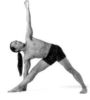

1. Practice two mini **Sun Salutations**, staying in Downward-Facing Dog for 5 breaths.

2. Practice two full **Sun Salutations**, staying in Downward-Facing Dog for 5 breaths.

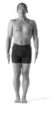

3. Practice **Mountain Pose** for 30 seconds.

4. Practice **Standing Forward Bend** for 1 minute.

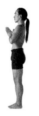

5. Practice **Triangle Pose** for 45 seconds on each side.

6. Practice **Standing Forward Bend** for 30 seconds.

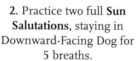

7. Practice **Extended Side Angle Pose** for 45 seconds on each side.

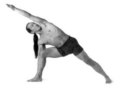

8. Practice **Standing Forward Bend** for 30 seconds.

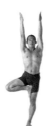

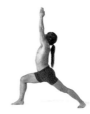

9. Practice **Tree Pose** for 45 seconds on each side.

10. Practice **Standing Forward Bend** for 30 seconds.

11. Practice **Warrior 1** for 45 seconds on each side.

12. Practice **Standing Forward Bend** for 30 seconds.

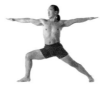

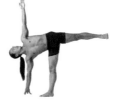

13. Practice **Warrior 2** for 45 seconds on each side.

14. Practice **Standing Forward Bend** for 30 seconds.

15. Practice **Half Moon Pose** for 30 seconds on each side.

16. Practice **Standing Forward Bend** for 30 seconds.

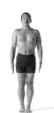

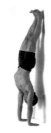

17. Practice **Pyramid Pose** for 45 seconds on each side.

18. Practice **Mountain Pose** for 30 seconds.

19. Practice **Wide Angle Standing Forward Bend** for 1 minute.

20. Practice **Handstand** for up to 30 seconds, two times.

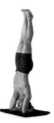

21. Practice **Headstand** for 2 to 5 minutes.

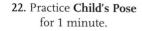

22. Practice **Child's Pose** for 1 minute.

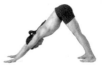

23. Practice **Downward-Facing Dog** for 1 minute.

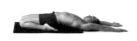

24. Practice **Reclined Hero Pose** for 1 to 2 minutes.

25. Practice **Camel Pose** for 30 seconds, two times.

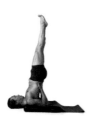

26. Practice **Shoulderstand** for 2 to 5 minutes (the same timing as or longer than Headstand).

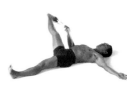

27. Practice the **Reclined Leg Stretch Series** for 1 minute for the straight-leg version, 15 seconds for the sit-up version, and 1 minute for the leg-to-the-side version on each side.

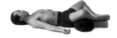

28. Relaxation and Breath Awareness. For 3 to 5 minutes, practice version 3 of **Supported Relaxation Pose** and focus on alternate nostril breathing.

Now use your right hand to block your left nostril and inhale through your right nostril. Then block your right nostril and exhale through your left. Inhale through your left nostril. Then block your left nostril and exhale through your right. This is a full cycle of *nadi sodhana* breath.

Repeat this cycle for 5 minutes.

29. Meditation. For 10 minutes, sit in **Hero Pose** and meditate on connecting with the earth. The work you did in the standing poses and the release and relaxation of your strong, activated legs allow you to connect to the earth through the roots of your legs and feet. Feel the powerful movements inside your legs converge into the lift of your spine. Let your arms augment the lift and movement of your upper spine.

One of my teachers once said that every posture in yoga has some aspect of a backbend within it. As you practice a sequence focused mainly on backbends, you will understand all the elements involved in opening your body in the backbends themselves and see that what my yoga teacher said is true. Yoga traditionally emphasizes supporting and opening the heart chakra, so whether you are in standing poses, backbends, or forward bends, always look for ways to feed and support your heart.

The sequence begins with Sun Salutations to integrate your mind and body with your breath. Holding Upward-Facing Dog, an obvious backbend, a little bit longer than the other poses in the Sun Salutations begins to open up your spine. Handstand follows to energize your entire body and to open up your shoulders. The standing poses activate your legs so that they can energetically support and help backbend your spine. Headstand then recenters your activity, taking all the energy from the salutations and standing poses into the center and core of your spine. You then move into the backbends, interspersed with Downward-Facing Dog, which elongates your spine, returns it to neutral

between the backbends, and calms your energetic body from the stimulation of the backbends.

The sequence of backbends itself moves from more controllable and elementary backbends to more energetic and demanding backbends. We intersperse Hero Pose in between the more demanding backbends to provide a moment of repose and observation while you keep your legs opening for the next backbend. After this vigorous backbend sequence, you move into Cobbler's Pose, giving your mind and body time to regroup in a fairly neutral, symmetrical, and contemplative pose. Simple Twist also returns you to neutral so that as you do Shoulderstand to cool your nervous system, you balance the practice. The Reclined Leg Stretch Series helps open up your back body, which you have used throughout the practice to support and open your front body. You end the practice with Wall Hang, which continues to release the muscles of your back body. As you move into Relaxation Pose, your body will still be affected by the backbends, giving you an understanding of what it might be like to be in the world with more vulnerability and openness in your throat, heart, and belly.

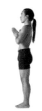

1. Practice two mini **Sun Salutations.**

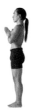

2. Practice four full **Sun Salutations,** staying in Upward-Facing Dog for 3 breaths.

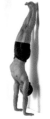

3. Practice **Handstand** for 30 seconds, two times.

4. Practice **Volcano Pose** for 1 minute.

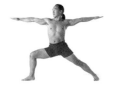

5. Practice **Warrior 2 Pose** for 1 minute on each side.

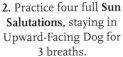

6. Practice **Standing Forward Bend** for 1 minute.

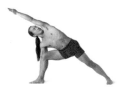

7. Practice **Extended Side Angle Pose** for 45 seconds on each side.

8. Practice **Standing Forward Bend** for 30 seconds.

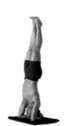

9. Practice **Warrior 1 Pose** for 1 minute on each side.

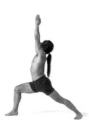

10. Practice **Headstand** for 1 to 3 minutes.

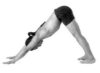

11. Practice **Downward-Facing Dog Pose** for 1 minute.

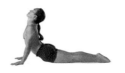

12. Practice **Cobra Pose** for 30 seconds, two times.

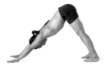

13. Practice **Downward-Facing Dog Pose** for 30 seconds.

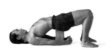

14. Practice **Supported Bridge Pose** for 1 to 2 minutes.

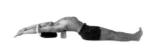

15. Practice **Passive Backbend** for 2 minutes.

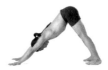

16. Practice **Downward-Facing Dog Pose** for 30 seconds.

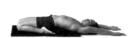

17. Practice **Reclined Hero Pose** for 1 to 2 minutes.

18. Practice **Bow Pose** for 15 seconds, two times.

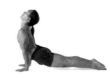

19. Practice **Upward-Facing Dog Pose** for 15 seconds.

20. Practice **Hero Pose** for 1 to 2 minutes.

21. Practice **Camel Pose** for 15 seconds.

22. Practice **Hero Pose** for 1 minute.

23. Practice **Upward-Facing Bow Pose**, three to five times, for 5 to 10 seconds.

24. Practice **Cobbler's Pose** for 2 minutes.

25. Practice **Simple Twist** for 30 seconds to 1 minute on each side.

26. Practice version 1 of **Happy Baby Pose** for 1 minute on each side.

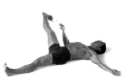

27. Practice **Shoulderstand** for 2 to 4 minutes.

28. Practice the **Reclined Leg Stretch Series** for 1 minute for the straight-leg version, 15 seconds for the sit-up version, and 1 minute for the leg-to-the-side version on each side.

29. Practice **Wall Hang** for 2 minutes.

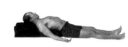

30. Relaxation and Breath Awareness. For 5 minutes, practice version 3 of **Supported Relaxation Pose**, focusing on full,

smooth inhalations and slow, complete exhalations as described on Day 6 of Week 7 (page 316).

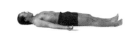

Afterward, practice classic **Relaxation Pose** for a few minutes, with free and natural breath.

31. Meditation. For 10 minutes, sit in **Seated Crossed-Legs Pose** at the wall and meditate on your open chest, wide collarbones, and the length of

your waist. This meditation follows a backbend practice, so the structure of your chest is already lifted and open. In this meditation, allow your heart to be

vulnerable and express itself freely. Center your mind—or what you consider to be your mind—in your heart. If you wish, focus on giving your loving

energy to someone or something in your life. Feel as though you know, feel, and relate to the world through your heart, and meditate on compassion.

DAY 3: FOCUS ON TWISTS

This sequence starts with four full Sun Salutations to wake up your entire body and engage your mind in the rhythm of your breath. In the Sun Salutations, you stay in Downward-Facing Dog so your breath will be more obvious and you can open up the backs of your legs. To prepare for twists, it is always useful to open up the backs of your legs and your hips, which create a strong but flexible foundation from which to spiral and turn. Next, you center yourself in Headstand so that you can observe how the foundation has been laid for moving into twists. The Core Strengthening Series then turns your attention to your core—your abdomen—as well as incorporating hip opening. As you move into the standing poses, you get a good sense of a gentle twisting from your core and from your legs.

In the twist sequence, you move from the most accessible twist into the more difficult twists, interspersed with Wide Angle Pose, Cobbler's Pose, and Staff Pose. These three neutral poses are both grounding and symmetrical, giving you time to digest and feel the effects of each twist. The last twist, Lord of the Fishes Pose, comes mainly from the opening of your outer hips, which creates a broad opening and vulnerability for your sacrum and lower back. This twist comes at the end because it creates this vulnerability, which is countered with Cobra Pose, a symmetrical backbend that reestablishes balance in your lower spine. Doing Cobra Pose twice creates symmetry and deepens your spine.

The last three poses provide restoration and relaxation. Since the twists cleanse your body and bring toxins from the organs into the blood stream, the three restorative poses give time for your body to clear the toxins away. The sequence ends with Supported Relaxation Pose so the backbending of your spine will further balance the broadening and vulnerability in your back body created by the twists.

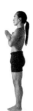

1. Practice four full **Sun Salutations**, staying in Downward-Facing Dog for 5 breaths.

2. Practice **Standing Forward Bend** for 1 to 2 minutes.

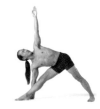

3. Practice **Triangle Pose** for 1 minute on each side.

4. Practice **Standing Forward Bend** for 30 seconds.

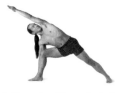

5. Practice **Extended Side Angle Pose** for 1 minute on each side.

6. Practice **Standing Forward Bend** for 30 seconds.

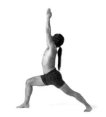

7. Practice **Warrior 1** for 30 seconds on each side.

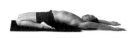

8. Practice **Reclined Hero Pose** for 1 to 2 minutes.

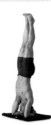

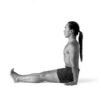

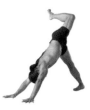

9. Practice **Headstand** for 1 to 3 minutes.

10. Practice **Child's Pose** for 1 minute.

11. Practice the **Core Strengthening Series** three times. On the last round, do a forward bend in Wide Angle Pose and in the last Cobbler's Pose for 1 minute each.

12. Practice version 3 of **One-Legged Downward-Facing Dog** for 15 to 30 seconds on each side.

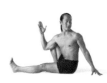

13. Practice version 2 of **Simple Twist** for 1 minute on each side.

14. Practice version 3 of **Simple Twist** if possible for 1 minute on each side.

15. Practice **Marichi's Twist 1** for 1 minute on each side.

16. Practice **Crossed-Legs Twist** for 30 seconds on each side, with Cobbler's Pose between sides and afterward for 30 seconds.

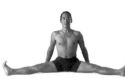

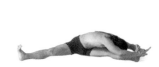

17. Practice **Staff Pose** for 1 minute.

18. Practice **Wide Angle Pose** for 1 minute.

19. Practice **Wide Angle Twist** for 1 minute on each side.

20. Practice **Cobbler's Pose** for 5 seconds.

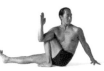

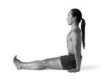

21. Practice **Staff Pose** for 30 seconds.

22. Practice **Marichi's Twist 3** for 1 minute on each side.

23. Practice **Staff Pose** for 15 seconds.

24. Practice **Lord of the Fishes** twist for 1 minute on each side.

25. Practice **Cobbler's Pose**, version 2 (with a bit of a backbend), for 30 seconds.

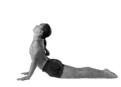

26. Practice **Cobra Pose** for 30 seconds, two times.

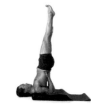

27. Practice **Shoulderstand** for 3 to 5 minutes.

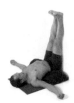

28. Practice **Legs Up the Wall Pose** for 3 to 5 minutes.

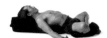

29. Practice **Reclined Cobbler's Pose** for 3 to 5 minutes.

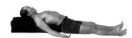

30. Relaxation and Breath Awareness. For 5 minutes, practice version 3 of **Supported Relaxation**

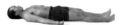

Pose, focusing on creating an even inhalation and exhalation as you begin to practice *ujjayi* breathing as

described on Day 6 of Week 7 (page 316).

For 2 minutes, practice classic **Relaxation Pose**.

31. Meditation. For 10 minutes, sit in **Hero Pose** against the wall, meditating on the evenness of the drop of your legs and the extension of both sides of your waist. Meditating after a twist practice helps you notice the cleansing effects of the poses. If you are sensitive, you may feel huge internal movements, like the surging of a river that has been swollen by a large rainstorm. You may feel as if the fluids of your body are cleansing the conduits, and if you allow yourself to relax during this fierceness, clarity will come. Sometimes as we meditate, the movements of our inner bodies create surprisingly strong sensations. Keep relaxing as much as possible during these times, scanning your body and observing your breath.

This sequence is designed to restore your nervous system and quiet your mind. It begins with Downward-Facing Dog, Standing Forward Bend, and Handstand, poses that warm you up for Headstand. From there you move to Headstand, which demands that your mind be present and begins to align your body around the central axis, the spine. Child's Pose and Downward-Facing Dog after Headstand ground your nervous system and release any tension from your neck. Then you practice Reclined Hero Pose and Restorative Backbend to open your front body. This also prepares you for Shoulderstand, which, except for the neck position, is considered a backbend. Shoulderstand and Plow Pose cool your nervous system. Reclined Leg Stretch Series follows to release your neck and to begin to open up your back body. This is a great pose to do before you do any seated forward bends because it stretches the backs of your legs while you maintain a neutral spine.

Now you move into the forward bend sequence, with a mind that is less goal oriented and more centered. You start with One-Legged Forward Bend because there is far less resistance in bending over one leg than both at the same time. This pose also incorporates a mild twist. Both factors allow you to open up one side of your back muscles more intensely than the other side, which allows for an easier first forward bend. Crossed-Legs Forward Bend follows to ease your back and rest your hamstrings. Repeating One-Legged Forward Bend after this allows you to get the benefit of repetition in easing your hamstrings. Cob-bler's Pose with a slight backbend comes next to counter any stressing of your lower back in the first few forward bends.

You now move into Seated Forward Bend, which creates resistance for most of us. But with your deep introspection from the earlier part of the practice, listen intently and slowly release. Seated Forward Bend is an opening for your entire back body, not just your lower back.

The next two forward bends, Cobbler's Pose and Wide Angle, incorporate both hamstring and hip opening, which release all the muscles of the insides and backs of your legs. Though these poses may seem more difficult, they create a bit of relief for your spine, allowing you to equalize it. Child's Pose is next because it stays within the basic shape of the forward bend but is fully supported by your legs. With that support, your back muscles further relax. So even though you may experience some surface agitation from the frustration of the forward bends, the deep inner waters of the body will be calm. To go from here into Restorative Relaxation Pose with your calves on the chair brings your back and spine back to neutral and adds awareness of how deeply you can rest on the ground now that you have opened up all the muscles of your back body.

We finish with Reclined Cobbler's Pose to reinitiate the natural curve of your lower back and to allow you to enjoy the depth of your restoration from the forward bends. Relaxation and meditation from this practice will probably be very deep.

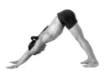

1. Practice **Downward-Facing Dog** for 2 minutes.

2. Practice **Standing Forward Bend** for 1 minute.

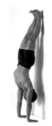

3. Practice **Handstand** for 30 seconds.

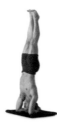

4. Practice **Headstand** for 1 to 4 minutes.

5. Practice **Child's Pose** for 1 minute.

6. Practice **Downward-Facing Dog** for 1 minute.

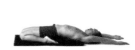

7. Practice **Reclined Hero Pose** for 1 to 2 minutes.

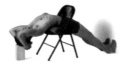

8. Practice version 3 of **Restorative Backbend** for 1 to 2 minutes.

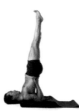

9. Practice **Shoulderstand** for 1 to 4 minutes (as long or longer than Headstand).

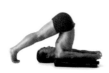

10. Practice **Plow Pose** for 2 minutes.

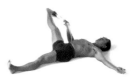

11. Practice **Reclined Leg Stretch Series** for 1 minute in the straight-leg version, 15 seconds in the sit-up version, and 1 minute in the leg-to-the-side version on each side.

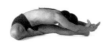

12. Practice **One-Legged Forward Bend** for 1 minute on each side.

13. Practice **Cross-Legged Forward Bend** for 1 minute on each side.

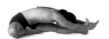

14. Practice **One-Legged Forward Bend** for 1 minute on each side.

15. Practice **Cobbler's Pose** with a slight backbend for 30 seconds.

16. Practice **Seated Forward Bend** for 1 to 2 minutes.

17. Practice **Cobbler's Forward Bend** for 30 seconds.

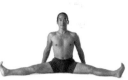

18. Practice **Wide Angle Pose** for 1 minute.

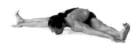

19. Practice **Wide Angle Pose Forward Bend** for 1 to 2 minutes.

20. Practice **Child's Pose** for 2 minutes.

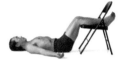

21. Practice version 2 of **Restorative Relaxation Pose** for 3 minutes.

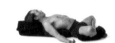

22. Practice version 3 of **Reclined Cobbler's Pose** for 3 minutes.

23. Relaxation and Breath Awareness. For 5 to 10 minutes, practice **Relaxation Pose.** Slightly extend the pause at the bottom of your exhalation.

24. Meditation. For 10 minutes, sit in **Seated Crossed-Legs Pose.** Meditate on the quietness and ease that the forward bends have brought to your nervous system. Also notice how your back muscles are more capable of supporting you with greater ease. The forward bends prepare you well for meditation because they have turned you inward to observe and feel yourself. Know that this is an infinite journey. Your mind and body can continue to fade into deeper and deeper quietness. Let this be the sanctuary that gives you deep physical, mental, and emotional rest.

When I do a practice that incorporates all the basic poses, my body hums in harmonious song. This extended practice was designed to let you feel the overall balance that comes from working in shapes that utilize all parts of your being in many different relationships to one another. When your body is this centered and balanced, you relax more deeply because of the innate trust that comes from these feelings.

This practice begins with Hero Pose to provide a couple of minutes for contemplation, allowing you to create a separation between what you have just been doing and the time and space you are giving your yoga practice. Use Hero Pose as a moment to turn inward, to observe how your body is feeling and what thoughts, emotions, and physical sensations are arising at the start of your practice. You next move on to three basic warm-up poses: Downward Facing Dog, Standing Forward Bend, and Handstand. With these poses, you essentially wake up your entire body, engage your mind, and open your heart. From here Mountain Pose gives you time to center yourself more fully in a pose that is so common to your daily life. The Sun Salutations then fully awaken and coordinate your body, breath, and mind. Mountain Pose again gives you a moment to see the influences of your movements and to incorporate them into your center.

The standing poses—interspersed with standing forward bends—completely awaken your legs and gather that wide, broad foundation into your spine and arms. From this fully awake state, you move into Headstand, which draws all of your awakened energy into your center. From here there is a gentle movement through an entire backbend sequence that brings you into your full vulnerability and openness and begins to address your fears, both physical and emotional, by challenging your spine and opening your heart. We then provide twists to balance out the backbends and to cleanse your inner organs.

With Shoulderstand, you begin to cool your nervous system. If any agitation was created by the vigor of the standing poses, the fire of Headstand, the vulnerability of the backbends, or the cleansing of the twists, you soothe your internal nervousness with the inward turning of Shoulderstand and Plow Pose.

The Reclined Leg Stretch Series releases your spine and your neck from the extensive movements in previous poses. It also sets you up for the forward bends that balance out the twists and backbends, as well as prepares you for dropping into a deep meditation and a deep relaxation.

1. Practice **Hero Pose** for 1 to 2 minutes.

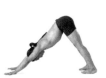

2. Practice **Downward-Facing Dog Pose** for 1 to 2 minutes.

3. Practice **Standing Forward Bend** for 1 minute.

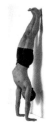

4. Practice **Handstand** for 30 seconds, two times.

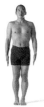

5. Practice **Mountain Pose** for 1 minute.

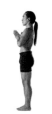

6. Practice two mini **Sun Salutations**, staying for 5 breaths in Downward-Facing Dog.

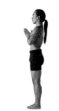

7. Practice two full **Sun Salutations**, staying for 5 breaths in Downward-Facing Dog.

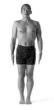

8. Practice **Mountain Pose** for 30 seconds.

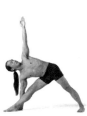

9. Practice **Triangle Pose** for 45 seconds on each side.

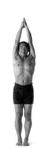

10. Practice **Volcano Pose** for 30 seconds.

11. Practice **Standing Forward Bend** for 30 seconds.

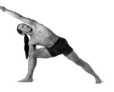

12. Practice **Extended Side Angle Pose** for 45 seconds on each side.

13. Practice **Standing Forward Bend** for 30 seconds.

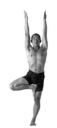

14. Practice **Tree Pose** for 45 seconds on each side.

15. Practice **Standing Forward Bend** for 30 seconds.

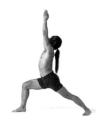

16. Practice **Warrior 1 Pose** for 45 seconds on each side.

17. Practice **Standing Forward Bend** for 30 seconds.

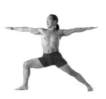

18. Practice **Warrior 2 Pose** for 45 seconds on each side.

19. Practice **Standing Forward Bend** for 30 seconds.

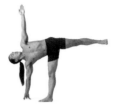

20. Practice **Half Moon Pose** for 30 seconds on each side.

21. Practice **Standing Forward Bend** for 30 seconds.

22. Practice **Standing Wide Angle Forward Bend** for 1 minute.

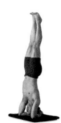

23. Practice **Headstand** for 1 to 5 minutes or any combination of Headstand variations adding up to 5 minutes.

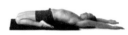

24. Practice **Reclined Hero Pose** for 1 to 2 minutes.

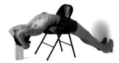

25. Practice version 3 of **Restorative Backbend** for 1 minute.

26. Practice **Downward-Facing Dog** for 1 minute.

27. Practice **Camel Pose** for 30 seconds.

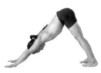

28. Practice **Downward-Facing Dog Pose** for 30 seconds.

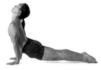

29. Practice **Upward-Facing Dog Pose** for 15 to 30 seconds.

30. Practice **Upward Bow Pose** for 5 seconds, one to five times.

31. Practice **Cobbler's Pose** for 30 seconds.

32. Practice **Simple Twist** for 1 minute on each side.

33. Practice **Cross-Legged Twist** for 1 minute on each side.

34. Practice **Marichi's Twist 1** for 1 minute on each side.

35. Practice **Cobbler's Pose** for 30 seconds.

36. Practice **Marichi's Twist 3** for 1 minute.

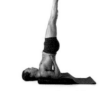

37. Practice **Shoulderstand** for 1 to 5 minutes (as long or longer than Headstand) or any combination of Shoulderstand variations adding up to more than 5 minutes.

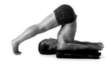

38. Practice **Plow Pose** for 1 to 3 minutes.

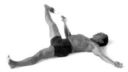

39. Practice the **Reclined Leg Stretch Series** for 1 minute in the straight-leg version, 15 seconds in the sit-up version, and 1 minute in the leg-to-the-side version on each side.

40. Practice **Seated Forward Bend** for 2 to 3 minutes.

41. Practice **One-Legged Forward Bend** for 1 minute.

42. Practice **Cross-Legged Forward Bend** for 1 minute.

43. Practice **Cobbler's Pose** with a slight backbend for 30 seconds.

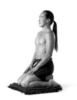

44. Meditation. For 10 minutes, sit in your favorite seated position. Scan your body from your head to the soles of your feet.

Typically when you scan your body, you will always check specific parts. But if you move slowly and methodically from the crown of your head to the soles of your feet, you can circumvent forming a habit. As you observe your body time and time again, you will invariably notice many minute changes. You will observe your mind fixating on certain feelings or thoughts, but continue to move right through these fixations by evenly scanning your entire being. You can let this scanning create natural, intuitive shifts in your posture that bring you closer toward the center of your natural balance and contentment.

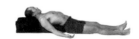

45. Relaxation and Breath Awareness. For 3 minutes, practice version 3 of **Supported Relaxation Pose.** Focus on inhaling smoothly and on letting your body go with your exhalations.

For 3 to 5 minutes, sit in **Seated Crossed-Legs Pose** and practice the *ujjayi* breath as described for Day 6 of Week 7 (page 316).

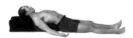

For 3 to 5 minutes, practice version 3 of **Supported Relaxation Pose** once more and let go as deeply and completely as possible.

DAY 6: BREATH AWARENESS AND MEDITATION

Breath Awareness

Go outside and take a walk. As you walk, practice releasing any observed tension. Walk with an open chest and very loose arms and legs. Feel your breath move easily through your body. Try to coordinate your breath with the rhythm of your walk.

Although it is not recommended that you do formal *pranayama* practices in your daily life, you can take the breath awareness techniques in this book outside the yoga room. In fact, one of the most important effects that my yoga practice has had on me is that I regularly observe my breath. Observing my breath allows me to key into shifting my posture and my mind toward a balance that is closer to center. As I center my body with an awareness of my breath, I can be more fully in the world. You may think that by observing your breath, for example, during a conversation, you might not be fully present. But I find the opposite to be true. If you center yourself by repeatedly observing your breath, and if you relax and open your heart and mind, then you will be a good listener. I believe that when you take breath awareness exercises into your daily life, your stress level will be greatly minimized and your ability to respond honestly and appropriately will be enhanced.

Meditation

For 10 minutes, sit in a chair, with your sitting bones on the front of the seat of the chair and your feet underneath your knees. Lightly press your thighs into the chair seat and your feet into the ground. Observe how this naturally lifts your chest and brings natural curves and elongation to your spine. Meditate on the energy moving through your entire body, from the soles of your feet pressing into the earth up through the conduits of your legs, into your pelvis and along the channel of your spine.

As you become familiar with seated meditation, you will realize that you can take this practice anywhere you go. You don't really need to be sitting and you don't really even need to be still. Meditation is more about a balance between inside and outside, an ease in your body, an acceptance of whatever is taking place, and an ability to be quiet and listen, an ability to receive and let go. Many of us sit all day, whether at work, in a car or bus, or in a restaurant or movie theater. At any of these times, you can periodically bring your mind back to your posture and your breath. You may think that these moments of meditation mean removing yourself from your social responsibilities, but I have always found that these moments of meditation sprinkled throughout the day are what allow me to be more present at work, with my family, with my friends, and with myself. Constantly reminding yourself to relax, to undulate with the beat of your heart and the fluidity of your breath, helps you center yourself through your body in the present moment. This is a wonderful foundation for true communication and a celebration of aliveness.

Anyone can see that if grasping and aversion were with us all day and night without ceasing, who could ever stand them? Under that condition, living things would either die or become insane. Instead, we survive because there are natural periods of coolness, of wholeness, and ease. In fact, they last longer than the fires of our grasping and fear. It is this that sustains us. We have periods of rest making us refreshed, alive, well. Why don't we feel thankful for this everyday Nirvana?

—Ajahn Buddhadasa

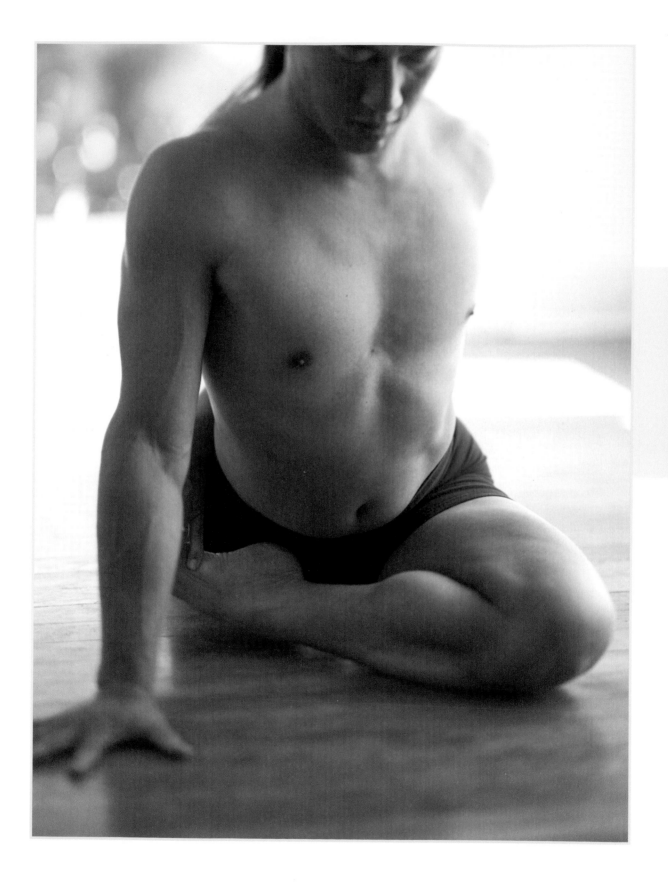

PART 3:

Customizing Your Practice

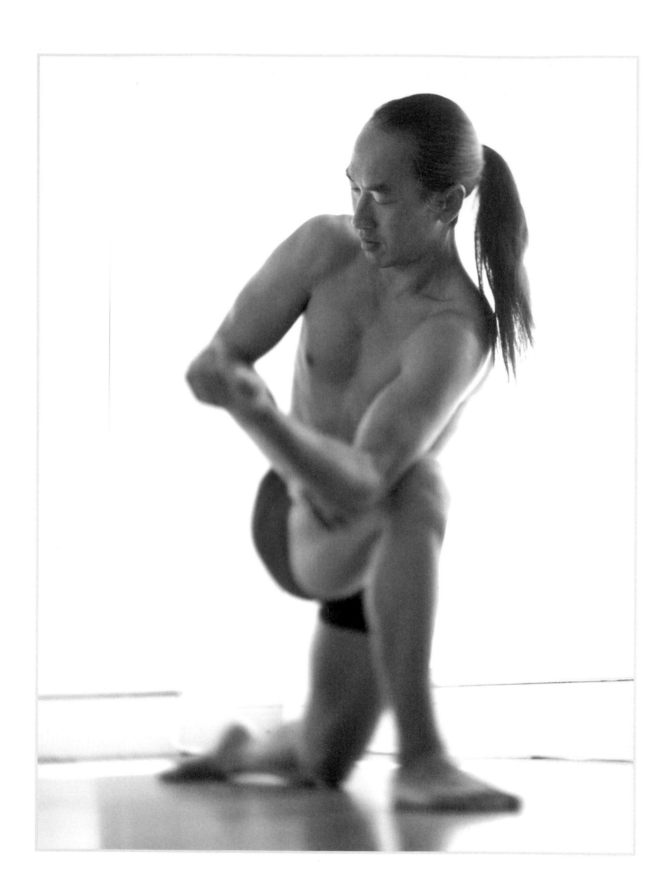

MOST OFTEN, PEOPLE ARE DOING YOGA FOR SOME SIMPLE REASON,
AND THEY PROGRESS INTO MORE INVOLVED, STEP-BY-STEP PRACTICES.
EACH STEP CAN BE ENJOYABLE, FITTED TO THE REALITY OF WHERE EACH PERSON IS NOW.
AS MY FATHER SAID, IF YOU GO STEP BY STEP, THERE WILL BE NO PROBLEMS. ENJOY EACH STEP.
—T. K. V. DESIKACHAR, *THE HEART OF YOGA*

Creating a Personal Practice

NOW THAT YOU'VE MADE IT THROUGH THE PROGRAM, YOU'RE PROBABLY WONDERING ABOUT WHAT TO do next. You want to keep practicing yoga at home, but what exactly should you practice?

If you are satisfied with continuing to practice sequences directly from this book, there are several ways you can do so:

- Repeat the entire program, starting again with Week 1. There is so much information presented during the eight-week program that repeating the program will be extremely beneficial for you, enabling you to absorb the daily lessons more deeply.
- Focus on practicing the seven essential balanced practices in this book, including the five balanced practices in Week 8, the Focus on Inversions Practice (Week 7, Day 5), and the Learning Restorative Backbend and Restorative Plow Pose Practice (Week 6, Day 4), and, if you are menstruating, A Moon Practice on page 360. These sequences provide enough variety to last you for some time and include all the poses needed to provide you with a balanced home practice.
- Browse through the book and choose any favorite practice to repeat, allowing yourself to be intuitive about what you feel like practicing on any given day.

But many of you will be ready to begin creating your own personal practice. Creating a personal practice means adapting your practice to suit your circumstances on any given day, whether that means tinkering around with the practices in this book or creating an entirely new sequence based on poses you love or poses that you want to explore in depth. Although some people are satisfied to continue to repeat the same yoga sequence or sequences for years at a time, many practitioners find that creating a personal practice is crucial to their ability to maintain their home practices and keep them thriving. In addition, learning how to adapt your practice to the kind of physical imbalances we all experience at one time or another—being sick, injured, or having lower back pain—will enable you to continue your practice during times of difficulty. In some cases, modifying your practice to accommodate a physical imbalance, particularly lower back pain, might even help alleviate your pain.

Therefore, this chapter provides information about how you can create your personal practice—hopefully without angst—by doing any or all of the following:

- Shorten or extend a practice in this book.
- Create the sequence that you love.
- Adapt your practice to your monthly cycle (for women).
- Modify your practice when you are sick.
- Modify your practice when you are injured.
- Modify your practice when you are having lower back pain.

However, the main ingredient to creating your personal practice is your ability to listen—to your body, breath, and mind and to the effects that the practices have on you. I will often make generalizations in this chapter, but it is up to you to determine whether you fit in any of these categories. Consider everything in this chapter as suggestions rather than hard-and-fast rules.

Shortening and Extending a Practice

The reality of your schedule means that you may have varying amounts of time available to practice yoga on different days. On Monday morning, you may have only 20 minutes to squeeze a practice into, while on some rainy Sunday afternoon you might have the free time for a leisurely two- or three-hour practice. To keep your practice thriving and to receive the full benefits of regular home practice, it is better to practice frequently for shorter periods of time, such as half an hour every day, rather than practicing once a week for two-and-a-half hours. Therefore, this section provides you with information about how to shorten the practices in this book for those days when time is scarce and how to extend the practices on those days when you have the luxury of a free morning or afternoon.

I like to do forward bends at work . . . and sometimes twists on the chair. Occasionally I will walk down the hall, look both ways to make sure no one is coming, and then go into a handstand or forearm balance. No one has caught me yet!

—Mark Silva

Shortening a Practice

The shortest practice is just to take one or two of your favorite poses and place them throughout your day.

WARMING UP. If your favorite poses require a prelude (that is, if they are too difficult to go into immediately), such as Headstand or deep backbends or forward bends, it is important to warm up by doing a few postures before them. Try a Downward-Facing Dog, a couple of Sun Salutations, or a Handstand to wake up your body and mind before moving on to those poses.

REDUCING TIMINGS. You can shorten any practice in this book by doing all the poses for shorter amounts of time. This is a very good way to get the full benefit from the practice and to learn a lot about sequencing in the process.

REMOVING POSES. Also, you can delete some of the poses from each section of any practice in this book (as shown below). For instance, you could cut out the two full Sun Salutations from a practice but leave in the two mini Sun Salutations. From the standing poses that are specified, you might cut out the last two in the practice and likewise for the backbends. For the Restorative Poses, you might cut out the beginning one, rather than the final Relaxation Pose. Because the practices have a natural order to them, when you are shortening the practices, it is best to cut out the more advanced poses, which are usually at the end of each section.

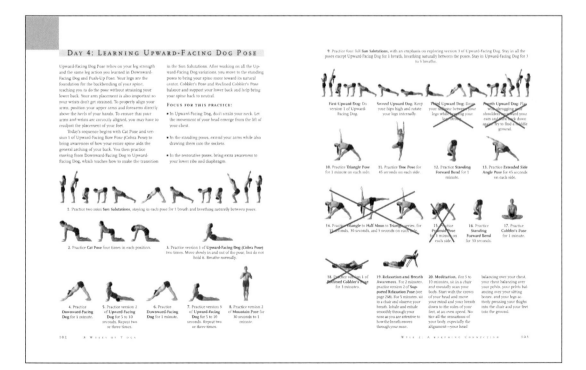

RESTORATIVE POSES. Many people will tend to shorten a practice by eliminating the restorative poses; however, this is not a good idea. It is very important to end your practice with at least one posture that provides restoration because this part of the sequence gives you time to digest the information you gained from the practice and provides a segue between your practice and what you have to do next. The sequences in this book have a natural completeness. Although you may be tempted to stop the practice halfway through, this is not advisable. If you must stop in the middle for some reason, try to finish with the restorative poses at the end of practice and end with Relaxation Pose as usual.

EXTENDING A PRACTICE

After you go through the eight weeks of yoga in the program, some of you will want to do longer practices than those in the book. You may be tempted to combine two entire practices back to back, but it is not recommended that you do this because the practices are complete sequences in and of themselves. Instead, you can try increasing the time you spend in each of the poses, repeating poses or sections of poses within a practice, or adding new poses to the practice.

INCREASING TIMINGS. When you are increasing the time you spend in the poses, you can do so freely for all poses in this book except for two twists: Marichi's Twist 3 and Lord of the Fishes Twist. You should generally not do these twists for longer than 1 minute on a side because of the stress they can put on your spine, nervous system, and digestive system.

EXTENDING HEADSTAND. If you decide to lengthen the time you stay in Headstand, you need to do so very gradually. Therefore, if you are doing one of the practices and are holding all the poses twice as long as the timings shown in the instructions, you should not, all of a sudden, double the amount of time you stay in Headstand. Instead, always increase the length of time you stay in Headstand in very small increments. For instance, if you are doing Headstand every day, I would recommend that you increase the length of your Headstand by approximately 15 seconds per week. Plus, you should not continue to increase the time in a linear way. You might have several months where you hold Headstand for the same amount of time, for instance, for 3 or 5 minutes. You can generally tell when you should do this by how your neck feels and how much ease there is in your breathing. If the length of time you spend in Headstand feels like it is going to compromise the ease of your neck or your breath, you are staying in the pose too long.

REPEATING POSES. You can lengthen any practice by repeating any of the poses in the sequence, except Headstand. For instance, if you wanted to go deeper into backbends, you could repeat all the backbends in the Focus on Backbends practice two or three times. Or, you could just pick a single backbend to focus on and repeat that backbend several times.

You can also repeat an entire sequence of poses, such as the backbend, forward bend, or twist section of a practice. For example, you might repeat the entire backbend sequence in the Focus on Backbends practice, from Cobra Pose to Upward-Facing Dog Pose, two or three times, including all the neutral poses between the backbends.

EXTENDING RESTORATIVE POSES. You can also extend a practice by lengthening the time you spend in the restorative poses as much as two or three times the amount given in the instructions. However, it is important not to fall asleep in restorative poses because you could injure yourself if you stay in the pose for an excessive amount of time. For example, staying too long in Reclined Cobbler's Pose could strain your adductor muscles. Therefore, if you know that you tend to fall asleep easily, be sure to set a timer that will wake you up if you do so.

PRACTICING TWICE A DAY. People often find it more convenient to practice two times in one day because they have limited time in the morning and limited time in the afternoon. When you practice twice a day, both your morning and afternoon or evening practices should include all the elements of a complete practice, with a beginning, middle, and end, finishing, as always, with Relaxation Pose.

In addition, it is generally more beneficial to do your strong, active practice in the morning, with a more restorative, quiet practice, including your inverted poses, in the afternoon. However, I occasionally like to switch this around and do a quiet, meditative practice in the morning and a vigorous practice, such as backbends, in the afternoon. Sometimes I'll do the same kind of practice twice in the day, with one a more restorative version of the other. For example, I might do an active backbend practice in the morning and a passive backbend practice in the evening. Often the body responds favorably to this and opens very deeply. Practicing twice in one day will allow you to see the cumulative effects of the first practice on the second practice.

Do not, however, repeat the Headstand and Shoulderstand on the same day. Reserve these for your second practice. Also, be sure to practice both Headstand and Shoulderstand within the same practice—don't split them up.

CREATING THE SEQUENCE THAT YOU LOVE

I hope that as you have practiced our eight-week program, you familiarized yourself with the poses that were introduced to you and that they brought you a deeper understanding of yourself. By continuing to become more intimate with the poses and by honing your sensitivity, you will become more intuitive about what your body and mind need that day. In general, however, certain types of poses will elicit specific effects on your emotional and physical body.

FORWARD BENDS. These poses have a quieting effect, allowing you to restore your body and your nervous system. They open and release your back body, which supports you throughout the entire day. They also turn your senses inward, creating a shell within which you can ruminate over things that have already taken place. This time of introspection allows you to focus on what is taking place within your body and mind at the present moment and, without a lot of new input, gives your nervous system a chance to rest. In therapeutic practices, you often do forward bends with your forehead or front body supported. Using a support for your head allows you to release tension from your neck because the weight of your head is carried and you can relax it completely. In addition, having your forehead and your front body rest on a support brings your attention to any binding in your front body, which you can then consciously release.

BACKBENDS. These poses awaken your nervous system and energize your entire body. They also open the heart chakra and—for many people—may even produce a sense of joy, uplifting the spirits and creating social, gregarious feelings. Because the poses leave you physically exposed and vulnerable and because you are working with your spine (your central nervous system), backbends may also elicit a sense of fear, which you will need to address in your practice.

After doing backbends, you may also feel you are emotionally exposed and vulnerable. This can create a chance for much deeper communication but also allows the difficult as well as the joyous to enter. Backbends reverse your habitual posture (which for most of us is somewhat rounded, hunched, and protected) and can bring you to a more centered place in your posture and in your emotional body.

STANDING POSES. Because these poses activate and open up your legs, they create a sense of presence, grounding, centering, and connection. They also give you an overall feeling of stability and strength, making you feel as if you can deal with whatever comes at you—standing on your own two feet. Standing poses, like backbends, energize your body, though they are more centering than backbends, which create vulnerability. Because you are standing on your feet, standing poses do not produce much fear or disorientation. They bring you into your body, allowing you to collect yourself and gather your consciousness, and from that sense of center begin to connect and relate. Standing poses also balance your body, opening up places that are tight and contracting places that are overly flexible, waking up areas that are dead and softening areas that are too active. This physical sense of balance will often engender an emotional centering as well.

TWISTS. These poses cleanse you emotionally and physically (although that effect is not always immediate). They leave you feeling as if you can let go of things that have set themselves deep inside your body, not just on your mind or on the surface of your heart, but that have embedded themselves in the tissues and vital organs of your body. During twists, you may feel a lot of resistance and agitation because you are confronting your limitations. And as you detoxify your physical and emotional body, you may initially feel stirred up and irritated. Yet what comes after this release is a feeling of clarity, which can be a joyous beginning or a liberating rebirth. Because twists tend to compress the diaphragm and cause a shortening of breath, they are easy poses in which to examine your breath. How can you breathe freely as you meet resistance?

INVERTED POSES. These poses change physical and emotional perspectives and can swiftly alter your mood from agitated and dispersed to quiet and centered. They demand your attention and presence of mind, but they also have a settling effect. Even though Headstand is stimulating to the circulatory and nervous systems, it also centers your mind and heart. Shoulderstand is more quieting and soothing than Headstand, but it, too, centers your mind and heart. In combination, Headstand and Shoulderstand are the two most emotionally balancing poses in the entire yoga practice. Plow Pose is both an inverted pose and a forward bend, so it combines the emotional effects of both types of poses. Handstand and Elbow Balance are very stimulating poses that alter your mood instantly from lethargy to alertness or from agitation to calmness.

RESTORATIVE POSES. These poses allow you to deal directly with your emotional body, magnifying your current emotional state. Because you are not distracted by physical sensations, you are asked to face whatever emotions are arising, which can at times be difficult. However, if you can allow for a sense of release and letting go, the overall affect of a restorative pose is a profound surrender. When you become experienced at observing your emotional body from these poses, you will become better at letting your emotions move freely without needing to protect yourself from feeling what you feel. This allows the emotions to move through their cycles more naturally so that the return to balance and equanimity can take place. The restorative poses can themselves be classified into restorative backbends, restorative forward bends, restorative twists, and so on. The restorative versions of a given type of pose have similar effects as the active versions of the same type of pose (for example, a restorative backbend has similar effects as an active backbend). It may surprise you to find that through the poses that seem like they require the least amount of effort, you may feel the strongest effects.

NEUTRAL POSES. These poses are transition poses that allow your body to find its natural balance after you do a sequence of poses that tend to take your body in a single direction, such as a series of backbends. After moving strongly in one direction, it is good to do one or more neutral poses before moving into an opposite direction (for example, between backbends and forward bends). Some examples of good neutral poses are Reclined Leg Stretch; Downward-Facing Dog (in the version that allows for a neutral spine); Staff Pose; Cobbler's Pose, with a bit of a backbend; Happy Baby Pose, version 1; Mountain Pose; Hero Pose; and Seated Crossed-Legs Pose.

A pose is "neutral" for you if your spine easily returns to its natural curves while you are in the posture. And you should always practice neutral poses in a way that allows for ease (such as using a prop or sitting against the wall). Neutral poses all enable you to observe the effects of the previous poses on your physical and emotional body. They also help center you and calm your nervous system.

Have you observed similar emotional reactions to these different types of poses in your own practice? By practicing Week 8 of the program, the week of balanced practices, you will begin to understand how the various types of poses affect you because each practice has a specific emphasis. By getting to know those practices well, you can learn how the various poses affect you physically, psychologically, and emotionally.

After doing the practices in this book, you will probably be able to make a list of all the poses that you love. For any such pose, maybe you love the pose itself or maybe you love the effects of the pose. Though it doesn't really matter why you do, it might be interesting to think about what it is that you enjoy. There might even be sequences of poses or full practices that you fully enjoy.

At this time, make your list of favorite poses and then identify poses that you love from each of the following categories:

- Standing poses
- Backbends
- Twists
- Forward bends
- Restoratives

Also, ask yourself:

1. What are the poses that I have the least resistance to, that at any time during the day I feel like dropping right into? (These are the poses that you might want to begin your practice with.)

2. Which poses are challenging for me but are also very exciting or something I may have always wanted to learn, such as Handstand or one of the backbends? (Some people have built a whole practice that they love around the pose they are challenged by or interested in learning.)

3. What is my favorite breath practice?

4. Did I enjoy any of the subjects of meditation?

Many of you may feel as if you can't get to a practice because it is too much like something you are *supposed* to do, and you don't practice the things that you love because you feel like you don't deserve them or you wonder if they are as beneficial as the things that are difficult. I know that this book is about moving toward balance and that I have said that the poses that are difficult for you or that challenge you are the poses that might bring you more into balance. However, I also believe that it is very beneficial to do a yoga practice that you really love and to which you have no resistance. I like to think of my own yoga practice as a treat for myself or just something I really look forward to doing. So I think it is especially important when you are beginning to create a practice for yourself to follow the path of least resistance.

To create the practice you love, start by identifying the poses that you want to include in your practice. You can then sequence them.

BEGINNING POSES. Traditionally, entry points to a practice include one or more of the following:

- Sun Salutations, mini Sun Salutations, or any other creative derivative
- Downward-Facing Dog
- Standing Forward Bend
- Handstand

However, if there is another pose or series of poses that make it more likely that you'll actually get to your mat, follow your intuition and start with those.

After selecting one or more beginning poses, choose one of your favorite standing poses and possibly let that be the invitation to do a few more standing poses. You might pick one of the sequences of standing poses shown in this book, or if you are working on a standing pose that is difficult for you, you might precede it with a simpler standing pose that is similar in nature.

After the standing poses, move on to one of your favorite backbends, again doing any necessary preparation. Realize that almost all the backbends can be done to varying degrees of depth, and it is important not to just jam yourself into a backbend thinking that you have to go to your maximum right away. I often tell people that the preparation for any posture is that posture done to a lesser degree.

If Headstand is one of your favorite poses, practice it either before or after the backbend.

After backbends, select a pose that is reclined or very neutral for the spine, such as Reclined Leg Stretch or Downward-Facing Dog.

Next choose one or more of your favorite twists. Then if you did Headstand (which should always be followed by Shoulderstand somewhere in your practice), or if Shoulderstand and Plow are among your favorites, add Shoulderstand and Plow after your twists. Finally, you can move on to one or more forward bends and end with your favorite restorative poses and Relaxation Pose.

In summary, the basic pattern for sequencing your favorite poses is as follows:

- Starting Pose
- Standing Poses
- *Neutral Pose*
- Headstand
- Backbends
- *Neutral Pose*
- Twists
- *Neutral Pose*
- Shoulderstand (and Plow)
- Forward Bends
- *Neutral Pose*
- Restorative Pose
- Relaxation Pose

Understand that this basic sequence is not the only good way to order your poses, but it is a very practical template. The more you become experienced with the poses, the more you can play around with this template and the more you can be intuitive about combining poses in many different sequences.

Realize, however, that changing the sequence in which you do yoga poses will have a strong effect on the poses that you do before and after any given pose, as well as a strong effect on how you feel after your practice. So it is mainly the degree to which you can listen to your body that allows you to be more free and intuitive with sequencing. I think you will find that after a certain amount of practice, the poses and the practices that you love may shift, even from day to day. So when you wake up or when you start a practice, give yourself a little time in meditation to listen to your body so that you will be able to do an appropriate practice for who you are in that moment. More and more often you will be able to follow your intuition to balance your body and your mind.

Your Monthly Cycle (for Women)

In many cultures, women treat their monthly periods as a time for resting and nurturing themselves. In this vein, many yoga teachers recommend that you alter your yoga practice during your periods. This section outlines specific recommendations for women based on the teachings of B. K. S. Iyengar and teachers trained in the Iyengar tradition. However, you should keep in mind that among long-time women practitioners, there is a wide variety of approaches to yoga practice during menstruation. Some women choose to practice very actively during their periods, while still avoiding certain poses, such as inversions, that they consider contraindicated. Other women think of their periods as a good opportunity to take the time to rest and nurture themselves. The best approach is probably to start out treating yourself gently, and then, if you wish, to incorporate a variety of different kinds of poses into your practice. As always, it is through experience and experimentation that you will find out what is most effective and preferable for you.

Poses to Avoid. The poses that almost all teachers recommend avoiding during your period are the inverted poses, for they are thought to impede your natural flow. Standing poses and active backbends are considered by many to be contraindicated because they are too energetic, and the general philosophy behind the practice during the menstrual period is that it is better to be more introspective and quiet during this time. Therefore, in general, it is recommended that you practice poses based more around receptivity than around effort. Extreme twists, extreme forward bends, and arm balances are also thought to be too intense due to the gripping and the closure of the abdominal and uterine cavities.

Menstrual Practice. A Moon Practice, which follows on page 360, will usually help relieve menstrual cramps. The folding forward into passive forward bends and the opening up into passive backbends creates a pumping in your body that is good for circulation and encourages your flow. This Moon Practice has evolved as a result of the experimentation of many long-time practitioners, so I highly recommend that you explore it. Yet at the same time, keep in mind that it might not work for you. By listening to your body and asking it what it wants and what it feels like doing, you will eventually be able to customize a practice that is most suitable for you.

A Moon Practice

This practices opens your body, folds it inward, and then opens it again, mildly massaging your body and encouraging your menstrual flow. The practice begins with two restorative poses, Reclined Cobbler's Pose and Reclined Hero Pose, which open your front body and are considered to encourage your flow. The forward bend series in this practice turns your energy inward and sometimes helps with menstrual cramps. The twisting action of Sideways Wide Angle Pose gently massages your inner organs, also encouraging your flow. The two passive backbends open your front body again after all your forward folding, encouraging your circulation and menstrual flow.

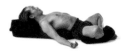

1. Practice version 3 of **Reclined Cobbler's Pose** for 3 to 5 minutes.

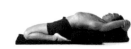

2. Practice version 2 of **Reclined Hero Pose** for 1 to 3 minutes.

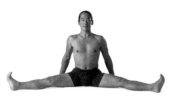

3. Practice **Wide Angle Pose** for 1 to 2 minutes.

4. Practice **Supported Child's Pose** for 2 to 3 minutes.

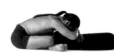

5. Practice version 1 of **Crossed-Legs Forward Bend** (supported) for 1 to 2 minutes per side.

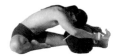

6. Practice version 2 of **One-Legged Forward Bend** for 1 to 2 minutes per side.

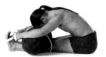

7. Practice version 2 of **Seated Forward Bend** for 1 to 3 minutes.

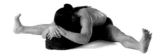

8. Practice version 2 of **Wide Angle Forward Bend** for 1 to 3 minutes.

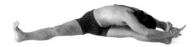

9. Practice **Sideways Wide Angle Pose** (optional: head on chair) for 1 minute per side.

10. Practice version 2 of **Cobbler's Forward Bend** for 1 to 2 minutes

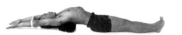

11. Practice **Passive Backbend** for 2 to 3 minutes.

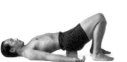

12. Practice version 1 of **Supported Bridge Pose** for 3 to 5 minutes.

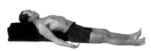

13. Practice version 3 of **Supported Relaxation Pose** for 3 to 5 minutes.

WHEN YOU ARE SICK

Many people wonder whether or not they should practice any yoga at all when they are sick with the flu, a cold, or some kind of virus. There are days when it is obvious that you can do very little with your body, but it is still an interesting time to observe your breath and try some of the different kinds of meditation taught in this book.

RESTORATIVE POSES. When you are up to it, restorative poses, such as Reclined Cobbler's Pose, Reclined Hero Pose, and Supported Relaxation Pose, can be very helpful. If nothing else, these poses change the position in which you are lying, which can help alleviate some of your physical discomfort and lift your spirits. Here are some poses to try:

- Child's Pose
- Reclined Leg Stretch
- Reclined Cobbler's Pose
- Reclined Hero Pose
- Reclined Twist
- Gentle twists while sitting in a chair
- Seated poses against the wall, including Cobbler's Pose, Staff Pose, Wide Angle Pose, and One-Legged Forward Bend
- Version 3 of Supported Relaxation Pose

POSES TO AVOID. Depending on the illness you have, you may need to avoid certain poses.

- For sinus infections, avoid inverted poses.
- For indigestion, avoid inverted poses and arm balances.
- For exhaustion, avoid holding the standing poses or active backbends for long periods of time, as this requires too much energy.

In general, the way you feel is going to dictate how much you can practice. However, sometimes when you are sick, the tendency to want to do nothing takes over and inertia sets in. These are the times to discipline yourself to focus your mind, to practice through visualization, breath awareness, and meditation, and to begin to move again, however mildly.

AS YOU RECOVER. When your body is recovering and you want to move around more, start by doing any yoga practice that appeals to you but in a very modified fashion, using props to support your body so you do not exhaust yourself and cause a relapse. In this way, your body will benefit from the poses without being overly taxed.

When You Are Injured

Many people give up their yoga practice entirely when they are injured. However, in my mind, this is not the most effective way to work with an injury. When an injury is not severe, you can find a range of motion within the yoga poses that can help you heal from your injury and rebuild your practice. Even if an injury prevents you from doing the full posture, this does not matter. Minimizing yoga poses while still understanding their general direction of movement is a significant practice. For instance, you might have a knee injury that does not allow you to bend your knee completely or bear your full weight on your knee joint. In this circumstance, you could take weight off your knee in some of the standing poses by supporting your pelvis on a chair, and you could then bend your front leg without bearing full weight on it.

As I get older, I realize there is usually some kind of difficulty—whether it is physical, emotional, intellectual, or psychological—that I have to deal with. If I shut down my practice in these times, I might never practice at all. Therefore, it is extremely important to learn how to modify your practice when you are injured or have some kind of physical difficulty.

Severe Injuries. Obviously there are injuries that are so severe you have no choice but to rest the injured area. But again, this does not mean that you have to give up yoga completely. In these times, practicing through visualization, working with your breath, practicing restorative poses, and meditating are all very beneficial.

(For lower back injuries, see page 364 for specific recommendations on how to deal with them within your yoga practice.)

Diagnosing an Injury

Initially when I start working with an injury, I try to do a variety of poses to help me further diagnose the injury. You will find that there are specific poses that seem to affect the injured area more directly. These are the poses that you will have to be extra careful with, though in my mind it is important to continue to do these poses in a minimal form in order to explore the injured area. For example, if I had a knee problem, I might try to take the shapes of all the standing poses while lying on my back. This would decrease the amount of weight on my legs and knees. But it would still allow me to explore the shapes and actions of the standing poses, and continue to work with the coordination of my leg joints and increase circulation, mindfulness, and strength. In the yoga practice, healing from an injury means continuing to explore your range of motion, promoting circulation, and bringing your mind to the area through body scanning and general mental focus.

There are injuries that occur outside of your yoga practice and injuries that result from the practice itself. In my own practice, I treat these injuries the same way. I determine which postures create difficulty and ask myself, How can I modify the poses to enable me to heal instead of injuring myself more? Injuries that occur in your yoga practice often occur due to a lack of understanding of a posture or because you are too aggressive and push yourself beyond your limits (for example, forcing your legs into Lotus Pose when your hips aren't open enough or pulling yourself too deeply into a forward bend). To avoid these types of injuries, focus on listening to the state of your body and your breath as you practice. If you come into a pose that is particularly difficult, instead of thinking you have to push through the resistance, you might ask yourself, How can I work differently and adjust my body to let my breath move more easily? And by listening deeply, how can I observe exactly where the resistance is and then let it go?

PRACTICING WITH AN INJURY

When you first start working with an injury, you cannot be sure whether your work is going to help or hurt. That is why it is always good to work cautiously and conservatively in the beginning. Within the next day or two after your experimentation, you can see the effects of your practice on the affected areas. Usually this analysis, observation, and reflection will help you intuit how to work further with your injury. Practicing while you are injured forces you to be more mindful and more careful. If you can take the element of fear out of the experimentation with your injuries and replace it with curiosity, keen observation, and a free breath, then you will not only help promote healing but also develop a more detached, less fearful approach. Complete avoidance of the injured area is sometimes the right course of action, but you should continue to work with different parts of your body as well as working with visualization and meditation.

JOINT PROBLEMS. When you have joint pain, back up until the pain is almost completely gone and then try to manipulate the joint—through engaging your muscles differently, rotating the joint, or slightly changing the position—until you reach a point where there is no pain. The alignment of any joint is extremely important but it is especially important for knee and elbow joints. Your shoulder and hip sockets should always feel centered, and all your joints should feel responsive and fluid, not jammed or locked. In addition, there should never be stress on one part of a joint with freedom in other parts; instead, the sensation should be evenly distributed around the entire joint. If you don't have this evenness, back up and move the joint until you find more equality. You should also consider how the given joint coordinates with other joints in your body. For example, your knee joint should coordinate with your ankle and hip joints. Often an injury to a joint or a pain in a joint is due to lack of coordination with adjoining joints. In this case, back up and play with a different coordination between the joint that is injured and adjacent joints. You may also wish to work with a qualified teacher.

WORKING WITH LOWER BACK PROBLEMS

Many people develop lower back problems at some point in their lives. These problems fall into the following three general categories:

- Intermittent pain that comes and goes within a day, week, or month
- Mild, but constant general aching
- Severe and chronic pain

Depending on your condition, you need to take a different approach to your yoga practice.

INTERMITTENT LOWER BACK PAIN. The interesting aspect of intermittent lower back pain is the constant question of why the pain comes. You might already know that there are specific positions or activities that create this intermittent pain. But I'm sure you're still interested in figuring out how to keep it from returning. The great thing about intermittent pain is that you know that there are times when you don't have it, so this means that something isn't chronically wrong or at least doesn't chronically show up. Usually with these kinds of pain, your yoga practice gives you much information about what brings the pain on and what keeps it at bay. By trying myriad different yoga poses and practices, you might be able to pinpoint which actual movements and positions cause your back to hurt. You might also find much quicker ways to get out of the pain and difficulty. Many people find that their emotional state is related to their lower back problems. If this is true for you, you can work with yoga practices to deal with your emotional state, such as any practice in this book that relives your stress by calming your nervous system.

MILD LOWER BACK PAIN. If you have been able to do most of the practices in this book and yet you have a mild back pain that sometimes gets better with the practices and other times is exacerbated by different practices, there are certain poses that you should begin to experiment with on a daily basis (see A Lower Back Practice on page 366). You should also continue to do all the practices in this book, but take special care and use the appropriate versions of the poses that release your back optimally. Also be very mindful not to be aggressive and to listen to what balances your body. You can use the different poses and sequences to investigate your difficulty and to figure out how to use the poses to help alleviate your pain and heal your back problems.

SEVERE LOWER BACK PAIN. If you have severe lower back pain and can barely walk or get out of bed, it is important to see a doctor to determine whether there are any serious injuries. Additionally, you have the option of working with alternative health practitioners who can give you exercises that may be better for you than just lying around and resting.

You can also try some of the poses in A Lower Back Practice on page 366 to see whether they help alleviate your pain. With any injury or problem there is going to be a time when you have to go on with your life and test it. You can try a mild twist, forward bend, back-bend, or standing pose as a way to begin to discover more about your condition. I also suggest meditating on your body in whatever position you are in by scanning from the crown of your head to the soles of your feet. Often when people are in severe pain, they want to avoid feeling their body at all, so there is a tendency to anesthetize or distract themselves. However, I believe it is extremely helpful to pay as much attention as possible to the sensations that are moving through your body.

INVESTIGATING PAIN. One way yoga will help you deal with different difficulties that arise in your lower back is that it will enable you to become less fearful about investigating pain and difficulty. I hope you will begin to feel that you can do some self-analysis and self-healing by using the lower back poses and the practice on page 366. Additionally, these crises provide good opportunities for learning more about yourself, whether about your injury or about how your mind and emotional body respond to difficulty. This part of the yoga practice is just as important as are the yoga poses, breath, and meditation.

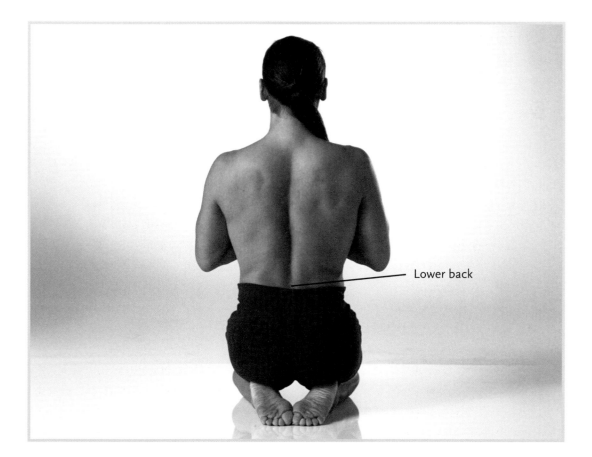

Lower back

A LOWER BACK PRACTICE

Try the poses in the following sequence in the order specified, and see how your lower back feels in each of the poses as well as how the sequence feels overall. If you do not have time to do the entire sequence, pick a couple of poses that feel the best to you and do those in the same order in which they are presented. You might even find that one or two of these poses are helpful during a work break or at the end or start of your day.

You can do the Lower Back Practice on its own or you can add it to the end of any yoga practice, immediately preceding the Relaxation Pose in that practice. You can also do it at the beginning of a practice or at any point during a practice when you feel like you have overworked or tweaked your lower back.

The practice begins with Supported Child's Pose to ease open your spine, allowing all the muscles of your lower back to widen, breathe, and relax. Reclined Leg Stretch follows to bring your lower back to a neutral position and gently release your back muscles, which are fully supported by the ground. This pose also helps stretch your hamstrings, which are often bound up from your lower back pain. Supported Standing Forward Bend normally puts your body into a somewhat vulnerable position. However, because this version is fully supported, your body can begin to reprogram itself by learning how to be in this position without having a spasm. Legs Up the Wall Pose then returns you to a fully supported neutral spine, adding a slight inversion to release your muscles even more and relax your nervous system.

The Passive Backbend and Restorative Backbend rebuild the natural curve in your lower back and restore and open your upper chest and neck. Version 1 of Supported Bridge Pose mildly opens your hip flexors and deeply relaxes your body and nervous system. Reclined Cobbler's Pose releases tightness around your abdomen (creating an ease in all your abdominal muscles and organs), encourages the natural curves of your lower back, and frees up your breath. Ending with any version of Relaxation Pose can help release much of the tension in your body created by your chronic lower back pain and will help soothe your nervous system.

1. Practice **Supported Child's Pose** for 1 to 3 minutes.

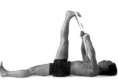

2. Practice version 1 of **Reclined Leg Stretch Pose** twice on each side for 1 minute each, focusing on maintaining the natural curve in your lower back.

3. Practice version 1 of **Supported Standing Forward Bend** for 1 to 3 minutes.

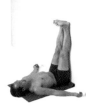

4. Practice version 1 or 2 of **Legs Up the Wall Pose** for 3 to 10 minutes. For version 2, you may need to move your buttocks slightly away from the wall.

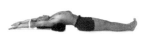

5. Practice **Passive Backbend** for 1 to 3 minutes.

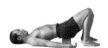

6. Practice version 1 of **Supported Bridge Pose** for 1 to 2 minutes.

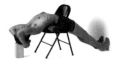

7. Practice version 1 or 3 of **Restorative Backbend** for 1 to 2 minutes.

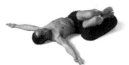

8. Practice version 1 of **Reclined Twist** for 1 minute per side.

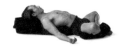

9. Practice version 3 of **Reclined Cobbler's Pose** for 2 to 10 minutes.

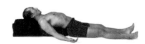

10. Practice **Relaxation Pose** or **Supported Relaxation Pose** for 2 to 5 minutes (any version of the six that feels best to you).

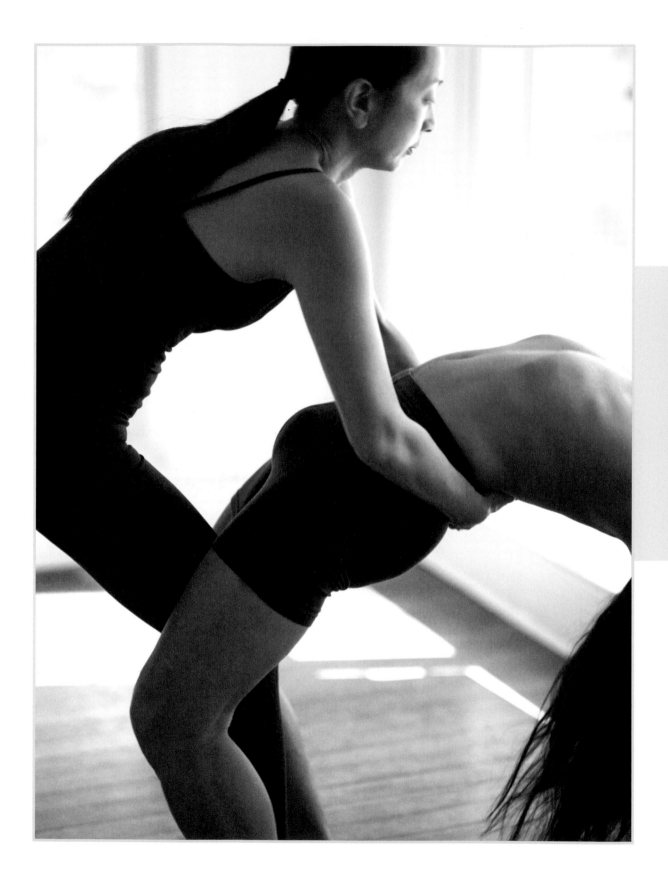

PART 4:

Keeping Your Practice Thriving

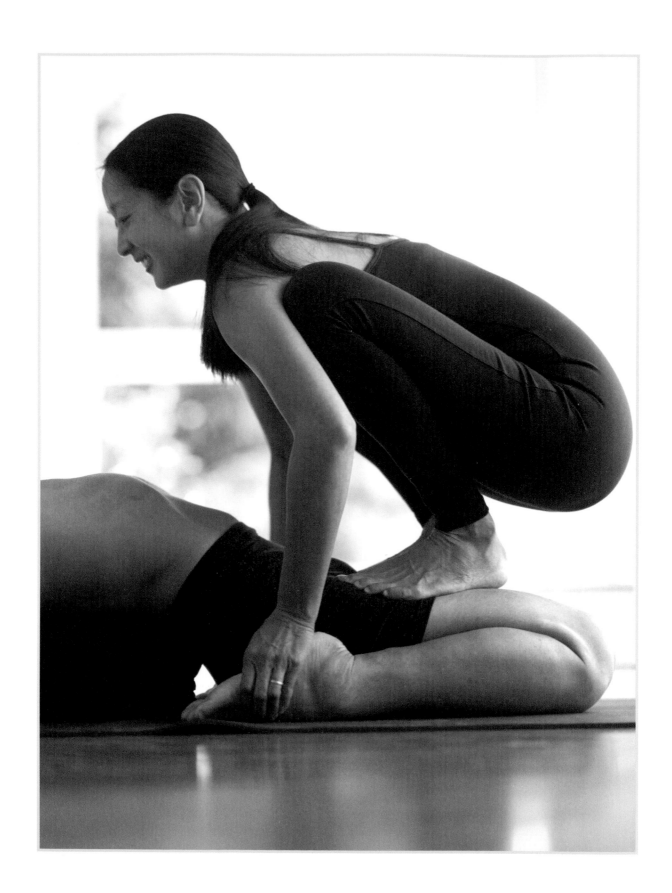

Feeding Your Practice

A YOGA PRACTICE, LIKE A LIVING THING, NEEDS CARE AND FEEDING IN ORDER TO FLOURISH. MOST LONG-time yoga practitioners have made special efforts to keep their practices thriving. You, too, will find that by taking active steps to feed your yoga practice, your commitment to yoga will deepen and your practice itself will become richer and richer. This chapter provides a wide range of detailed suggestions for feeding your practice in the following ways:

- Taking classes and workshops
- Reading yoga books
- Challenging yourself
- Practicing yoga with a friend
- Establishing consistency and ritual
- Making the practice your own
- Accepting the natural ebb and flow of your practice

Depending on your particular personality and how developed your practice is, you may find that some of these suggestions are relevant for you at this time while others are not. As you read through this chapter, identify those recommendations that seem most helpful at this time. You can always return to this chapter at any time in the future when you need inspiration and are ready for some new suggestions.

TAKING CLASSES AND WORKSHOPS

One of the most effective things you can do to keep your practice thriving is to find a regular teacher from whom you can take a weekly class. Taking a weekly class provides you with ideas that you can take home, such as new poses and sequences to try, and helps keep you inspired. A good teacher can also help you by providing alignment tips and observations about your particular body and your practice that can enable you to find more steadiness and ease in your poses. Your teacher can teach you to observe habits that you might not notice on your own and can help you learn how to break them, enabling you to balance your body as well as your practice.

FINDING A TEACHER. If you don't already have a yoga teacher whom you love, take your time to find one. Rather than simply going to the studio nearest you or taking from the teacher whose schedule fits yours, it is worthwhile to look for someone who is experienced and well trained, and whose teaching style and personality you find inspiring.

When you look for a teacher, it is a good idea to learn something about the training your potential teachers have undergone. Some teachers have studied yoga in rigorous two- or three-year Advanced Study programs or have done in-depth study in India, and they have a solid foundation in anatomy and philosophy as well as well-honed teaching skills. On the other hand, there are teachers who have simply taken a two-week crash course or who have not even received any formal training. While the type of training a particular teacher has undergone does not necessarily guarantee he or she will be a good (or a bad) teacher, a well-trained teacher may be able to offer you more in the long run.

You should also consider the teaching style and personality of your teachers. To put it simply, who inspires you? Some people prefer a gentle, nurturing teacher while others want someone to set them on fire. Some people prefer a physically or technically oriented class while others want a class with a more meditative or spiritual orientation. Some people want a teacher who will provide them with straightforward feedback so that they can look at the way they work more deeply. And some people simply want a teacher who has a good sense of humor. In the end, you should study with someone whose classes you look forward to and who helps keep you enthusiastic about yoga and your home practice.

WORKSHOPS. Taking workshops from visiting teachers will motivate you to deepen your practice and provide you with new ideas to take home with you. Some of the most inspiring yoga teachers from America as well as from Australia, Europe, and India teach workshops throughout the United States, and taking classes from them can fire up your practice as well as introduce you to approaches to yoga that are not taught locally. In addition, many local teachers offer workshops that give you a chance to delve more deeply into certain aspects of the yoga practice, such as inverted poses, backbends, restorative yoga, *pranayama*, meditation, or philosophy, which you may not have a chance to work with in depth in your regular classes. To supplement the programs in this book, workshops in the following areas are particularly recommended:

- Inverted poses
- Restorative yoga
- Yoga for women
- Therapeutic yoga
- Meditation
- *Pranayama*
- Yoga philosophy

RETREATS AND INTENSIVE PROGRAMS. Yoga retreats and intensive programs can help you deepen your practice by allowing you to feel the cumulative effects of well-rounded daily practice. Also, immersing yourself in yoga without the distractions of your daily life allows you to focus on aspects of your practice that you don't typically explore at home, and you may find yourself taking giant leaps. For many people, going on a retreat is what launches their home practice.

The following suggestions are several different ways to incorporate what you learn in a class, workshop, or retreat into your home practice.

SEQUENCES. If you go through a sequence you particularly enjoy or that seems especially intriguing, write it down immediately after the class or ask your teacher afterward to go over it with you. You can then add that sequence to your repertoire for home practice, exactly as the teacher designed it, or you can customize it to fit your needs.

> When I first really started practicing was after my first retreat. When I got home, I felt like I was going through withdrawal not having yoga as part of the day. It felt weird not to do yoga—I was craving it! So I thought, well, why don't I just try doing it at home and see how that goes. That eventually evolved into a morning practice, which is actually a great way for me to start my day.
>
> —DEBBI HERSH

ALIGNMENT. Many teachers design their classes to focus on aspects of alignment, such as keeping your knee over your foot in standing poses or centering your arm in the shoulder socket. In your home practice, it can be very interesting to take this focal point and incorporate it into your own sequences, either into the balanced practices in this book or into practices that you design. For example, if your teacher has been focusing on the alignment of your knees in standing poses in your classes, you could integrate that work into the Focus On Standing Poses practice in Week 8. Your teacher may also make specific recommendations to you as an individual about how you can improve your alignment, and, again, you can incorporate those suggestions into your practice. For example, if your teacher observes that your head is always in front of your heart, you could work with the alignment of your head and neck in every practice that you do. This is one of the best ways to break old habits and bring yourself more into balance.

NEW POSES. There are thousands of yoga poses, and some of us even have teachers who make up new ones! It's always fun to play with new poses at home, and you can easily incorporate them into your home practice by classifying them as standing poses, backbends, twists, forward bends, inverted poses, arm balances, or restorative poses and then inserting them into a suitable point in any of the practices in this book, as explained under "Extending a Practice" on page 352. For example, Revolved Triangle Pose is a standing pose that you can add toward the end of any standing pose sequence.

It's amazing how much more you hear and understand what your yoga teachers are talking about in class when you practice the poses and concepts at home. It causes me to think, looking back on it, that I was sleep-walking through it all the years before I started practicing on my own.

—LOUISA SPIER

HOMEWORK. You can also explicitly ask your teacher for homework. What does he or she recommend that you work on in your daily practice? Perhaps your teacher will recommend certain poses that will be helpful to you in opening up certain parts of your body or will recommend that you take on some new challenges.

Taking what you learn from a yoga teacher into your home practice allows you to bring variety into your practice and keep it from stagnating. By exploring and experimenting on your own, you deepen your understanding of what you experienced during class and evolve your practice in interesting and surprising ways. It takes time for all of us to embody the knowledge we acquire during class.

READING YOGA BOOKS

Reading yoga books can motivate you to continue practicing as well as provide you with a wealth of new information about the yoga practice. There are many fascinating figures in the yoga world, both in India and in the West, whose life stories and approaches to yoga can provide inspiration.

YOGA POSES AND SEQUENCES. You can also use yoga books to find new yoga poses and sequences to incorporate into your home practice, either based on the teachings of B. K. S. Iyengar (the style taught in this book) or from other yoga traditions, such as Ashtanga Vinyasa, Viniyoga, and Kundalini yoga.

PRANAYAMA AND MEDITATION. Books are a good way for you to deepen your understanding of breath awareness, *pranayama,* or meditation.

YOGA PHILOSOPHY. Yoga is thousands of years old, and the philosophy of yoga is rich and thought provoking. If you are interested in learning more, you can read some of the source texts (such as *Yoga Sutras* and *Bhagavad Gita*) or some of the many books that detail the history and philosophy of yoga. You may also wish to ask your yoga teacher for his or her recommendations, so you can learn more about that teacher's personal approach to yoga.

CHALLENGING YOURSELF

Surprisingly, many people find that working on their own on the poses they hate—poses that are very difficult, that scare them, or that they cannot even do yet—is what keeps their practices thriving. Challenging yourself can help you from getting bored or stuck in a rut (you'll probably be feeling excited, scared, or apprehensive instead). And tackling difficult things can be a rewarding experience, even if you don't make rapid progress. As a matter of fact, one fellow practitioner's entire home practice evolved out of her determination to try to learn the poses that were the most difficult for her.

It can be exhilarating to face the things that you have been avoiding. And your practice can become like a laboratory where you can experiment with your fears and difficulties with certain poses. You can then go on to use those experiences to help you deal with your fears and difficulties outside the yoga room.

Challenging yourself also leads you toward doing things you are not familiar with, which provides a more balanced practice. For example, you may have been avoiding backbends because they are the poses you have the most difficult time with, but it is very likely that they are difficult for you because they are so unfamiliar to your body. By focusing on them in your practice, you balance your body and your practice.

In general, you should build up gradually to difficult or scary poses. For example, in Headstand, you're dealing with your neck and spinal column, and you're balancing

Lately I've been working on one particular area that has been plaguing me for years and that is the most difficult, challenging, upsetting pose for me—that being backbends, specifically drop backs. I finally just decided, okay, this is something I'm going to get beyond. It is extremely exhilarating and liberating to tackle something you've been afraid of and to get through it and realize it isn't as scary as you originally thought. It is also interesting to me to figure out what habits and tendencies are making this so difficult. I find it really fascinating to work through those and to discover unproductive habits that are preventing me from doing, or even trying, a pose. Instead of falling into my habitual way, I try to find a different way to approach it, to see if something else could work.

—DEBBI HERSH

in a very unfamiliar way, so it is good to progress gradually and address your fear in incremental ways. If you go too far, too fast, all you do is hold your breath, clench, and shut down. This state is not helpful because you can't navigate through it to learn anything. The reason to do yoga poses with ease is so you have some ability to observe more deeply and respond more appropriately to open and balance the posture.

For this reason, in the eight-week program, Weeks 5 and 7 (Handstand and Headstand weeks) are designed so that you can continue to practice versions 1 or 2 of the challenging poses for as long as you need to and then return to tackling version 3 (the full pose) months or even years from now. Feel free to use this same strategy for any pose that you find difficult, whether it is Reclined Hero Pose, Pyramid Pose, or Upward Bow Pose.

PRACTICING WITH A FRIEND

This section describes in detail why and how to practice yoga with a friend because for many people having a practice partner (or several practice partners) is the single most important factor in their ability to maintain an ongoing home yoga practice. Rodney frequently acknowledges the fact that there is no way he would have maintained the depth of commitment to his practice over the last 10 years if he didn't practice almost every day with his friend Ian. For Nina, practicing once a week with her friend Jason not only helps her renew her dedication to her solo practice, but also having his support and encouragement while she was working with an injury helped her keep up her practice during that difficult time.

Bonnie and I started practicing yoga together 12 years ago when there were no yoga teachers in our small community. We would spot each other for Handstand, Upward Bow, and Forearm Balance. We would incorporate many of the things we learned together on yoga retreats into our sessions. Many times, our rhythms would be in sync, and we would both crave an hour of quiet, restorative yoga poses. Other times we would get distracted talking about family of origin issues, politics, children, husbands, patients, and any of a host of problems.

—JOLENE MONHEIM

Those of you who find practicing alone is difficult, either because you spend too much time alone already or because you are simply very gregarious, may find that having a practice partner can help get you out of bed and into your yoga clothes. Knowing someone is coming to meet you (or that you need to meet someone) is a strong motivation to get you to the yoga room. And for those of you who live in a part of the country where there are no yoga teachers, having a practice partner may make the difference between having a practice and not having one.

Your practice partner can be anyone in your life. Married couples practice together, friends practice with friends, parents practice with children, teachers practice with students, and people become friends because they practice together. You do not have to have the same levels of yoga experience or even be practicing the same style of yoga. All that matters is that you and your partner honor your commitment to yoga and to each other by being reliable about meeting each other for your practice dates.

Depending on your preferences and those of your partner, as well as on your mood on any particular day, there are many different ways you and your partner can practice together.

LEAD EACH OTHER. If you and your partner want to practice the same sequence of poses together, one partner can lead the other through a practice (or a part of a practice). The sequence of poses that you practice can be one that you design specifically for that day for the two of you, one that you get from a book (such as this book or *Light on Yoga* by B. K. S. Iyengar), or one that you learned in a class or workshop. The person who is leading the practice can lead verbally, by naming each pose as it comes up in the sequence, or one person can simply follow the other by copying the leader. One partner may even wish to teach the other partner something he or she learned recently in a class or share insights that he or she came up with during solo practice.

My favorite practice used to be Friday afternoons with three other teachers. We started out doing the routines in the back of Light on Yoga. *Then we started playing a sequencing game— we wrote a pose on a piece of paper, lots of them, like charades. You drew three poses and had to sequence them. It was so much fun! This usually led to, "Well, can you do it this way? How can we get from here to there?" It was a truly creative time.*

— SUSAN OREM

CHALLENGE EACH OTHER. For many of us, it is often difficult to practice the poses that are the most challenging when we are alone. Having the companionship of a partner (not to mention that peer pressure thing) can enable you to focus on aspects of your practice that you normally avoid. And chances are that you and your partner will not find the same poses equally challenging. So you can strike a deal with your partner, such as, "I'll help you practice those backbends you hate if you help me focus on my forward bends." Maybe you can even teach your friend how to love (or at least come to terms with) the poses that you love but that he or she hates and vice versa. Or perhaps both of you are finding it difficult to focus on a particular aspect of your practices, such as meditation or breath awareness. In this case, you and your partner can encourage and support each other in moving into new areas.

ADJUST EACH OTHER. Manual adjustments and partner poses can deepen your understanding of yoga poses and can teach you to find greater ease and steadiness in a pose that is difficult for you. For example, having your partner pull your thighs back into your hamstrings in Downward-Facing Dog gives you a visceral understanding of how the pose *can* feel and in what direction your pose should move. See "Partner Poses and Adjustments" on page 379 for some of our favorites.

KEEP EACH OTHER COMPANY. You may not even need to do more with your partner than simply practice in the same room. Practicing side by side with a friend or family member can be very sweet, whether you talk or are completely silent. You can talk about yoga as you practice, whether about yoga philosophy or things you've learned recently about yoga poses. (When you are in love with yoga, it can be quite a relief sometimes to talk about it with someone who doesn't think you're weird or nerdy— or who can at least laugh with you about being weird or nerdy—especially if your family and friends don't share your interests.) Or simply talk about anything you wish— yes, it turns out that is what many of us really do.

Practicing regularly with one partic- ular friend—and trying to practice with other friends of mine—helps feed my practice just because it's good to have company. I don't need that on a day-to-day basis. I actually like being pretty solitary in my practice. But it's really nice just to have company some- times, the same way it's nice to have company when you go for a walk.

—JASON CRANDELL

Meditating silently with friends is not only enjoyable, but having company can inspire you to sit longer for a change (or to sit at all). Meditating in a group also helps you harness your mind and encourages you not to distract yourself with every little thing that arises. In addition, the energy created by a group of individuals meditating together can take each in- dividual much deeper into the meditation.

YOGA COMMUNITY. Having a friend or a group of friends who are also yoga practi- tioners can help you maintain your practice even if you just meet for coffee after class or exchange e-mail messages. Obviously, you can tell each other about teachers you recom- mend, upcoming workshops you think might be interesting, books you've been reading, or things you learned recently in class. But having other yoga practitioners to talk with can be especially helpful when you get stuck or feel discouraged. Maybe your friends will have specific recommendations for you based on their own experiences or maybe they will simply remind you of why you do yoga in the first place.

When the eight-week program in this book was taught as a series course at Piedmont Yoga Studio, half the class was spent on teaching the new poses for the coming week and half the class on group conversation. Many students said afterward that the most useful and inspiring part of the class was the group conversation. Hearing what fellow classmates were going through helped them put their own struggles into perspective (true confes- sions!), and listening to how their fellow students solved various problems in their home practices taught them as much as talking with their teachers.

These days, because of yoga's popularity, some yoga studios are becoming community centers as well as places to take classes. When Rodney and Donna designed the new Pied- mont Yoga Studio, they consciously included several public areas, such as a lounge and a meditation room, because they believe that as much learning takes place outside the yoga room as inside it.

Partner Poses and Adjustments

This section contains instructions on how to do a few of our favorite partner adjustments and partner poses. Having someone touch you enables you to bring mindfulness to an area that is either overworking or collapsed and teaches you how certain poses can be done with more evenness. At first, you may feel somewhat awkward and unskilled touching each other. However, if you play around at least a couple of times during each practice, you will find that touch adds a wonderful dimension to your practice. The following adjustments are a small sample of the many possibilities for partnering each other.

COMMUNICATING. When you work with a partner, it is important to communicate frequently. Keep asking the person who is doing the pose, How does this feel? Have your partner tell you whether he or she wants you to pull more, less, or in a different direction. The photographs of partner adjustments in this section clearly indicate the direction to pull or push. But the amount you should pull or push will change from moment to moment. Start with a mild touch and begin to increase the intensity while you observe the results of your action. If your partner continues to respond by giving in to your touch, you can increase the intensity. When you feel your partner resisting, back up, maybe changing your grip or the angle from which you are applying the pressure.

OBSERVING. In some adjustments, you will touch your partner lightly where you want your partner to breathe. In other adjustments, you will pull or push more strongly to create space where there is compression or congestion. While giving the adjustment, observe how the breath is moving into your partner's body and how even the pose looks. Then, as you adjust your partner, ask whether that adjustment is bringing your partner more toward balance. In all adjustments, the person receiving the adjustment should get a feeling of relief and ease. After you finish adjusting your partner, back off slowly and see whether your partner can maintain the opening or balance on his or her own.

STRAP AROUND THE THIGHS. In this adjustment, you pull your partner's thighs back into the hamstrings. This creates traction on your partner's spine to relieve compression in the lower back and takes weight off your partner's shoulders and arms, creating a sense of elongation. Most importantly it teaches your partner the general direction of

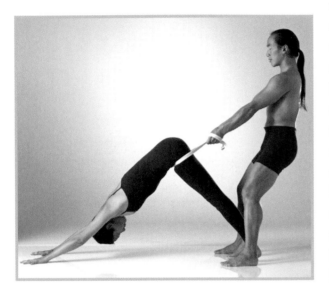

movement in the posture. Place the strap at the very top of the thighs, where they meet the pelvis, and wrap the strap around your hands so your fingers don't have to overwork to hold on to it and you can pull strongly. Draw the strap back at the angle of the torso, pulling diagonally upward and back. Ground your legs around your partner's, so that as you pull back, you bend your legs and use your own weight to create the pull. Pull as strongly as you can unless your partner's hands start sliding toward the feet or lifting off the ground.

PUSHING THE SACRUM BACK. In this adjustment, you press your partner's sacrum into the body and toward the sitting bones. This allows your partner to fully utilize the legs because your partner's weight shifts onto the feet. This adjustment creates length and relief in the lower back, with a sense of grounding through the legs and heels and lightness in the hands, spine, and shoulders. Place the heels of your hands at the top of your partner's buttocks, where they meet the lower back. If needed, readjust your hands so that you can

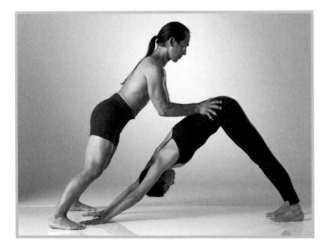

feel the ridge under the top of the sacrum with the heels of your hands. Splay your fingers around the buttocks so you can move the muscles strongly in the direction of the sitting bones. Bend both your arms and legs so you can push your partner's hips using the strength of your legs. Push as strongly as you can unless your partner's hands begin to slip toward the feet or lift off the ground. Breathe and feel the grounding of your legs moving into your hands.

RECLINED LEG STRETCH ADJUSTMENT

PULLING TOP OF THIGH ONTO HAMSTRING. In this adjustment, you pull the top of your partner's raised leg toward the hamstring as you push the very top of the bottom leg toward the ground (also into the hamstring). This adjustment relieves compression in the hip joint and lower back and allows your partner to breathe more completely throughout the torso. Place your hand on the top leg so that when you pull back, you pull the thighbone toward the

hamstring with a slight external rotation. Place your hand on the bottom leg so that it rotates your partner's bottom leg inward as you press down. Be sensitive about creating an even pressure on both legs so your partner can sense the relationship between the two legs as well as the length of the lower back and the space between the thighs and pelvis. Ask your partner what amount of pull and push feels good.

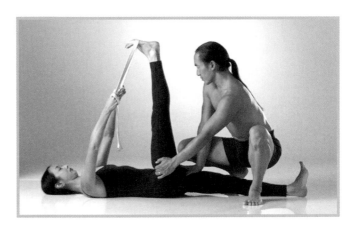

CHILD'S POSE ADJUSTMENTS

PRESSING DOWN ON THE SACRUM. In this adjustment, you press your partner's sacrum down into the body and toward the sitting bones to release the muscles of the lower back and allow the legs to fold more deeply. This adjustment also helps your partner release

the neck and head more completely because the sacrum and the pelvis are anchored down toward the heels. Stand over your partner's head so that you can press the buttocks flesh toward the sitting bones. Start with a light press to make sure that your partner's knees, lower back, ankles, and feet feel comfortable when you begin to apply pressure. If these areas feel fine, apply more pressure. Usually your partner will enjoy a strong push, but as always it is best to ask periodically. Instead of just pushing with your arms, use the weight of your body on your arms as the source of power.

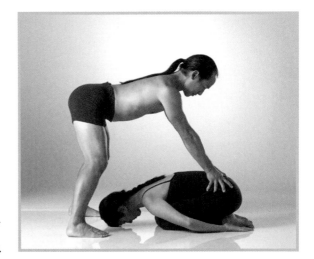

BACKBEND OVER PARTNER. In this partner pose, you do a backbend over your partner's Child's Pose. This is beneficial for both partners. The weight of the top person enables the person in Child's Pose to fold more deeply. And the person doing the backbend receives a very even, mild backbend, which softly opens the spine and chest. Begin by sitting behind your partner and lining your sitting bones and sacrum up with your partner's. Then, as you lie back over your partner, make sure the weight of your hips and legs draws your partner's buttocks flesh down toward the sitting bones while the weight of your chest and head elongates your partner's upper back and head in the opposite direction of the buttocks. Move into the backbend very carefully and slowly, lowering your vertebrae one at a

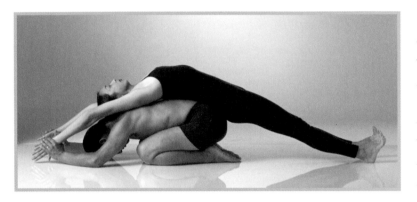

time onto your partner's. Once your spine is draped over your partner's, extend your legs and arms to form a backbend.

To come out of the pose, have your partner (the bottom person) push slowly up and raise his or her torso as you slide off.

STAFF POSE ADJUSTMENT

SITTING BACK TO BACK. In this partner pose, you sit back to back with your partner in Staff Pose to provide each other with the support to sit upright and to bring awareness to your upper bodies. With this awareness, you can learn how to sit upright in Staff Pose without overusing the muscles of your backs. To get into this pose, both partners lean slightly forward and scoot their sitting bones back toward their partner's.

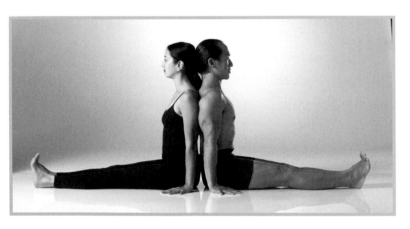

Then both of you can slowly sit up in Staff Pose, adjusting your posture so that you both sit as upright as possible. It may take a little bit of movement back and forth for both of you to get comfortable. Enjoy feeling and breathing into this alive, organic back rest.

COBBLER'S POSE ADJUSTMENT

SITTING BACK TO BACK. This partner pose is essentially the same as the Staff Pose adjustment described on the opposite page. You sit back to back with your partner in Cobbler's Pose to provide each other with the support to sit upright and to bring awareness to your upper bodies. With this awareness, you can learn how to sit upright in Cobbler's Pose without overusing the muscles of your backs. To get into this pose, both partners lean slightly forward and scoot their sitting bones back toward their partner's. Then both of you can slowly sit up in Cobbler's Pose, adjusting your posture so that you both sit as upright as possible. It may take a little bit of movement back and forth for both of you to get comfortable. Allow the warmth of your partner's body to help you relax your back muscles and learn to sit upright through a sense of release and extension rather than struggle.

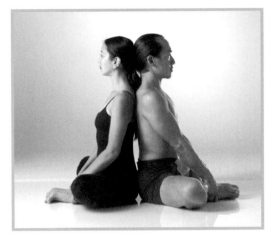

SEATED WIDE-ANGLE POSE ADJUSTMENT

GROUNDING THE THIGHS. In this adjustment, you ground your partner's thighs so your partner can sit up more easily. Anchoring your partner's thighs also allows your partner's breath to move more easily down toward the base of the pelvis. This adjustment teaches your partner not to overuse the back muscles as it brings an understanding of the connection between the grounding of the legs and the ease of the spine. Place your hands at the very top of your partner's thighs, with the heels of your hands in your partner's hip creases. First, move the quadriceps toward the knees to release any binding of the muscles from the hip socket. Then ground the thighbones as much as possible down into the hamstrings. Press directly down toward the floor as your partner keeps his or her knees and toes pointing directly up toward the ceiling. If you wish, you can do this adjustment while creating a back rest for your partner, using your chest, your knees, or even your back.

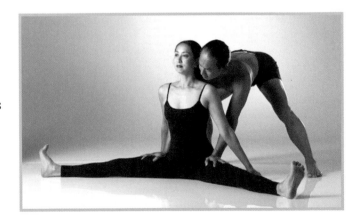

WARRIOR 2 ADJUSTMENT

DRAWING THE ARMS. In this adjustment, you draw your partner's arms away from center so your partner can feel the alignment and lightness of the arms. This adjustment

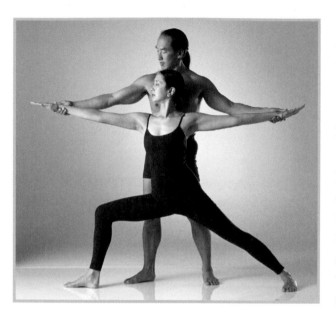

also helps open your partner's chest from the front and back. Start by holding your partner's wrists, forearms, or the heels of the hands and then draw the arms away from center. As you do this, encourage your partner to expand from his or her center rather than from the shoulder sockets. Also, encourage your partner to release the base of the neck and any excess tension in the tops of the shoulders. Lift your partner's hands slightly higher than parallel to the ground so your partner has the feeling that the waist is lifting up into the outstretched arms.

WARRIOR 1 ADJUSTMENT

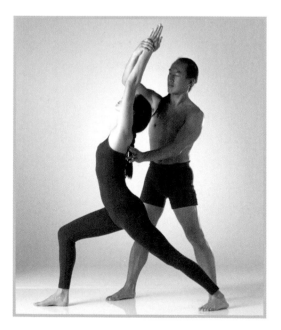

LIFTING THE ARMS, WRISTS, AND HANDS. In this adjustment, you use one hand to firm your partner's shoulder blades into the back body, helping your partner to integrate the reach of the arms with the lift of the chest. With your other hand, you lift your partner's wrists, hands, and arms upward out of the lower back. With this adjustment, your partner will understand the role of the arms in facilitating the full extension of the spine. This work also helps to fully open the upper chest, so the neck and the head can easily release backward. Don't be afraid to give your partner a strong lift, though you should ensure first that your partner's arms are connected in their sockets.

SEATED TWIST ADJUSTMENT

HANDS ON THE BELLY AND LOWER BACK. In this adjustment, you place one hand on your partner's belly and the other on the lower back to get your partner to release tension in those areas and to help your partner initiate the twist from the lower rather than upper body. As you give this adjustment, be very sensitive to when and how much your partner should turn. Just by touching your partner in the lower back and belly, you may help him or her release the tension in those areas. When you feel your partner's presence of mind in these areas, you can help initiate your partner's turn on an exhalation. Both of you should refrain from using too much force. Use your hands as ears and eyes for observation. Often there will be a natural gateway in which the twist will easily occur. See if you can both be sensitive enough to wait for the gateway to open and then twist more deeply.

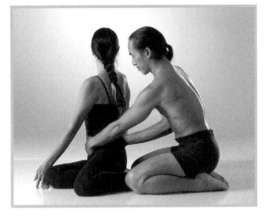

UPWARD BOW ASSIST

HELPING YOUR PARTNER UP. In this adjustment, you help your partner move into Upward Bow Pose. This assist is helpful if your partner cannot get into the pose on his or her own or to help relieve some of the intensity of the pose, especially at the wrists. By giving your partner's hands some height, you also take some intensity out of the lower back and emphasize more opening in the upper chest. This assist also encourages your partner to put more weight on the feet (the general direction in which the pose should head).

Start by having your partner place his or her hands on your ankles. Then place your hands underneath your partner's upper back so your fingers almost touch the spine. Your arms will help harness your partner's arms so the elbows don't splay out to the sides. When your partner begins to lift up, bend your legs so you can lift your partner using your legs and not your lower back. While trying not to hinder the movement of your partner's arms

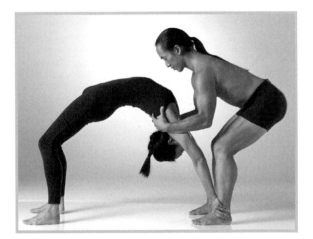

and shoulder blades, lift your partner's upper back to help him or her extend upward into Upward Bow. This adjustment is a bit more complicated than the other adjustments in this chapter and is dependent on the proper timing. Be sure to lift your partner's chest just as he or she begins to raise the hips, so that your partner's arms extend just slightly after the legs extend.

As your partner uses his or her legs to lift into the backbend, tell your partner to move the weight of the pelvis more over the legs, instead of pushing the pelvis toward the head and chest. If your partner's shoulders hurt while doing this pose, bring your partner down partway so he or she can move the shoulders and arms around before trying to re-extend the elbows. This adjustment may take a bit of time to master, but if you keep helping each other, you'll both learn to appreciate this wonderful partner pose.

ESTABLISHING CONSISTENCY AND RITUAL

Cultivating the habit of doing yoga at the same time each day and, if possible, rarely skipping your practice can help you establish a consistent practice that is completely integrated into your daily life. Eventually you will find you *crave* your practice, both physically and emotionally. (Some practitioners even find that if they skip practice for a few days, they start to dream about doing yoga.) If you have a hard time getting yourself to your mat, tell yourself you can do just one pose (such as Downward-Facing Dog). Often you will find that once you do a pose or two, your momentum picks up and carries you through a longer practice.

Sometimes, of course, practice can feel flat. You really don't feel like going to your mat at all. My philosophy is to hear that emotion and practice anyway. Once I get going, my enthusiasm grows. It's like trying to get a kid to take a bath: They don't want to get into the tub, but once they're in, they don't want to get out.

—TIMOTHY MCCALL

Practicing yoga every day may mean that you always go through a sequence that includes yoga poses as well as meditation and breath awareness or that you simply meditate or practice breath awareness on those days when your schedule is especially demanding.

For newer practitioners, it may be unrealistic to try to practice five or six days a week. For you, a good strategy may be to start by resolving to practice three days a week, and then allowing your practice to evolve over time as your commitment deepens. However, whether your goal is to practice three or six days a week, it is worthwhile to stick with your plan long enough to develop a real relationship with yoga.

PERCEIVED OBSTACLES. If there is an obstacle in your life that makes it hard for you to practice consistently, question it. Maybe you think you are lazy, but maybe you really are just tired, tired from trying to do too much. In this case, you need to ask yourself, What can I subtract from my life? One of the main reasons that people don't continue to practice is that they always think about adding more to their lives, rather than figuring out what they can remove. You have to be pragmatic and maybe even a little ruthless. If you really value the benefits that you are receiving from your yoga practice, focus on removing something from your life that's not serving you well.

CREATING A RITUAL. For some people, performing a ritual before they practice or making the practice itself into a ritual can help them establish consistency and maintain their inspiration. Your ritual need not be elaborate; you can light a candle or incense, play certain music, or spend a few minutes meditating. For years, Rodney and Ian used to start their early morning yoga practice by solving the word jumble in the *San Francisco Chronicle* before doing their first poses.

For some of us, it is enough to simply put on our designated yoga clothes and roll out our yoga mats.

My home yoga practice takes place in the quiet of my kitchen floor at 5:30 in the morning. I go into the kitchen wearing a T-shirt and sweatpants. I light a candle by the window. I always begin with two sets of sun salutations. By that time, my body is more awake and ready for the rest of the practice.

—VALERIE JEW

MAKING THE PRACTICE YOUR OWN

To keep your practice thriving, you must, at some point, transition from always doing practices straight out of a book or video to taking charge of your practice and making it your own.

INTUITION. Start to trust your intuition. Ask yourself, What do I feel like doing today? There are so many different practices in yoga that you can usually find something to suit your mood and your physical state. In the end, you're doing the practice for yourself, so there is no need to think about practicing the "right" or "wrong" way. Simply practice in the way that fits your body, your personality, and your current emotional state.

Sometimes trusting your intuition means *not knowing* and staring blankly into your body as you wonder what to practice. This is a good time to meditate until something arises. The ability to relax while you are in a state of "not knowing" is itself a very important part of the yoga practice.

For many years, my home practice was uninspired and I did not get from my home practice what I got from yoga classes. That all changed when I took the eight-week series course at Piedmont Yoga Studio based on the program in this book. One day, near the end of the program, when I was practicing at home, I thought to myself, "This is MINE!" Meaning, the yoga had come from within ME and was no longer some perfunctory thing I did because I "should" have a home yoga practice.

—MELITTA RORTY

CREATIVITY. Allow yourself to be creative in your approach to your practice. This can mean mixing different styles of yoga within your practice, using your coffee table as a yoga prop, or finding some weird way to trick yourself into doing a pose that you hate. For example, maybe you're afraid to kick up into Handstand but want to practice it at home without a partner, so you eventually figure out that you can crawl up one side of a narrow hallway and bring your legs across to the other wall and—voilà!—you're in Handstand. Or perhaps you find that when you are doing a supported forward bend, the chair is too high for your head, the bolster is too low, but that small end table in your bedroom is just right. The point is for you to create a practice that suits you as an individual, and the more creativity you bring to the practice, the more the practice will become your own.

My practice has evolved a lot. The first couple of years I pretty much just did the equivalent of an intro asana class at home every day and I didn't do pranayama. Then as I learned more and went deeper into my own practice, I started branching out and getting more adventurous. For example, I do a lot of what Richard Freeman jokingly calls "illegal yoga poses." I make stuff up. And my apartment is basically one big prop.

—TIMOTHY McCALL

ACCEPTING THE NATURAL EBB AND FLOW OF YOUR PRACTICE

There is a natural ebb and flow to everyone's practice. Internal or external circumstances, such as being on a trip, having a houseguest, being overloaded with work, going through emotional difficulty, being sick, and so on, can cause your practice to ebb temporarily. Learn to accept this natural ebb without panicking.

Indirectly I feed my practice now by seeing, allowing, and embracing more ebb and flow in my practice and not having a sense of guilt if I take a few days off. Because I don't want to have that kind of relationship with my practice. I don't want it to be just another thing that I have to do. I want to want to do it.

—JASON CRANDELL

If you drop the practice for a few days or even a few weeks, that doesn't mean it's over forever. When you are ready, simply find your way back to it. Try giving yourself a break by starting again with the poses and sequences that you love. The more often you go through this cycle, the more you will be able to trust that your practice will eventually flow again.

For some long-time practitioners, practice may even ebb for long periods of time, such as after the birth of a child. Again, this does not mean it is over forever.

Now, looking back 13 years after the birth of my first child, I realize that the cycle of my yoga practice is not 24 hours, or even weekly or monthly, but is spread out over my lifetime.

Putting my practice into a larger perspective, I realize that yoga is so deeply ingrained in my life that it's not going anywhere; it just looks different at the various stages of my life.

—DONNA FONE

For all of us—whether we are able to practice consistently, day in and day out, for 25 years or whether our daily practice ebbs and flows during the different stages of our lives—there will be times when practice feels flat and uninspired. Realize that this, too, is part of a natural cycle, like the waxing and waning of the moon.

B. K. S. Iyengar says somewhere that a yoga practice waxes and wanes like the moon. What he means is that sometimes our work is bright and shiny, like the full moon, while at other times it feels dark, as when the moon is new. This has certainly been my experience over the last quarter-century. To me, "dark" means there's no connection to the self, no juice (rasa), and the sequence of the practice doesn't flow naturally, but clunks along. It's duhkha, *which literally means "having a bad axle hole (kha)," and which translates as suffering. I'm certainly practicing, no matter how I feel, but in the dark, without the illuminating presence of the self shining through the body/mind. The dark can last for a day, a week, a month, or years. It's how we handle these dark times that reveals our true commitment to the self.*

I've tried to remain emotionally balanced, remembering how Krishna counsels Arjuna in The Bhagavad Gita *(2.47–48, translation by Juan Mascaro):*

Set thy heart upon thy work, but never on its reward. Work not for a reward; but never cease to do thy work. Do thy work in the peace of Yoga and, free from selfish desires, be not moved in success or failure. Yoga is evenness of mind—a peace that is ever the same.

—RICHARD ROSEN

Acknowledgments

There is something about books that seems to bring the best out in people. It turns out that when you say you are writing one, all kinds of people offer their assistance—many of them just for the fun of it. And the work that these people do is always their best, too, whether they are carefully reviewing your manuscript or writing an honest, heartfelt report on their weekly yoga practice. So, while we are not quite as surprised as we were last time at the number of people it took to create a book, we are once again quite amazed at the number of people who gave so freely of their time. We are immensely grateful both to have received help again from several old friends as well as to have received assistance from many new people we met only recently.

We would like to start by thanking our agent, Richard Pine, who helped us develop the concept for this book and saw us through the entire process of its creation. Thank you, Richard, for your integrity, your kindness, and your support.

We would also like to thank everyone at Rodale, especially our editor, Margot Schupf; our project editor, Nancy N. Bailey; our designer, Trish Field; and our layout designer, Donna Bellis, for giving us so much of your time, expertise, and personal attention and for helping us to create a book we could be proud of.

Rod would like to take this time to bow gratefully to the Iyengars and all the yoga teachers and students from whom he has absorbed invaluable love, *shakti,* and knowledge. *Namaste.*

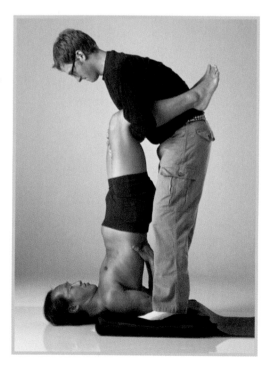

He also gives big thanks to his friend and fellow early morning practitioner, Ian Swensen, who was once again side by side on the yoga mat with him, philosophizing, complaining, snoring, practicing, and meditating. Without Ian, half the yoga insights in this book would not have been possible, for Rod would never have gotten out of bed.

Then there's Jason Crandell.

No other single person gave us as so much of his time and expertise, not to mention emotional support. Jason reviewed the entire book, tested many of the practices, assisted at the photo shoot, and did much of the grueling work of entering photo ID numbers into the manuscript. In addition, he helped teach the eight-week program as a course at Piedmont Yoga Studio and was always available (and interested!) to discuss issues and concerns, whether large or small. "Thank you" seems too small an expression in some ways, but, well, thank you, Jason.

Baxter Bell also helped out with this book in a large number of ways. He helped teach the eight-week program to our first group of volunteers and reviewed significant parts of the book, providing us with both yoga and medical expertise. Thank you, Baxter, for all of that and also for your continuing friendship and support.

Nina is especially grateful to have had help again from Melitta Rorty, her long-time friend and yoga buddy. Thank you, Melitta, for reviewing chapters, for providing editorial suggestions, and for always being there to talk anything (and everything) over with.

And thank you to Quinn Gibson for his help proofing the text. You've always been great company, Quinn, but who knew that one day you'd become so useful!

We would also like to thank the "guinea pigs" in our three Home Practice courses, who tested the sequences in the program and provided us with invaluable information about the realities of home practice. Your sincerity about the yoga practice kept us inspired, and your honest observations about the program enabled us to continue to refine and improve it.

Thank you to the following people for testing additional practices: Karen Flynn, Chrisandra Fox, and Shosannah Marks.

Thank you to the following people for allowing us to interview them about their home practices: Vickie Russell Bell, Jason Crandell, Wendy Edelstein, Donna Fone, Hilary Fox, Debbi Hersh, Valerie Jew, Timothy McCall, Susan Orem, Melitta Rorty, Richard Rosen, Louisa Spier, Mark Silva, and Vanessa Silva.

Thank you to Richard Rosen for sharing your wonderful book collection with us and for taking time to talk about your favorites.

Thank you to our photographer, Michal Venera, and his assistant, John Bedell, for beautiful photographs, not to mention interesting conversation and really great vegetarian sandwiches.

And thank you once again to Donna Fone for modeling with Rod in the partner photographs and for assisting at the photo shoot. As always, you were there when we needed you, and you gave us your time graciously and unstintingly.

Thanks to Elnora Lee and John Hall of Color 2000 for photographic wisdom and support.

And, finally, we would like to thank our families for their continuing support and for tolerating our sometimes rather weird working schedules. Rod wants to thank Donna especially for her support in helping to hold up the magical illusion of Rod's yoga world by working to keep their children, their business, and their home in impeccable tune and abundant aliveness.

(And should we embarrass Nina's husband, Brad, by publicly admitting that he was not only actually supportive this time around, but that he started a home yoga practice after testing the eight-week program? What was it that he said? "I'm not stupid. I know a good thing when I see it.")

Index